OPHTHALMOLOGY

OPTICS & REFRA

OPHTHALMOLOGY BOARD REVIEW

OPTICS & REFRACTION

Brent J. MacInnis, M.D.
Clinical Associate Professor of Ophthalmology
University of Ottawa
Ottawa, Canada

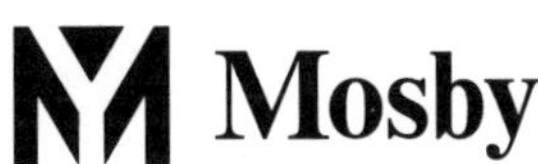

St. Louis Baltimore Boston Chicago London Madrid Philadelphia Sydney Toronto

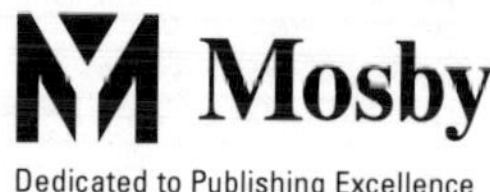

Editor: Laurel Craven
Developmental Editor: Dana Battaglia
Project Manager: Carol Sullivan Wiseman
[illegible]

Printed in the United States of America
Composition by University Graphics, Inc.
Printing/binding by Maple-Vail Book Manufacturing Group

Mosby–Year Book, Inc.
11830 Westline Industrial Drive
St. Louis, MO 63146

International Standard Book Number 0-8016-7999-0

93 94 95 96 97 / 9 8 7 6 5 4 3 2 1

Special thanks to Lesley and Melanie
without whose love, neglect, reciprocal verbal abuse,
patience, and skill this work simply would not be.

Preface

This manual is intended to bridge, not abridge, *Optics and Refraction.* A widening information gap exists between "bare bones" texts and complete "works" that can easily overwhelm. The American Academy manual provides excellent direction and instruction on the core material necessary for a solid foundation in clinical optics. Classic works, such as Duane's, the "Duke," or Michaels', provide encyclopedic reference sources for detailed solutions and explanations to complex problems. For the resident-in-training, this manual fills the gap and provides an understandable yet complete treatment of fundamental principles and clinical pearls geared for the clinician by a clinician. Explanations are rendered in a format comprehensible to anyone with college entry-level physics. No double integral calculus graces these pages! In Part I, subject material is addressed in a fashion appropriate for review before OKAP, board, or recertification examinations. Part II contains a unique collection of multiple choice problems on optics and refraction. Part III provides answers with graphic solutions. This approach circumvents the frustration felt when an answer is derived at odds with the letter answer tucked away at the back of the book. The complete solutions provided show where and why the answer is right or wrong. This immediate feedback is a valuable form of self-tutorial. This three-part combination format is invaluable as a preexamination and self-assessment review.

At times, explanations require the scientific equivalent of "literary license" to make a concept understood. I apologize if this is offensive to some. Often it is the only way that I could understand it well enough to attempt to teach it! I am a practicing clinician not a nuclear physicist. These practical and relevant explanations explain the principles behind what we do every day.

I have intentionally chosen to identify by name rather than by reference those individuals I feel deserve credit for a particularly unique idea, pearl, procedure, or instrument. Seldom have I seen a resident refer to the reference section of the optics texts, let alone clamor to the library to retrieve originals. At least this way the authors/originators get instant credit for their cleverness.

I must also acknowledge the driving force behind the framework of many of the questions in Part II. Melanie MacInnis worked to ensure completeness of the subject material and its correspondence to Part I. She deserves much of the final credit, if final credit is due.

We often teach as we were taught. I would be remiss if I did not recognize the major influence of David Guyton on this work. Many years ago, as a fellow with Dave, I listened and watched and learned a great deal. As a premedical undergraduate, Dave was a summa cum laude graduate in physics. Dave has a truly unique perspective. We have all benefitted from his equally unique contributions to ophthalmology. I hope I have given him his due.

Paul Boeder, Kenneth Ogle, Melvin Rubin, Jack Holladay, David Michaels, and many, many others have made major contributions to how we understand optics. I am like a translator, as I try to understand their brilliance and explain it in ways we less-gifted mortals can comprehend. I hope I have succeeded.

Inevitably, errors of commission and omission will surface. Similarly, differences in approach to solutions will often give rise to a different answer. The graphic solutions clearly yield the source of difference and our possible source of error. We are always open to feedback and welcome your comments or questions.

Good luck in your studies.

Brent J. MacInnis

Contents

How to Use This Review Book

Part I condenses the principles of *Optics and Refraction.* It contains an amazing amount of information in a few pages. With each successive read, another pearl will emerge that was missed the time before. To truly meet the claim as a "review," even those topics with less "appeal" have been addressed. There is enough information included in these pages alone to pass any written or oral examination.

Part II contains 754 multiple-choice questions based on the text. Most important, the solutions are given in detailed and graphic form, explaining how and why the answer is correct. The derivation of the answer is included when it adds to the understanding of the underlying principle. It is cross-referenced to Part I for ease of use and further explanation. When a permutation arises that is not covered in the text, another reference is provided if the topic is important enough. Part II can be used as a stand-alone review once the basic principles have been mastered from Part I.

A serious attempt has been made to incorporate the usual and not-so-usual permutations and combinations one encounters in all examination formats. This completeness separates this review from course reviews and handouts given out at Board Review courses. This text forms a useful complement to such courses and similarly these courses beautifully complement this text. Mastery of the contents of both will guarantee success at any level of examination.

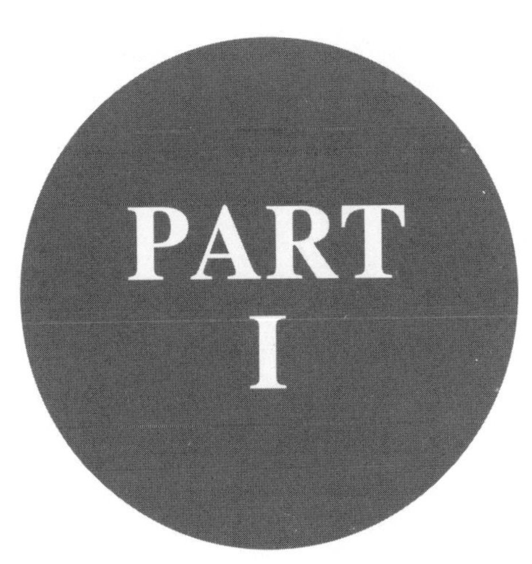

THEORY

CHAPTER 1: THE BASICS

PROPERTIES OF LIGHT

Light in small doses is well tolerated; so is optics. Too much light is toxic; too much optics is only nauseating. To understand the nature of phototoxicity, it is necessary to understand some of the basic properties of light. Unfortunately, no single theory can explain all optical phenomena. Light behaves one way one minute and another way the next. To reconcile these varied properties and apparent inconsistencies, optics is artificially divided into various domains, e.g., physical, quantum, geometric, or physiologic. This is nothing more than the easiest and most convenient way to explain very complex behaviours of light.

Light is energy with particulate (photon), bundle (quantum), and wave properties. Quantum optics deals with light as both a particle and a wave. Like a proton or electron, a photon has particulate properties that make it capable of being emitted or absorbed. Yet each photon is a wave with a defined length (λ) and quantum of energy for that wavelength. It is so diverse that its length can vary from 0.0001 to 30,000 m and each "step"alters its energy. A photon of wavelength 100 nm has 12.50 eV per photon, one of 193 nm has 6.4 eV per photon, i.e., the shorter the wavelength, the greater the amount of energy per photon. This fact is essential in understanding why shorter wavelength light, e.g., ultraviolet, has greater potential for photic damage.

Visible light is a very narrow range of the electromagnetic spectrum (380 to 780 nm). Invisible light may not stimulate photoreceptors but still may be absorbed and do damage. Gamma rays and x-rays have very short wavelengths (10^{-14}, 10^{-10} nm) and thus extraordinary amounts of energy per photon. Absorption of their energy is the basis of their therapeutic efficiency and toxicity. Television and radio waves have wavelengths greater than 1 m and hence carry very little energy, often approaching a level of insignificance equal to their content.

The most attention has been devoted to ultraviolet (UV) phototoxicity (280 to 400 nm). The current list of ocular disorders triggered, implicated in causing, or caused by UV phototoxicity includes the following:

1. Basal cell carcinoma of the eyelid skin, conjunctiva
2. Pingueculae, pterygia
3. Phototoxic keratitis, herpes simplex, recurrent corneal erosion
4. Uveitis
5. Cataracts
6. Age-realted macular degeneration, solar retinopathy, cystoid macular edema, pigmentary retinopathy with photosensitization

The proposed mechanisms for damage vary for acute to chronic exposure. These can be acute thermal effects or chronic photochemical damage induced by free radicals produced by oxidative metabolism. Absorption of UV photons produces excited singlets and metastable triplets of oxygen that are toxic to protein binding RNA and DNA within the cell. Photic damage is normally followed by repair. This is diminished with age, photosensitizing agents, susceptible genetic predisposition, increased exposure, temperature, and probably a multitude of other factors. Certainly the eye is a prime candidate for phototoxicity having the highest demand for both oxygen and light for its function. This mounting evidence promotes UV filtration for us all but especially those at higher risk, i.e., those with aphakia, with pseudophakia without UV-blocking implants, exposed to occupational hazards (e.g., dental-curing compounds),taking photosensitizing drugs (e.g., PUVA, phenothiazines, tetracycline, etc), and with any of the previously listed disorders.

Infrared radiation is emitted by arc lamps, molten glass, and metal and infrared lamps. It is implicated in "glass blowers' " cataracts and other chorioretinal thermal injuries.

PHYSICAL OPTICS AND WAVE THEORY

Physical optics examines light as energy particles, which are emitted by light sources and absorbed by other substances. Wave theory describes a sinusoidal wave within the electromagnetic spectrum that has a wavelength (λ), velocity (*c*), and frequency (*v*). These wave properties are useful in the understanding of how light interacts with itself, different media, and various surfaces. It is necessary to invoke wave theory to understand the naturally occurring phenomena of interference, diffraction, and polarization. The basic concept of vergence is the unifying concept between wave theory and geometric optics. Geometric optics deals with the formation of images by rays of light acted on by lenses, prisms, and mirrors.

From Fig. 1-1 it can be seen that the sinusoidal curve has peaks (maxima) and troughs (minima). These occur with a certain amplitude and separation (wave-

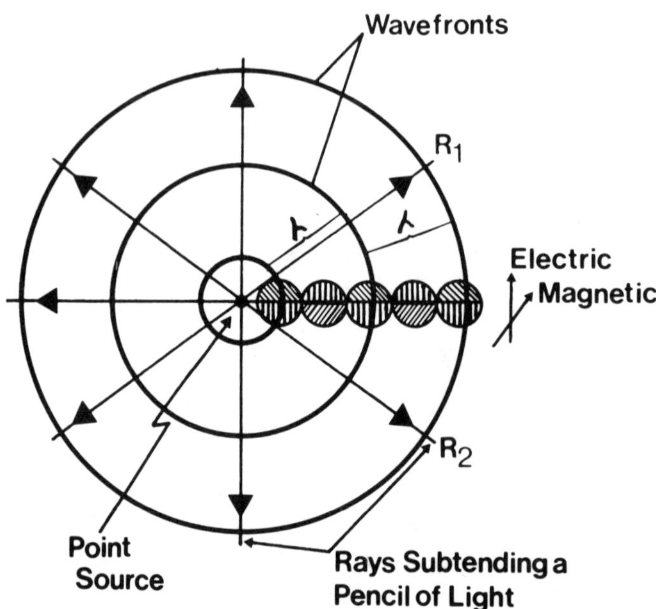

Fig. 1-1 The electric field is propagated perpendicular to the magnetic field. The wavelength is measured crest to crest or trough to trough. The radius of curvature of the wavefront (*r*) is a measure of the vergence of the advancing wavefront, not the divergence of the pencil R_1-R_2.

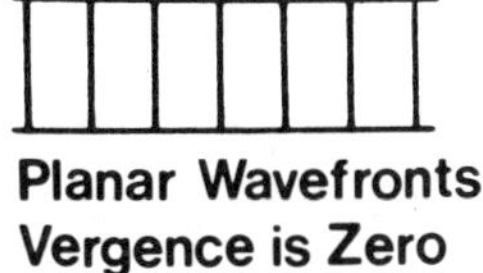

Planar Wavefronts
Vergence is Zero

Fig. 1-2

length). These maxima create an advancing wavefront emanating from a point source. This, of course, is a three-dimensional projection from the source. The configuration of the wavefront is such that in one plane an electric field exists and perpendicular to this plane a magnetic field is propagated. The direction of the propagating electromagnetic wavefront can be depicted unidimensionally as a ray, e.g.,R_1 or R_2. If all other rays outside R_1-R_2 are prevented from emerging, a front resembling a three-dimensional pencil of rays bounded by $R_1$and R_2 in Fig. 1-1 is created. The wavefronts within the pencil each have a radius of curvature that increases as the distance from the source increases.

As the distance from the source increases, the radius of the curvature of the wavefront increases to infinity until it is an advancing plane that is perpendicular to the optical axis. At this point the power of vergence of the wavefront is defined as zero. The pencil of light, as delineated by the two-dimensional rays, is thus infinitely far from the source and contains planar wavefronts whose vergence is zero (Fig. 1-2).

CONVERGENCE, DIVERGENCE, AND THE DIOPTER

All naturally occurring wavefronts are diverging as they emerge from a source as in Fig. 1-1. The amount of divergence of a pencil is not defined as the angle subtended by its limiting rays but rather by the radius of curvature of the wavefront. As already noted the radius of curvature increases with increasing distance from the source. This relationship between the distance from the source and the divergence of the wavefront is employed as a measure of the vergence or power of the pencil. The radius of curvature can be described as the radius of the circle that would yield the arc with that curvature. Rather than the radius of curvature, the reciprocal of the radius of curvature in meters is used as the unit of vergence. This is the *diopter:*

$$1 \text{ Diopter} = \frac{1}{1 \text{ Meter}}$$

By convention, divergence is given in *minus* vergence power and convergence is given in *plus* vergence power (Figs. 1-3 and 1-4).

Convergent wavefronts are seldom found spontaneously in nature but are the result of an alteration of a planar or divergent wavefront by a refractive or reflective medium. In geometric optics the configuration of the wavefront in three dimensions is difficult to depict diagrammatically. Instead, a two-dimensional plane of a pencil bounded by limiting rays is employed and the true configuration is implied with each ray trace.

The distance an object is located from a refracting or reflecting surface is again

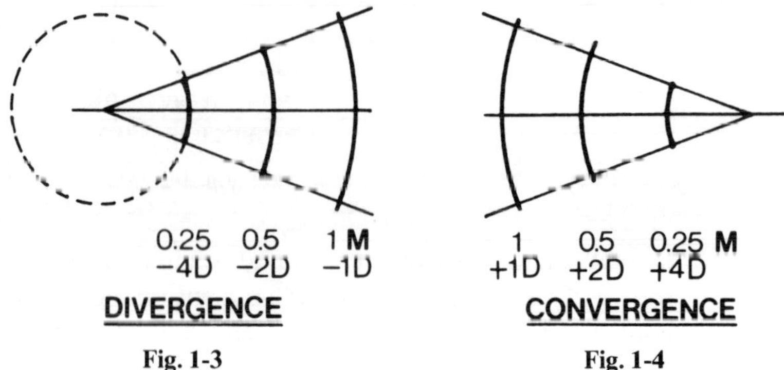

Fig. 1-3

Fig. 1-4

representative of its radius of curvature at that surface. This distance (u) is related to the object vergence (U) by the reciprocal $\frac{1}{u}$, i.e., $U = \frac{1}{u}$ diopters. An optically active surface alters this vergence by reflecting or refracting these incident rays so that the emergent rays are either more divergent, convergent, or planar. This implies the surface has a *power,* which is denoted D. This power in diopters is fortuitously *additive* to the object vergence to give a resultant image vergence (V). The image is located at the image distance "v."

$$V = \frac{1}{v}$$

This relationship can be expressed in the familiar form:

$$U + D = V$$

This simple relationship with minor modifications will hold true for lenses, mirrors, and the interface between any two media with a smooth refracting or reflecting surface. All that need be known is the derivation of the power (D) for whatever system one is dealing with and the index of refraction of the object and image media.

For thin lenses in air this is a simple matter. If parallel rays strike the lens, the power (D) of the lens will then be equal to the vergence added, i.e., the vergence of the image rays leaving the lens (Fig. 1-5).

$$U + D = V$$

$$0 + D = V$$

$$D = V$$

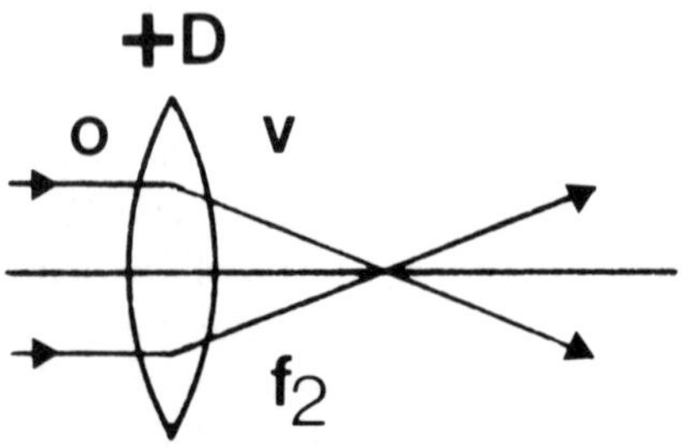

+D

O V

f_2

Fig. 1-5

Since the vergence is expressed in diopters, the reciprocal is naturally a distance. In this special circumstance ($U = 0$) this value is the *focal length* (f) of the lens. Hence $D = \frac{1}{f}$. In Fig. 1-5 the lens adds vergence power to form image rays, which are convergent. This is, by convention, a *plus* lens. It is noted that the focal length defines a *focal point* to which image rays are convergent. With a plus lens this lies to the right of the lens.

In a diverging lens, the focal point lies to the left of the lens and the lens is given, by convention, a *minus* power (Fig. 1-6): $D = \frac{1}{-f}$.

SIMPLE LENS FORMULAE

With this knowledge, the simple lens formula becomes an interchangeable entity as follows:

$$\boxed{U + D = V} = \boxed{\frac{1}{u} + \frac{1}{f} = \frac{1}{v}}$$

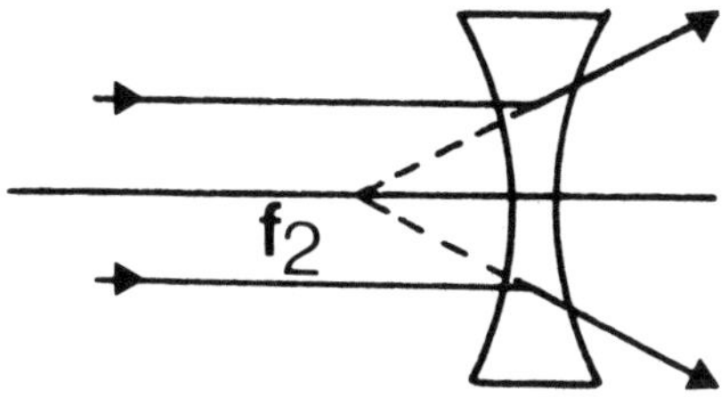

Fig. 1-6

It has been noted that the power of the lens has altered the vergence of incoming rays to yield a new wavefront, which comes to a point or stigmatic focus. This relationship holds true only for a spherical lens whose power is the same in all meridians. As will be explained later, different powers in two principal meridians create an *astigmatic* system with two *focal lines* instead of one focal point.

Every now and again physical optics must creep in and spoil everything! In the earlier discussion about lenses, the lenses were qualified as infinitely *thin* and immersed in *air*. Consider first the latter qualifier.

Intuitively it can be reasoned that if light encounters any medium other than air or a vacuum, it will be slowed down, i.e., its velocity is reduced. The amount it is reduced is a function of the nature of the medium and it defines the *index of refraction* (n) of that medium.

$$n = \frac{\text{Velocity of light in a vacuum } (c)}{\text{Velocity of light in the medium } (v)}$$

Since the velocity in the medium is always slower than the reference standard in a vacuum, it follows that n will always be greater than unity (1). For virtually all optical considerations in North America, the index is calculated for *yellow* ($\lambda = 589$ nm) light, since the velocity is wavelength dependent. This may vary from continent to continent.

This relationship can be given by the formula:

$c = \lambda \nu$ where: c = velocity of light (3.00×10^{10} cm/sec)
λ = wavelength of light
ν = frequency of light

The velocity of light in a vacuum is a constant. This implies that when $c = \lambda\nu$, any change in the frequency is accompanied by an equal and opposite change in the wavelength. When one speaks of *frequency doubling,* for example, with the YAG laser, this is equivalent to halving the wavelength, i.e., 1064 nm infrared would become a visible 532 nm. Using various harmonics, one could theoretically manipulate the wavelength with various crystals to have a single laser deliver over a wide range of wavelengths for different functions.

When changing media, the frequency of light is constant. To maintain the above relationship ($c = \lambda\nu$), if the velocity (c) of the light is slower, the wavelength (λ) must be reduced. The amount reduced depends on the index of the medium. This yields the *reduced* wavelength.

$$\lambda_M = \frac{\lambda}{n}$$

Reduced wavelength describes the reduced distance measured in a medium. Vergences on the other hand are mathematically the inverse of the image and object distance. Being the inverse, reducing the distance will increase the vergence. In a medium, a reduced distance increases the vergence of the wavefront. Although numerically it is increased, the"concept" of reduced distances has led to the name "reduced vergence." It would be more aptly called "corrected" vergence.

For example:

$$\text{Image vergence} = \frac{1}{\text{Image distance}} \text{ or } V = \frac{1}{v}$$

In a medium of n, v is reduced to $\frac{v}{n}$:

$$V = \frac{1}{v/n}$$

$$\text{or} \quad nV = \frac{1}{v}$$

$$n \text{ is always} > 1$$

The reduced vergence nV is numerically greater than V, the vergence in air.

In reality this is a normalized vergence rather than a reduced vergence. The concept is important when there exists an interface between media of differing index of refraction. For example, in visual imagery, this is used to consider the effects of the cornea, aqueous, lens, and vitreous on the final image distance relative to the retina.

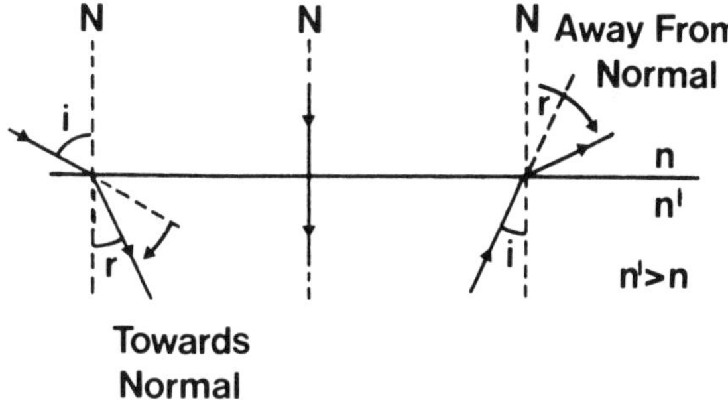

Fig. 1-7 As light travels from a less dense to a more dense medium, it is refracted toward the normal.

REFRACTION AND SNELL'S LAW

The reduced velocity of the light on encountering a denser medium is accompanied by bending or *refraction* of the light if the incident rays are not normal to the surface. The relationship of the refracted to the incident ray may be trigonometrically determined. This relationship is described by Snell's law:

$n \sin i = n' \sin r$ where: i = angle of incidence as measured from the normal
r = angle refracted as measured from the normal

As seen in Fig. 1-7, as an incident ray travels from a less dense to a more dense medium, it is refracted toward the normal and it remains in the same plane defined by the incident ray and the normal. If it is coincident with the normal, it is slowed but not refracted. If emerging from a more dense to a less dense medium, it is refracted away from the normal. This is the basic law of refraction and it illustrates the great impact of changing media.

REFLECTION AND CRITICAL ANGLE

A special circumstance occurs in passing from a more dense to a less dense medium (Fig. 1-8). As the incident angle increases, the angle of refraction will eventually be 90° to the normal, i.e., parallel to the interface between the two media. Clearly any further increase in the angle of incidence will result in a "refracted" ray that is contained within the same medium, i.e., it is *reflected* and not refracted. This phenomenon is referred to as *total internal reflection*. The angle after which all light is reflected is the *critical angle*. This angle can be determined for the interface between any two media by using Snell's law.

$n \sin i_c = n' \sin 90°$ where: i_c = the critical angle and the refracted angle is 90°

$$\sin i_c = \frac{n'}{n} \times 1$$

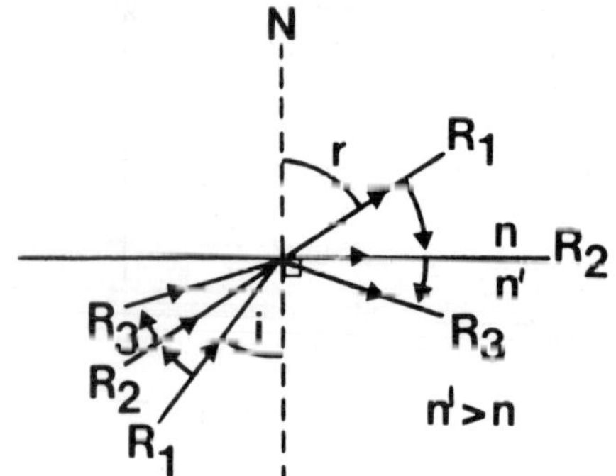

Fig. 1-8 Light beyond the critical angle of incidence is internally reflected.

It becomes important to manipulate this critical angle optically for several clinically useful techniques.

When trying to evaluate the internal structure of the anterior chamber angle of the eye, the light attempting to emerge from the cornea to the observer is incident on the tear cornea interface at an angle superseding the critical angle.

$$\sin i_c = \frac{n'}{n} = \frac{1}{4/3} = \frac{3}{4} = 0.75$$

$$i_c = 48°$$

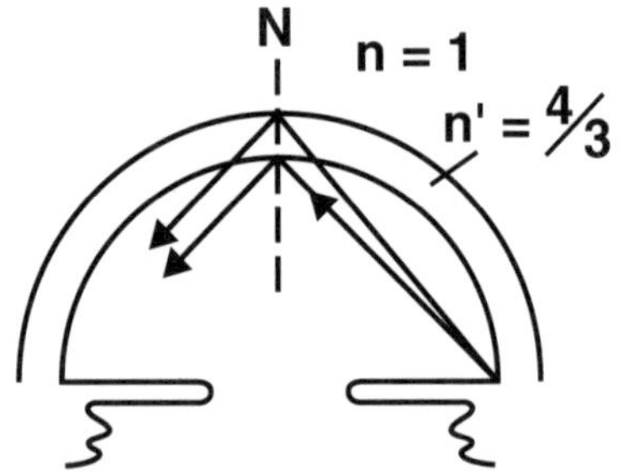

Fig. 1-9

In Fig. 1-9 a ray is depicted that is greater than the critical angle (48°), and thus it is reflected internally. This implies that these structures are inaccessible to ordinary viewing. To overcome this, the critical angle can be increased by contact lenses and methylcellulose. In this fashion an incident angle of almost 90° can be achieved before total internal reflection occurs. In this way *gonioscopy* or the clinical visual examination of the angle is possible. Conversely, the property of total internal reflection can be used to advantage. Fiberoptic bundles and reversing and reflecting prisms operate on this premise (Fig. 1-10).

This form of reflection is governed by the same law of reflection that affects any stationary smooth reflecting surface. Since reflection "traps" light in the incident medium, the incident and refractive media are the same. Thus the angle of incidence ($>i$) is equal to the angle of reflection ($>r$) and no consideration of the refractive index is required (Fig. 1-11).

VERGENCE FORMULAE

There is some debate as to the nomenclature surrounding mirrors. Some systems name concave mirrors as minus mirrors in view of their configuration similar to concave minus lenses. Similarly, convex mirrors would be called plus mirrors.

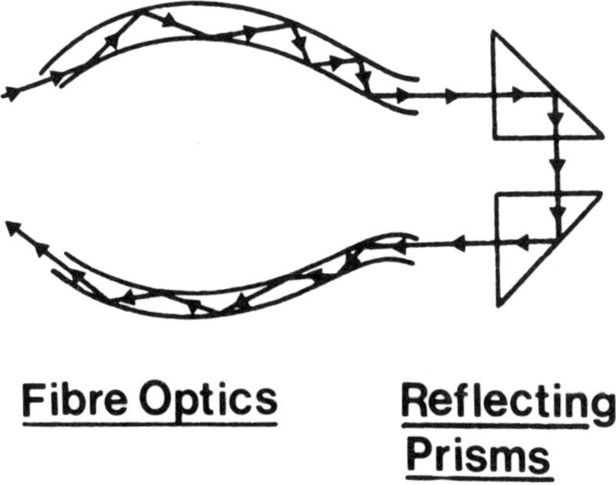

Fig. 1-10

It is less confusing if the effect on vergence is used as the parameter defining whether the mirror is plus or minus. A plus mirror would add positive vergence in the same way plus lenses add positive vergence. With this convention plus mirrors are concave and minus mirrors are convex. This latter method will be used for the remainder of the text.

Fig. 1-11, *b* and *c*, illustrate the fact that concave (plus) and convex (minus) mirrors not only obey the basic law of reflection but also affect the vergence of the incident light. To achieve this, the mirror must by definition have power.

Similar to lenses, the power $(D) = \frac{1}{f}$ for the mirror. In mirror parlance, however, the focal length is often given in terms of the radius of curvature (in meters). The relationship is such that the focal length is equal to one half the radius of curvature.

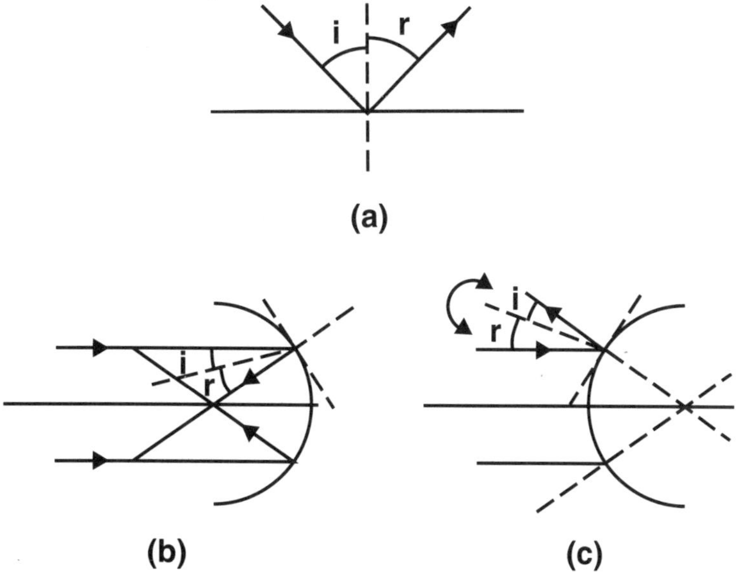

Fig. 1-11 In a plane mirror (**a**) the $>i = >r$. A concave mirror (**b**) adds positive vergence (plus) and convex mirrors (**c**) add negative vergence (minus).

$$f_m = \frac{1}{2} \times r_m = \frac{r_m}{2}$$

where: f_m = focal length of the mirror
r_m = radius of curvature of the mirror

$$D_m = \frac{1}{f_m} = \frac{1}{r_m/2} = \frac{2}{r_m}$$

If the focal point is to the left of the mirror, the mirror is convergent and thus r is positive (plus). Similarly for a divergent, convex mirror, r_m is negative or minus. With this convention of power determination, the vergence formula $U + D_m = V$ becomes $U + \frac{2}{r_m} = V$. This can be applied similarly to the simple lens formula.

A plane mirror is one whose power is zero and hence the image and object vergence are the same. The minus image vergence indicates that the image lies behind the mirror at the same distance as the object.

Reflection occurs not only with mirrors. The interface between two media of different indices of refraction is capable of reflection *and* refraction (Fig. 1-12). This is the single smooth reflecting or refracting surface. As stated, the process of reflection being confined to one medium obeys the law of stationary reflection. In going from one medium to the next there is a change in vergence and therefore refracting power to the surface. This power has been derived and is $D_s = \frac{n' - n}{r}$. The difference in media dictates the use of reduced vergence.

$$nU + D_s = n'V \quad \text{(The sign convention is the same as for mirrors.)}$$

$$\text{or} \quad nU + \frac{n' - n}{r} = n'V$$

Thus, for any reflecting or refracting surface, the vergence relationships can be derived from one of the three basic formulae. Unfortunately, this is only applicable to thin lenses and the lens thickness is not considered. These considerations become important in real optical systems and will be dealt with later.

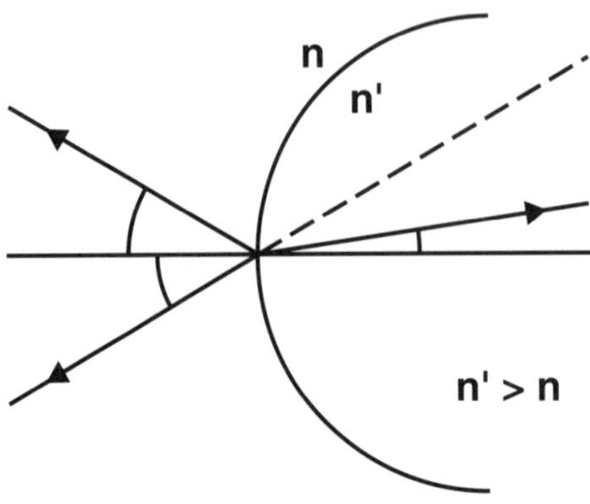

Fig. 1-12 Light can be reflected or refracted at the interface between two media.

Basic Vegence Formulae

Simple lens	$U + D = V$
Mirror or reflecting surface	$U + \frac{2}{r_m} = V$
Refracting surface	$nU + \left(\frac{n' - n}{r}\right) = n'V$

where: U = vergence of object rays at the lens
D = lens power
V = vergence of image rays emerging from the lens
r_m = radius of curvature of the mirror
n, n' = indices of refraction of the media at an interface
r = radius of curvature of the interface

REAL AND VIRTUAL OBJECTS AND IMAGES

Until now, consideration has only been given to the object vergence and the determination and effects of lens power on this object vergence. The ultimate purpose of this exercise is to form an image. The vergence formulae facilitate the derivation of *where* the image is found for a given optical system but the character of that image, i.e., whether it is considered real or virtual, erect or inverted has not as yet been considered. Real space versus virtual space is a consideration not only for objects but also for images.

Light from an object can be anywhere and can have any vergence. It can be on the incoming left side of a plus lens or it can be the image of a previous lens and can be on the outgoing right side of the same lens. The incoming rays are object rays that strike the optical system from the left, since by convention we always use the direction of light as going from left to right (Fig. 1-13). The outgoing rays are image rays that emerge from the right side of the optical system.

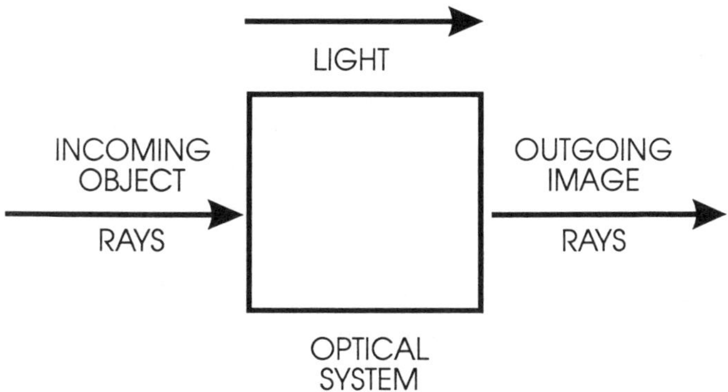

Fig. 1-13 Real objects can give real or virtual images depending on the optical system.

A real object is on the same side as the incoming object rays. A real image is on the same side as the outgoing image rays (Fig. 1-14).

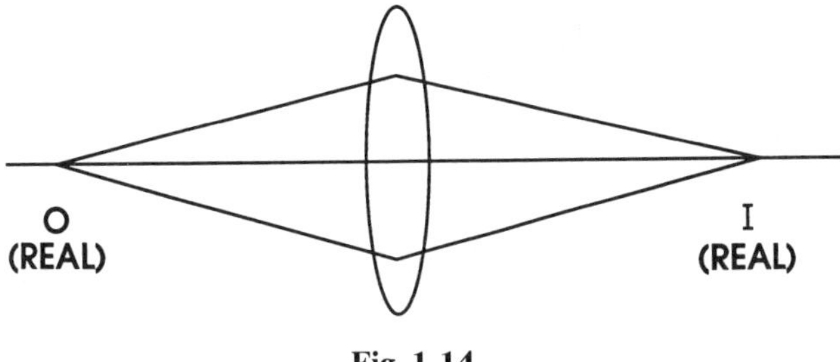

Fig. 1-14

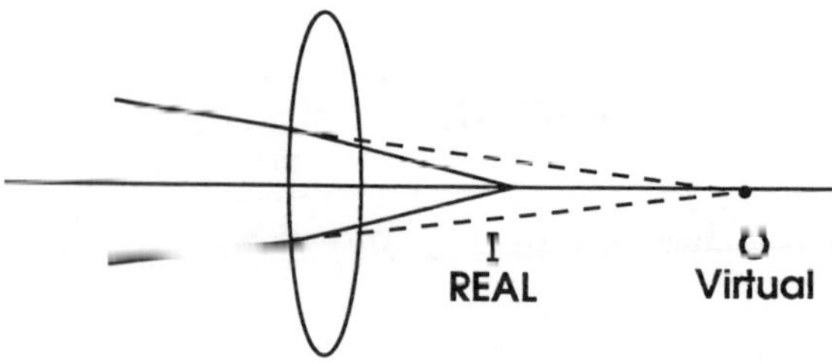

Fig. 1-15

A virtual object is on the opposite side as the incoming object rays. It is depicted on a ray trace by dotted lines representing imaginary extensions through the optical system to the object (Fig. 1-15).

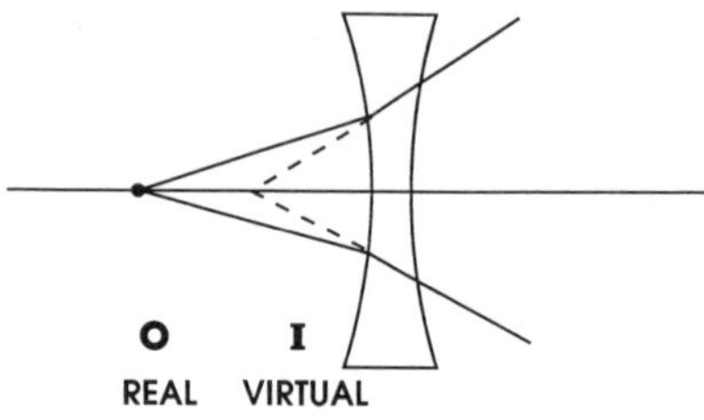

Fig. 1-16

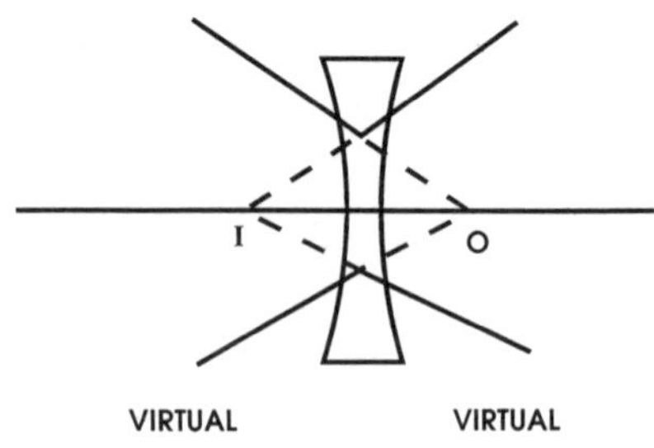

Fig. 1-17

A virtual image is on the opposite side as the outgoing image rays (Fig. 1-16).

A virtual object may also have a virtual image (Fig. 1-17).

A *real* image is one that is capable of being "captured" on a screen (if the screen blocks the source of illumination such as in the case of the indirect ophthalmoscope, the image is still real, although not "capturable" with that system). A *virtual* image is one that is not capable of being projected onto a screen through an intervening lens or mirror.

A real image lies on the opposite side of a lens to the incoming light for real objects. For a mirror, a real image of a real object lies on the same side as the incoming light. (Fig. 1-18) Conversely a virtual image of a real object lies on the same side as the incoming light with a lens but the opposite side with a mirror. Although this may seem confusing at first some further clarity will be derived when ray tracing is discussed. From Fig. 1-18, it can be seen that the image and object space can overlap and occupy the same side of the lens or mirror, e.g., in the case of a plus mirror the image and object space are to the same side as the incoming light and each extends infinitely far.

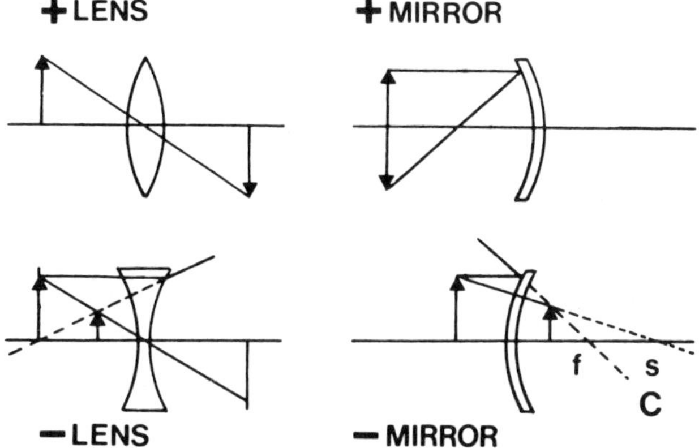

Fig. 1-18 Real objects can give real or virtual images depending on the optical system.

RAY TRACING

The image size, orientation, and position can be determined by a combination of ray tracing and vergence formulae. To understand the technique of ray tracing several important aspects of optical systems are necessary.

The optical axis passes through the center of curvature of both optical surfaces of a thin lens and is thus perpendicular to both surfaces. Although not uniquely defined, the optical axis of a mirror, for ray tracing purposes, passes through the center of curvature of the mirror (Fig. 1-19).

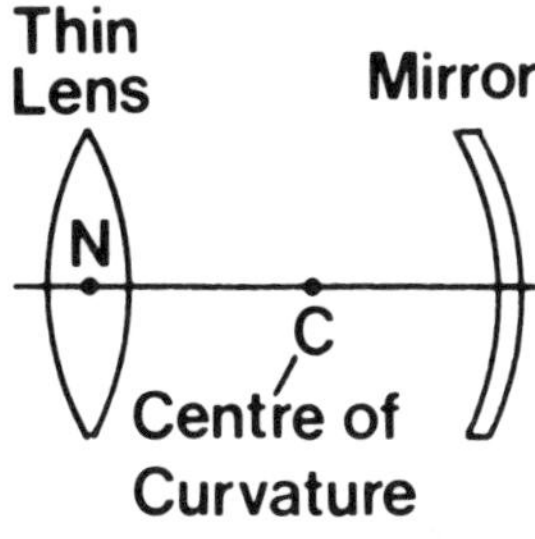

Fig. 1-19

The center of curvature of a mirror and the nodal point of a thin lens are very useful points. Rays passing through these points are not deviated, irrespective of their inclination to the optical axis. A ray from the tip of an extended object through these points is thus undeviated and forms a very useful ray—the *central ray* (Fig. 1-20).

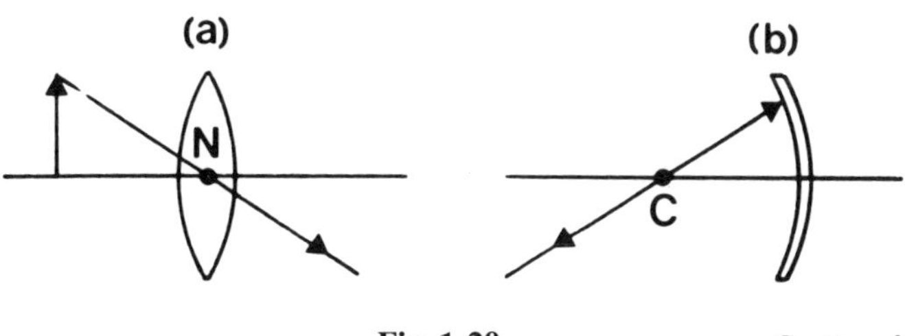

Fig. 1-20

Continued.

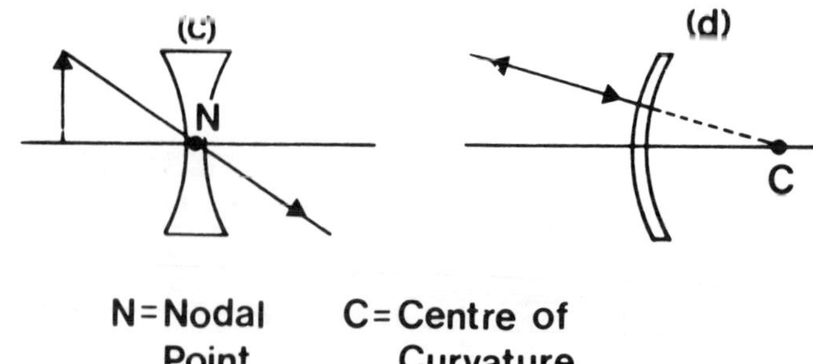

Fig. 1-20, cont'd.

The primary focal point is that *object* point for an image located at infinity, i.e., having an image vergence $V = 0$ on leaving the lens (Figs. 1-21 and 1-22).

For a plus lens:

$$U + D = 0$$

$$U = -D$$

$$U = \frac{-1}{f}$$

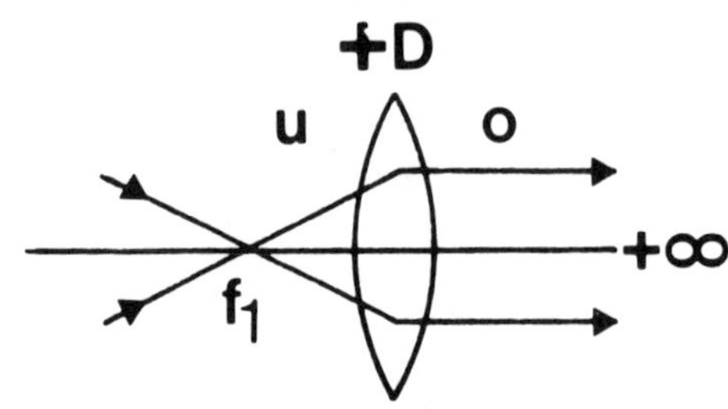

Fig. 1-21

For a minus lens:

$$U + (-D) = 0$$

$$U = D$$

$$U = \frac{1}{f}$$

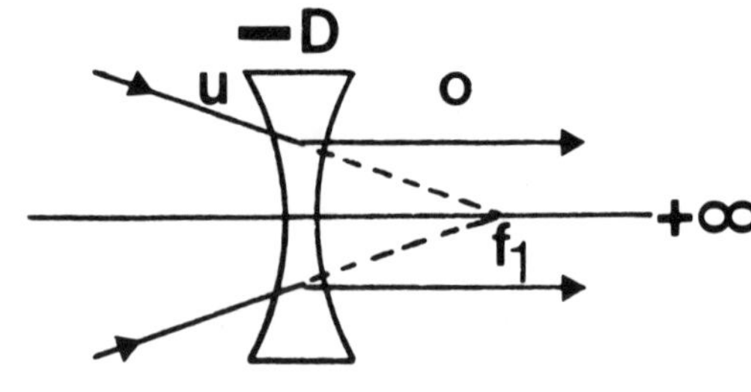

Fig. 1-22

The secondary focal point is the *image* point for an object located at infinity, i.e., having an object vergence $U = 0$ at the lens.

For a plus lens:

$$0 + D = V$$

$$D = V$$

$$\frac{1}{f} = V$$

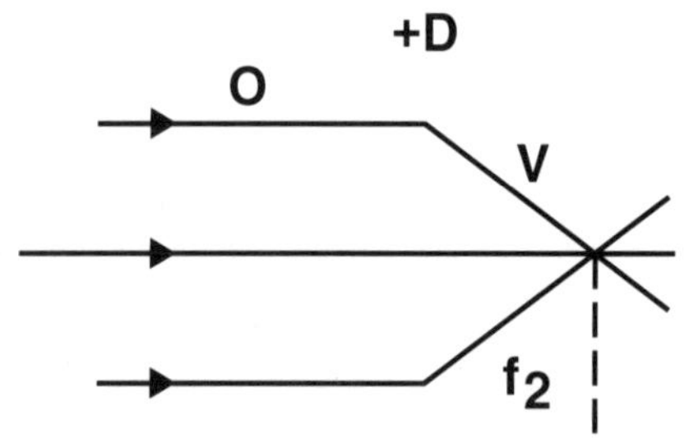

Fig. 1-23

For a minus lens:

$$0 + (-D) = V$$

$$-D = V$$

$$\frac{-1}{f} = V$$

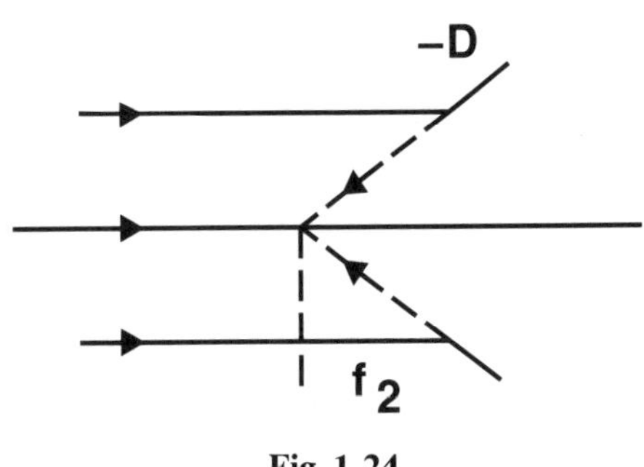

Fig. 1-24

These focal points are examples of *conjugate* points; if the direction of the light is reversed, the position of the object and image is reversed. The concept of conjugacy becomes exceedingly important in the understanding of retinoscopy and the correction of the ametropias.

Since mirrors are reflecting surfaces, the two focal points are superimposed leaving a single focal point with which to deal.

In any optical system of thin lenses or mirrors, the images formed can be characterized and localized by a *ray trace.* Each system contains three constant rays: the central ray, the parallel object ray passing through the secondary focal point, and the ray from the object passing through the primary focal point and emerging parallel to the optical axis. For simplicity's sake, the central ray and the ray through f_2 will always suffice. Consider the examples in Fig. 1-25.

When performing ray tracings, two special situations seem to provide inordinate difficulty for the initiate.

The convergent (plus) mirror as depicted in Fig. 1-25, *c*, exhibits variable imagery with different object positions relative to the focal point and center of curvature. (Convex lenses also change imagery when inside the anterior focal point.) If

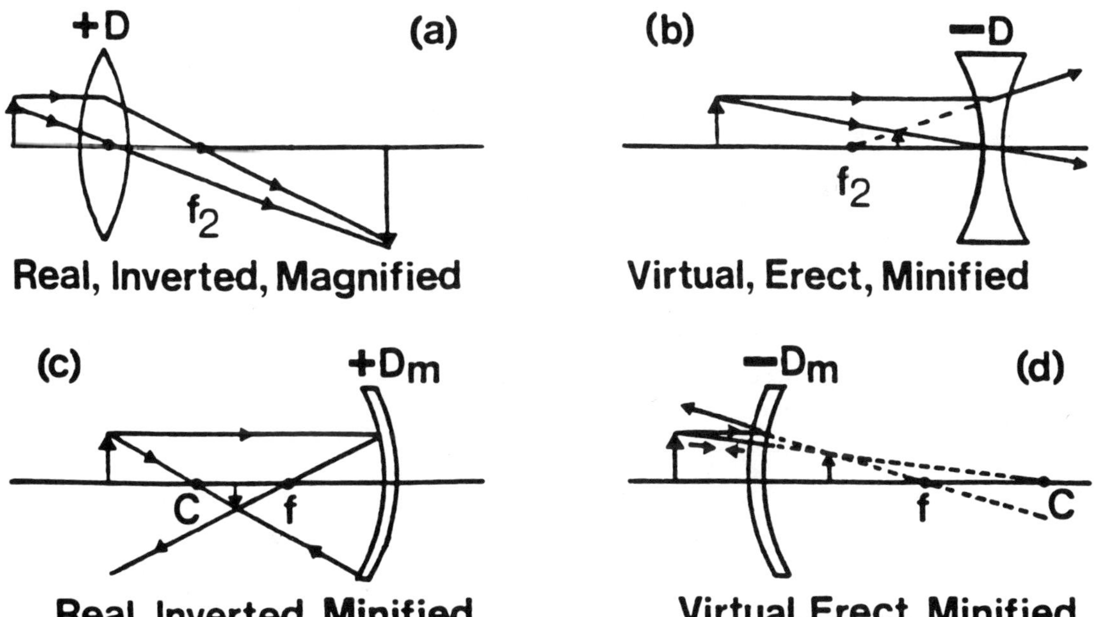

Fig. 1-25

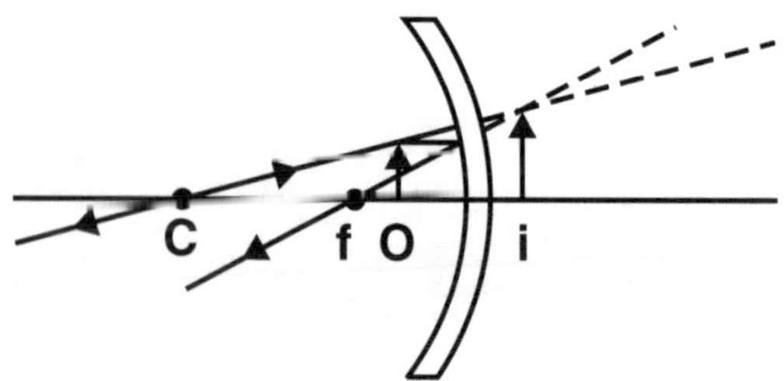

Fig. 1-26

one remembers Fig. 1-25, *c*, and Fig. 1-26, the varying intermediate determinations are more easily derived.

The other confusing situation is that of a plane mirror. The power $\frac{(2)}{r}$ is zero so that

$$U + D_m = V \text{ becomes } U + 0 = V \text{ or } \frac{1}{u} = \frac{1}{v}$$

This rightly implies that the object and image distance are equidistant from the mirror. The image lies to the right of the mirror and is therefore a virtual image. As explained below with equal object and image vergence (and distance) the image size is the same as the object size, i.e., the magnification is 1×.

Although the magnification of a plane mirror is 1×, there is a *perspective* change in size as one moves closer to and further away from the mirror. As one approaches the mirror, the image appears larger, although the object is always the same size. Conversely, one looks smaller from further away. This is because the *true* magnification of the system is calculated by using the object and image distance relative to the *mirror.* The *perceived* magnification is relative to the observer distance to the image.

$$\text{Magnification} = \frac{v}{u} = \frac{0.5}{0.5} = 1\times$$

But to the observer (O), the image appears to be 1 m away from him or her.

$$\text{Perception} = \frac{u}{u + v} = \frac{0.5}{1} = 0.5\times$$

i.e., to the observer the image appears half as big.

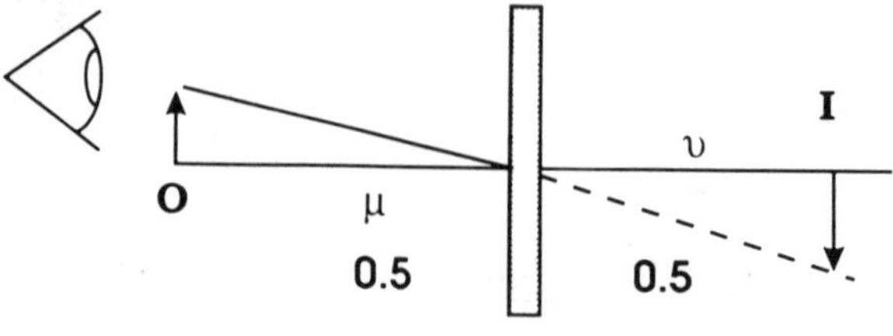

Fig. 1-27

The image is upright but is reversed left to right (a quick glance in the mirror in the morning will verify the reversal for the doubters in the crowd). The ray trace is unique in that a plane mirror has no radius or center of curvature through which to trace. The necessary rays are determined by the position of the *viewing* eye and a perpendicular drawn at the lower extent of the object to bisect the mirror or bisecting the object to extend to the lowest extent of the mirror (Fig. 1-28 and Fig. 1-29).

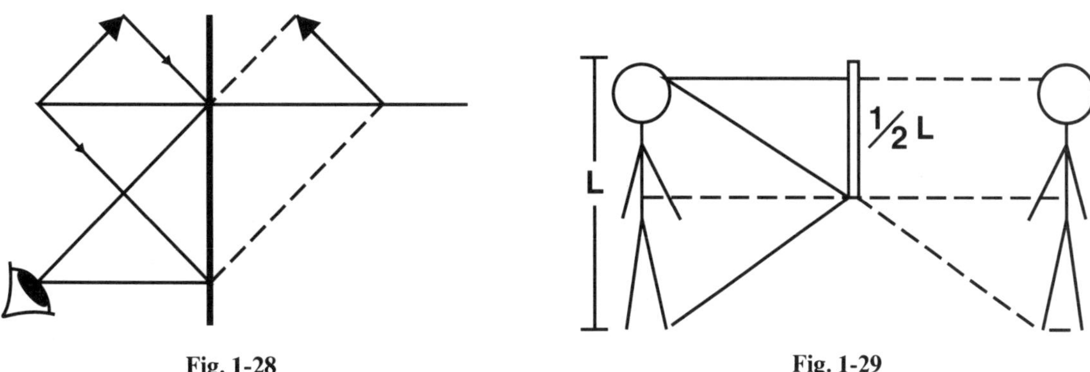

Fig. 1-28 **Fig. 1-29**

As can be seen from Fig. 1-29 the field of view is double the size of the mirror so that a mirror only one-half one's height is required to obtain a full-length view.

Thus far the determination of the position, orientation, reality, or virtuality of the image have been covered, but the size can only be estimated from the diagrams.

Fig. 1-30 on inspection reveals two similar triangles so that:

$$\frac{\text{Image size (I)}}{\text{Object size (O)}} = \frac{v}{u} = \frac{U}{V}$$

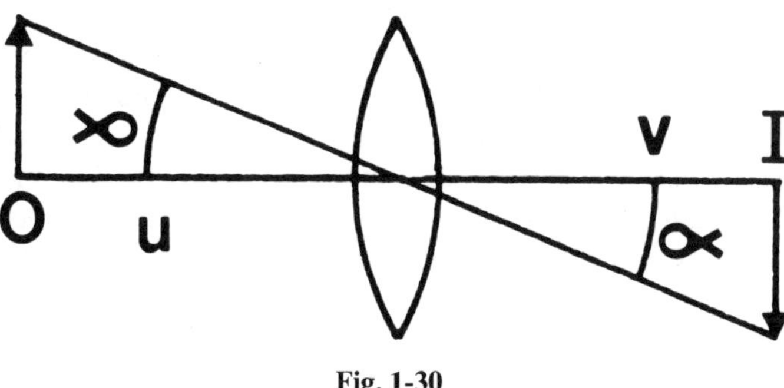

Fig. 1-30

This is synonymous with the entity called linear or lateral magnification. As shall be seen later, this is only one aspect of magnification, for axial and angular magnification must be given consideration when dealing with optical systems.

Consideration of the effects of a single thin lens on the formation of an image has been given so far but the effect of two or more thin lenses used in combination has been remiss. If multiple lens systems are dealt with in such a way as to consider each lens in turn, a very simplified scheme is derived. In this manner the image from the first lens becomes the object for the second lens and so forth.

Consider the following illustrative example:

An object is placed 50 cm from a +4.00 D lens. A second −2.00 D lens is situated 25 cm from the first. Where will the final image be located?

Solution:

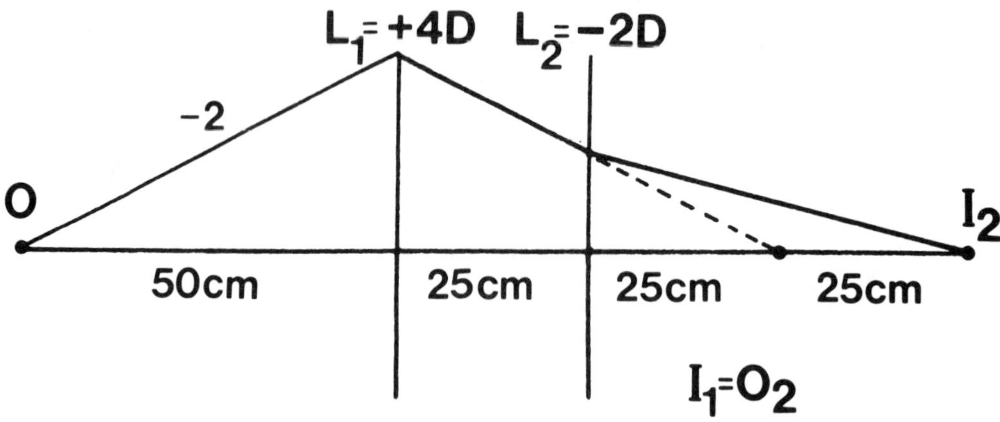

The object is located 50 cm to the left of L_1 so that the object vergence at the lens is $U = \frac{1}{u} = \frac{1}{-0.5} = -2.00$ D. $U + D = V$ yields $V = -2 + (+4) =$ $+2.00$ D; thus $v = \frac{1}{2} = 0.5$ m or 50 cm to the right of L_1. This image now becomes the object for L_2, but since it lies to the right of L_2, it is a virtual object for L_2. The new object distance is 25 cm to the right of L_2 and convergent on it. Thus $U_2 = \frac{1}{u_2} = \frac{1}{0.25} = +4.00$ D. $U_2 + D_2 = V_2$ yields $+4 - 2 = +2.00 \text{ D} = \frac{100}{2} = 50$ cm. The image is thus a real image 50 cm to the right of L_2. As is easily appreciable, this can get very cumbersome for a very complicated multilens system. For this reason the concept of principal planes was developed.

With the use of an optical bench or another method for determining the power of the entire system, an "incoming" and an "outgoing" plane can be constructed. This effectively reduces the system to two focal points (and planes) and two principal planes. Ray diagrams can then be constructed ignoring everything in between the two principal planes. The two focal planes, as determined from the power determination, are measured from the principal planes. Two nodal points also exist so that a ray entering the system encounters the first nodal point and it emerges from the second undeviated but displaced by the distance between nodal points (Fig. 1-31).

This, in essence, has reduced a multiple thin lens system to a single thick lens. To measure the TRUE power of a lens the location of the principal planes must be known. Since this is not known commonly in a real lens, the measurement is taken from the back surface of the lens—the so-called back vertex power or posterior vertex power. This is derived with the anterior lens surface facing the examiner at the lens meter.

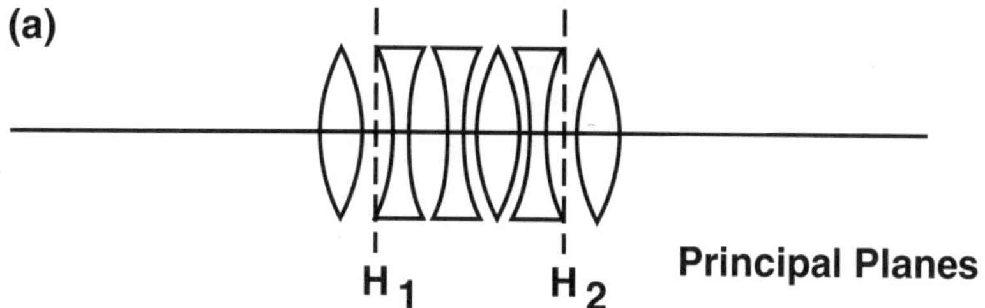

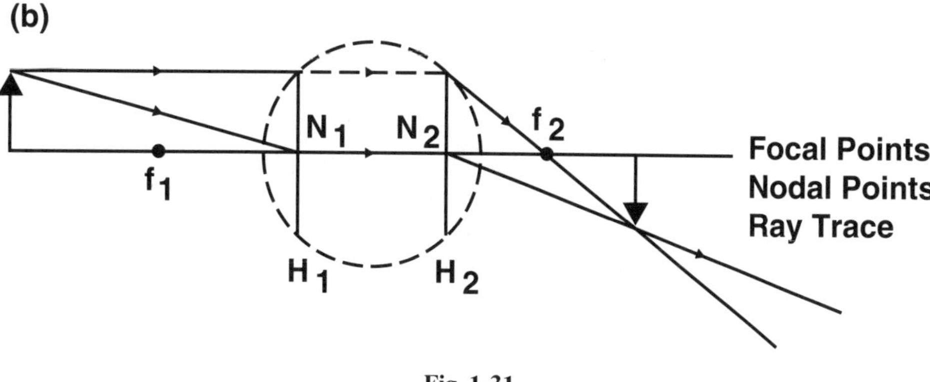

Fig. 1-31

VERTEX POWER AND DISTANCE AND LENS EFFECTIVITY

The factors that alter the vertex power so that it is simply not the sum of the two surface powers are the thickness of the lens and the index of refraction (as one would expect intuitively). The approximation is:

$$D_v = D_1 + D_2 + \frac{t}{n} D_1^2$$

where: t = thickness
n = index of refraction

The value of $\frac{t}{n} D_1^2$ is usually small unless a high plus lens of low refractive index is used. Under these conditions an 0.25 to 0.50 D adjustment may be required to the sum of the two surfaces.

Back vertex power is not to be confused with *lens effectivity*. This entity is simply a function of the distance of the lens from the desired point of focus. It is related to the clinical entity of *vertex distance* or the distance of the correcting lens from the eye.

Consider the situation depicted in Fig. 1-32. It is desired to focus an image at point *I*. If a +4.00 D lens is selected it must be placed 25 cm away. Similarly a

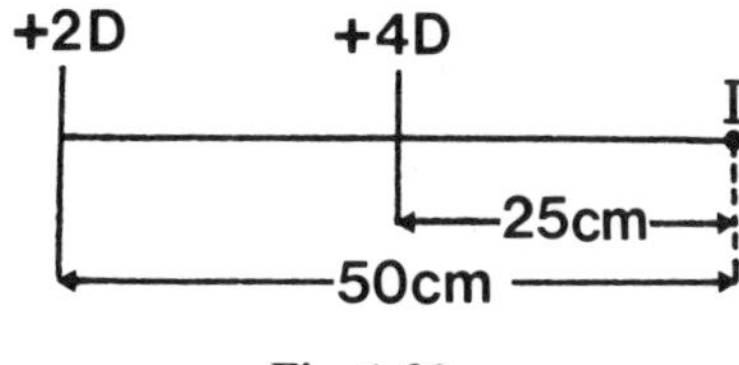

Fig. 1-32

+2.00 D lens could just as easily be selected but must be positioned at 50 cm to perform the same optical task.

When dealing with correcting spectacles, the power required will vary according to the vertex distance. As can be seen from Fig. 1-32, as one approaches the desired point of imagery, the more plus (or less minus) power is required. The useful mnemonic "CAP" represents this "closer add plus" vignette. The clinical implications of these principles will resurface in the discussion on the correction of aphakia and contact lenses.

It should also be recalled that the power determination of lenses is performed in air. From the discussion on reduced vergences, recall the profound effect of the refractive media on the system. The effective power of the lens is profoundly affected by the media in which it is immersed. A prime example of this phenomenon is the intraocular lens implant. Consider how the power might change when measured in air relative to that in the ocular media.

The amount of change is proportional to the differences in the refractive indices between the intraocular lens and air relative to the difference between the intraocular lens and the aqueous:

$$D_{air} = \frac{(n_{IOL} - n_{air})/r}{(n_{IOL} - n_{AQ})/r} = \frac{n_{IOL} - n_{air}}{n_{IOL} - n_{AQ}}$$

A posterior chamber intraocular lens implant power calculation (using axial length and keratometry) reveals that a +19.50 D implant is required. What should this lens measure in air when packaged ($n = 1.5$ for the implant)?

$$\begin{aligned} D_{air} &= \frac{D_{air}}{D_{aqueous}} \times D_{aqueous} \\ &= \frac{n_{IOL} - n_{air}}{n_{IOL} - n_{aqueous}} \times +19.50\text{ D} \\ &= \frac{1.5 - 1.0}{1.5 - 1.33} \times 19.5 \\ &= +57.30\text{ D} \end{aligned}$$

Thus the measured power in air is almost 3× that in aqueous.

Please see Part II: Problems and Part III: Solutions for typical examination questions pertaining to the material in this chapter.

CHAPTER 2: LENS ABERRATIONS

Thick lenses, unlike their utopian counterpart thin lenses, are subject to many aberrations that affect the quality of the image.

SPHERICAL ABERRATION

Spherical aberration is shape dependent. As rays approach the periphery of a lens, they are subject to increased prismatic effect and more power, so a blur interval occurs along the axis (Fig. 2-1). Aspheric surfaces for hyperopic and aphakic lenses greatly improve the spherical aberration of high-power lenses. In lower powered lenses this does not achieve great significance.

Spherical aberration is also manifest in the naturally occurring optical system of the eye. Physiologically, three factors are responsible for reducing this phenomenon:

1. The size of the pupil acts as an aperture, eliminating peripheral rays to some extent.
2. The peripheral cornea has a flatter radius of curvature, which decreases its refracting power peripherally.
3. The nucleus of the crystalline lens has a slightly higher index of refraction, which increases the refraction of axial rays.

These compensatory features are illustrated in Fig. 2-2.

Although this physiologically corrects the majority of spherical aberration of the eye, with larger pupils (as occurs at night or in reduced illumination) more rays gain access to the periphery of the lens. These are refracted more and contribute to the phenomenon of night myopia. As will be seen later, this is only a minor contribution to the dark focus.

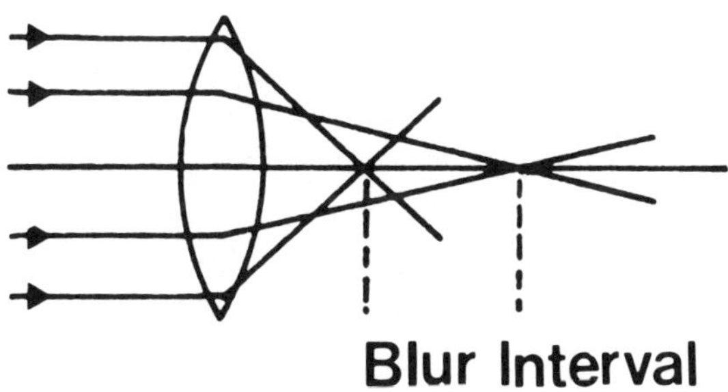

Fig. 2-1 Spherical aberration.

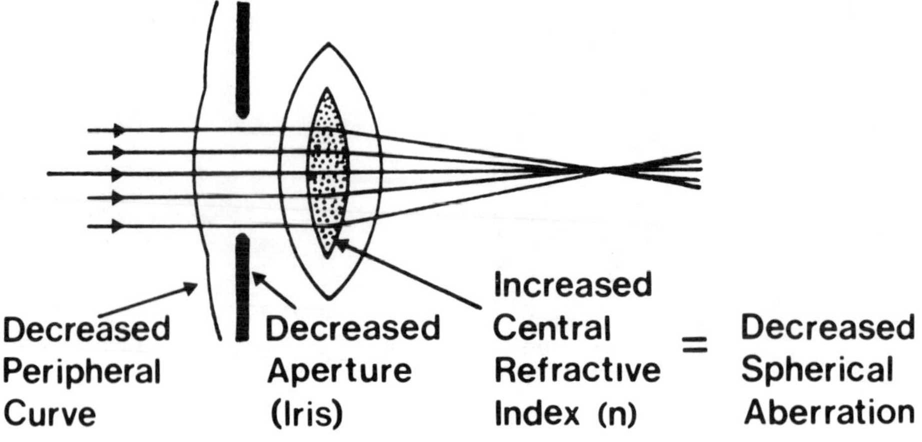

Fig. 2-2

COMA

Coma is a related aberration except that it concerns *off axis* peripheral rays causing a comet-shaped image deformity to nonaxial portions of the image (Fig. 2-3). This contributes very little to aberrations of visual imagery.

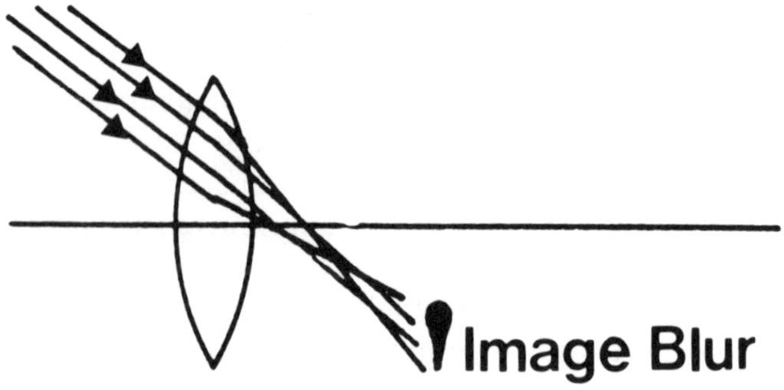

Fig. 2-3 Coma.

ASTIGMATISM OF OBLIQUE INCIDENCE

Astigmatism of oblique incidence is a similarly related phenomenon but it is attributable to oblique rays encountering different toricities at the front and back surface of the lens (Fig. 2-4). Since these surfaces have different radii of curvature, the dotted square in Fig. 2-4 has different powers in different meridians and is thus a spherocylinder. This results in an astigmatic image with two focal lines and an astigmatic interval in which the image is variably blurred. The effect creates a curved rather than a flat image, and this aberration is the *curvature of field.* This is the only advantageous aberration when dealing with the eye. When flat images for cameras and projectors are required, this is obviously of no advantage.

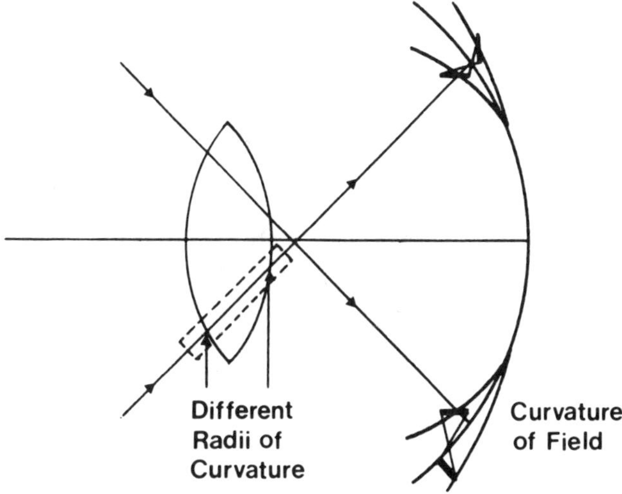

Fig. 2-4 Astigmatism of oblique incidence and curvature of field.

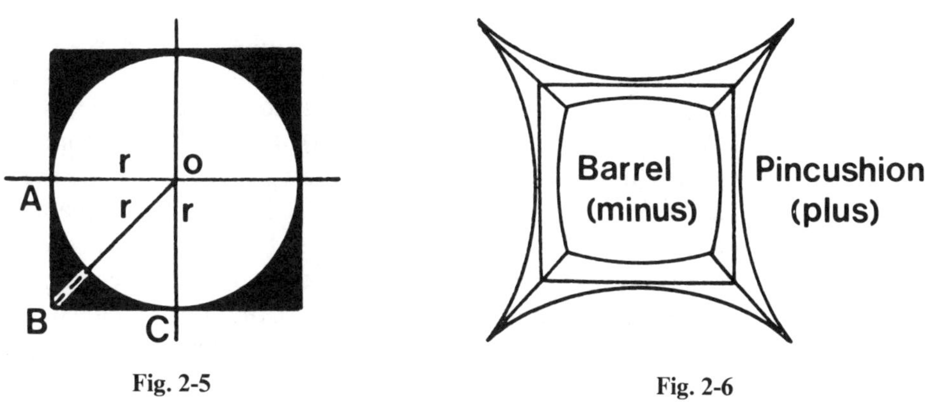

Fig. 2-5

Fig. 2-6

DISTORTION

Distortion is another aberration of thick lenses. It concerns the distortion of straight edges of square objects. If one looks at the square depicted in Fig. 2-5, it is evident that the dotted line on *OB* represents the distance that point *B* is further from the center than points *A* or *C*. Since a square is an extended object, image-forming rays from the corners have to go through a more peripheral part of the lens before gaining access to the eye through the pupil. Just as with spherical aberration, an increased spherical power in the periphery minifies or magnifies the corners more than the sides since they enter more peripherally. This results in *pincushion distortion* in plus lenses (Fig. 2-6). Minification of the corners in minus lenses results in *barrel distortion.*

CHROMATIC ABERRATION

Another aberration is that known as *chromatic* aberration. White light is composed of all the colors in the visible spectrum. Each wavelength (λ) of the com-

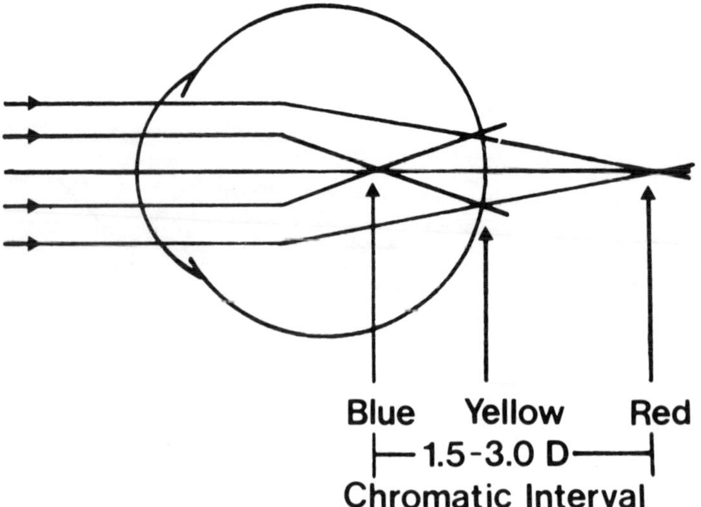

Fig. 2-7 Chromatic aberration.

ponent parts has a different index of refraction. As stated earlier, yellow light is considered the standard for which the various indices are calculated. The fact that each λ has a different *n* affects the refraction of that wavelength (since from Snell's law $n \sin i = n' \sin r$). Blue (shortest λ) light is refracted more than red light (longest λ). This describes a chromatic interval (Fig. 2-7) in the eye of approximately 1.50 to 3.00 D, which is individually variable. In the emmetropic eye the yellow, or middle portion of the spectrum is in best focus. If the eye has too much plus power (myopia), red would be in better focus than green or blue. Similarly, if the eye has too little plus power (hyperopia), the green or blue would be more clearly seen. This is the basis of the clinical test in refraction called the *duochrome or bichrome test,* which is covered in greater detail later.

An easy way to remember the aberrations is the mnemonic ABCs:

A, Astigmatism of oblique incidence

B, Barrel and pincushion

C, Coma, Chromatic, Curvature of field

S, Spherical

When asked to describe the problems associated with thick lenses, one must include magnification, minification and visual field scotomata in addition to the ABCs.

Please see Part II: Problems and Part III: Solutions for typical examination questions pertaining to the material in this chapter.

CHAPTER 3: PRISMS

When one thinks of the dispersion of light into its spectral components, one thinks of the classic property of *prisms* and not lenses.

PLANE PARALLEL PLATE

Before considering prisms, it is instructive to examine the effects of a plane parallel plate on light. As already seen, light travelling from a less dense to a more dense medium is refracted toward the normal (Snell's law). On emerging from the second interface another change of refractive index occurs and again the light is refracted, but this time away from the normal and *parallel* to the incident ray. This ray is thus *displaced* but not deviated from its initial path (Fig. 3-1).

In a prism the denser medium has a nonparallel, wedge-shaped configuration. Light is refracted in a similar fashion (according to Snell's law) as the parallel plate, but the emergent ray is not only displaced but also *deviated* from its original pathway (Fig. 3-2). The prism thus has power. The unit of power is the *prism diopter.* A prism diopter (symbolized P.D. or Δ) is the apparent displacement of a ray (in centimeters) at 1 m (Fig. 3-3). $1 \text{ P.D.} = \frac{1 \text{ cm}}{1 \text{ m}}$.

For example, if the image of an object is displaced 2 cm at ⅓ m, the prismatic effect is 6 P.D. Notice that light is always deviated toward the base of the prism. The base is used as the orienting surface to describe the power. The prism noted above would be specified as base down. If presented with both a horizontal and a vertical prism at the same time, a single representative prism corresponding to the vector sum of the individual components is formed (Fig. 3-4).

This is derived by the Pythagorean theorem or by measurement of the vector resultant on a "to scale" diagram. The angle is measured with a protractor (for example, a trial lens frame or phoropter) or calculated trigonometrically. The eye and position of the base must also be specified as in the caption below the diagram in Fig. 3-4, or the orientation may be reversed.

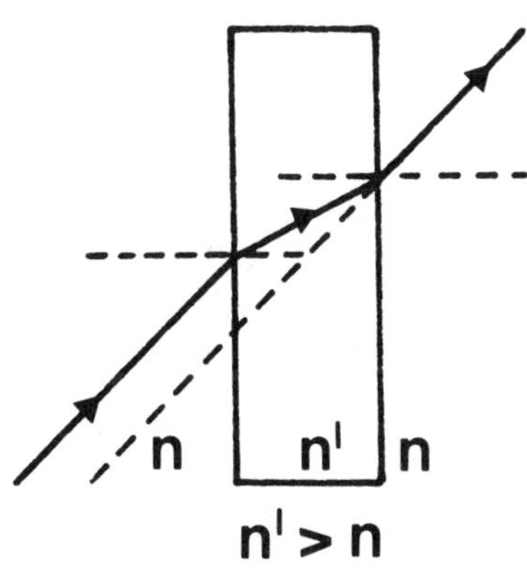

Fig. 3-1

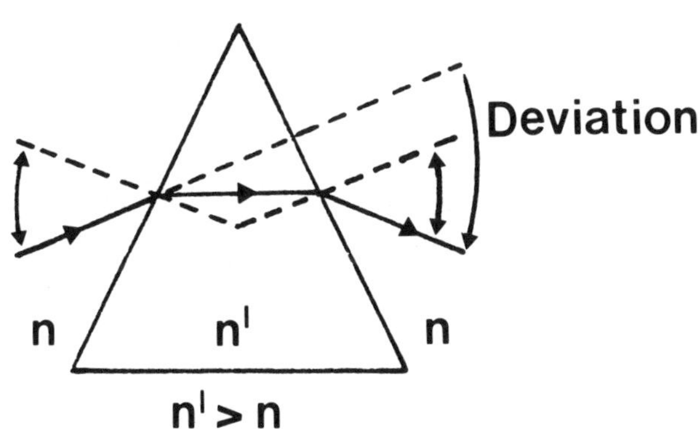

Fig. 3-2

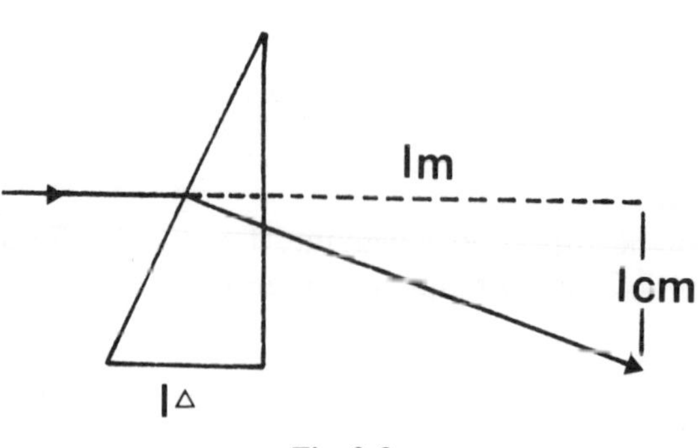

Fig. 3-3

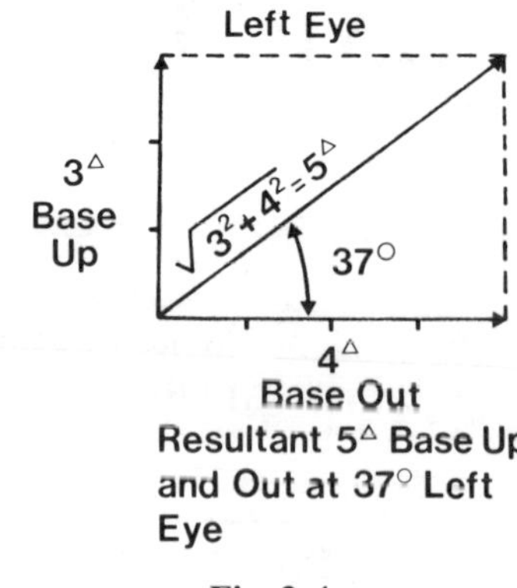

Fig. 3-4

PRISM DEVIATION

Another aspect of prisms frequently spoken about is the minimum and maximum deviation. Quite simply, the minimum angle of deviation is achieved at an inclination where equal deviation occurs at both surfaces (Fig. 3-5). The maximum is achieved with the tilt of the prism until the incident ray just enters the surface. The minimum deviation is clinically important, for it is in this position that *plastic* prisms are calibrated. When eye deviations are measured, the back surface of the plastic prism should be held in the *frontal* plane, parallel with the forehead if the measured deviation is to correspond with the calibration. *Glass* prisms, on the other hand, are calibrated with the incident light perpendicular to one of the surfaces—*Prentice* position (Fig. 3-6). This means that no matter what the position of the eye, the prism must be held such that one surface is normal to the visual axis. If not, the measured value will not correspond to the calibrated value. Thompson and Guyton have found that a glass prism held improperly with the back surface in the frontal plane position will decrease the prismatic effect; for example, 40 P.D. glass prism will exert only 32 P.D. effect (80%).

These authors have also considered this phenomenon in relation to stacking prisms to obtain an intermediate power when the trial prism set is lacking a desired power, e.g., 45 P.D. The emergent light from the first prism is incident on the stacked second prism by an already deviated amount. This new incident angle is far removed from the minimum angle for plastic prisms or the Prentice position

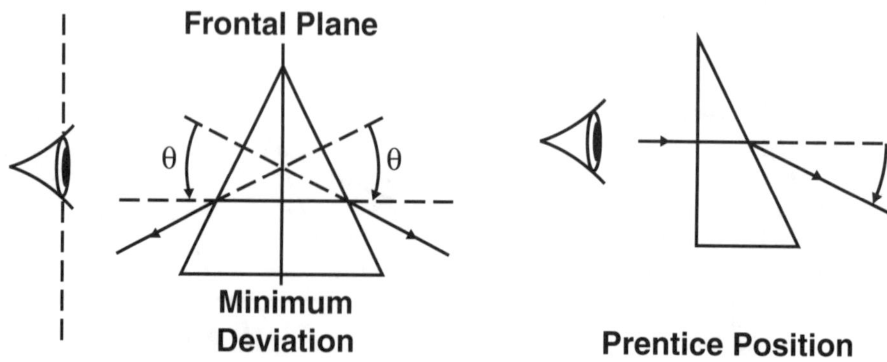

Fig. 3-5 Plastic prism.

Fig. 3-6 Glass prism.

for glass prisms. This results in a completely different deviation than the calibrated sum of the two prisms. This becomes significant even in the 5 P.D. to 10 P.D. range when added to larger (30 P.D. +) prisms, as is frequently performed clinically, e.g., 40 P.D. + 5 P.D. = 58 P.D. To avert this artefact, the prisms can be added to each eye separately in the desired amount, or a loose prism over one eye and a rotary prism over the other eye can be used. *The stacked combination of two prisms in the same direction should never be done.* The combination of horizontal and vertical prisms produces no significant artefact and is a clinically useful method of measuring deviations.

CIRCULAR MEASURE AND THE ANGLE OF DEVIATION

Other measures of *circular* measure are used occasionally and interrelate with the prism diopter, such as radians and degrees.

A radian is the angle θ measured when the length of the arc of rotation (AB) is equal to the radius (r) (Fig. 3-7). To convert radians to degrees is easy. Imagine the arc AB rotating a full 360° to complete the circumference of a circle (2π radian $= 2\pi\, r$)

$$2\pi \text{ radian} = 360°$$

$$1 \text{ radian} = \frac{360°}{2\pi}$$

$$\approx 57°18'$$

$$\text{or } 1° \approx 0.01745 \text{ radian}$$

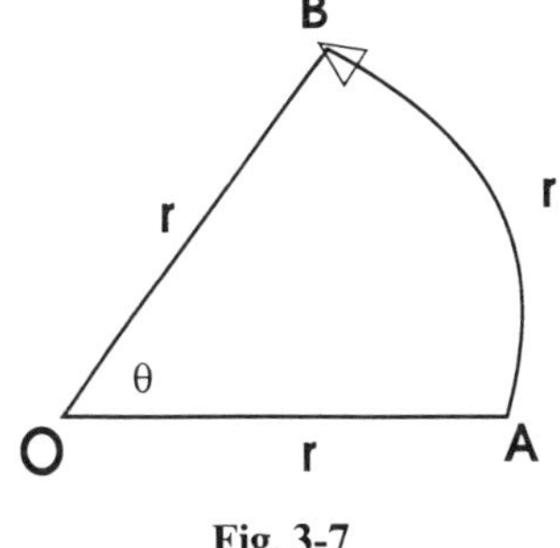

Fig. 3-7

In the SI (Système Internationale), the radian and milliradian (1/1000 radian) are the only recognized units of circular measure.

Angle β in Fig. 3-8 has as its tangent the length of the opposite over adjacent sides, so that:

$$\tan \beta = \frac{10}{100} = 0.1$$

$$100 \tan \beta = 100 \times 0.1 = 10 \text{ P.D.}$$

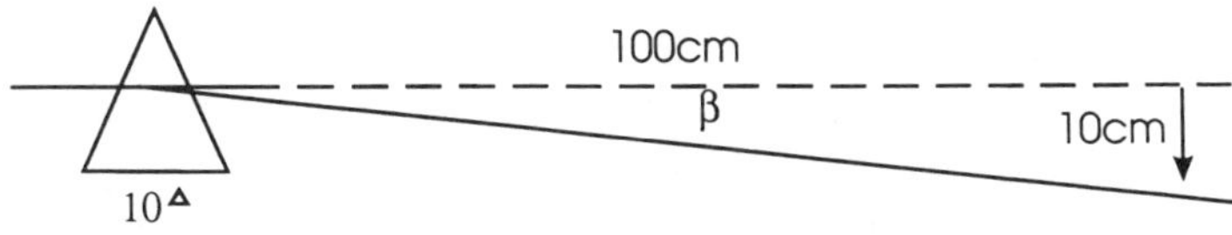

Fig. 3-8

Table 3-1

Angle in Degrees (β)	Tangent	Angle in Prism Diopters (100 tan β)
2°	0.0349	3.49 P.D.
10°	0.1763	17.63 P.D.
20°	0.3640	36.40 P.D.

An angle β, then, is expressed in prism diopters simply by multiplying its tangent by 100. This is not a unit, linear scale in that the tangents increase faster than the angles.

Angle β is the *angle of deviation* and, as can be seen by inspection, is approximately related by the tangent to the prism diopter. So for small angles:

$$1° \approx 2 \text{ P.D.}$$

APPROXIMATION FORMULA

The approximation formula 1° = 2 P.D. becomes less accurate after approximately 45 P.D. This is not equivalent to the apex angle, and the two should not be confused. The apex or apical angle (γ) (Fig. 3-9) can be approximated by several formulae, e.g.,

$$\tan \gamma = \frac{\sin d}{n - \cos d} \qquad \text{where: } \gamma = \text{apical angle}, \quad d = \text{deviation}$$

(a)

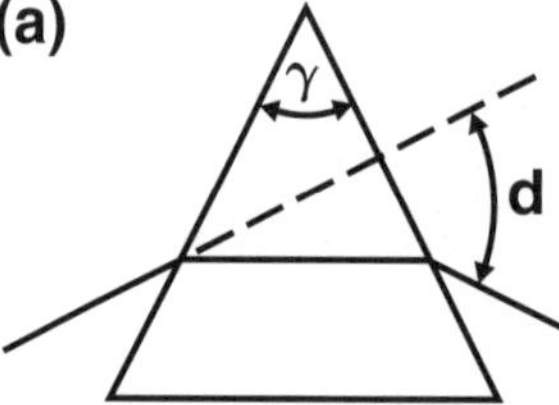

(b)

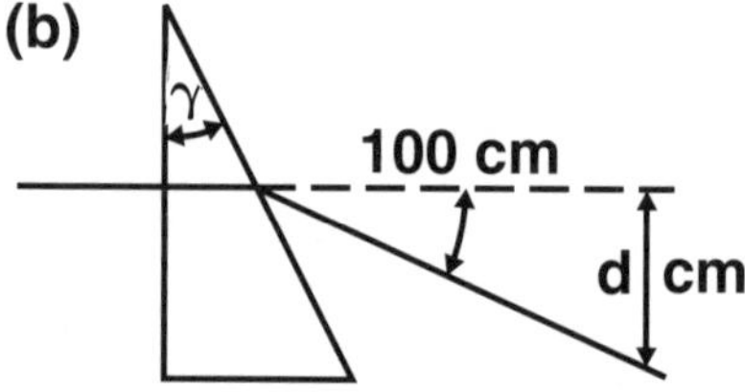

Fig. 3-9

In ophthalmic optics the prism diopter is used almost exclusively to define the prism and calibrate it. During actually grinding of the prism the apical angle and the base width do become important and are used to verify its strength.

A limit is reached when the emergent ray is deviated 90° from the incident ray (Fig. 3-10). The prism would have an infinite prism diopter value, since it would never intersect this axis at 100 cm. Hence 90° $= \infty$P.D. In other words, the light is reflected and not refracted.

Like any optical device, a prism also affects the image of the system. Light is always deviated toward the base of the prism. When one is looking through a

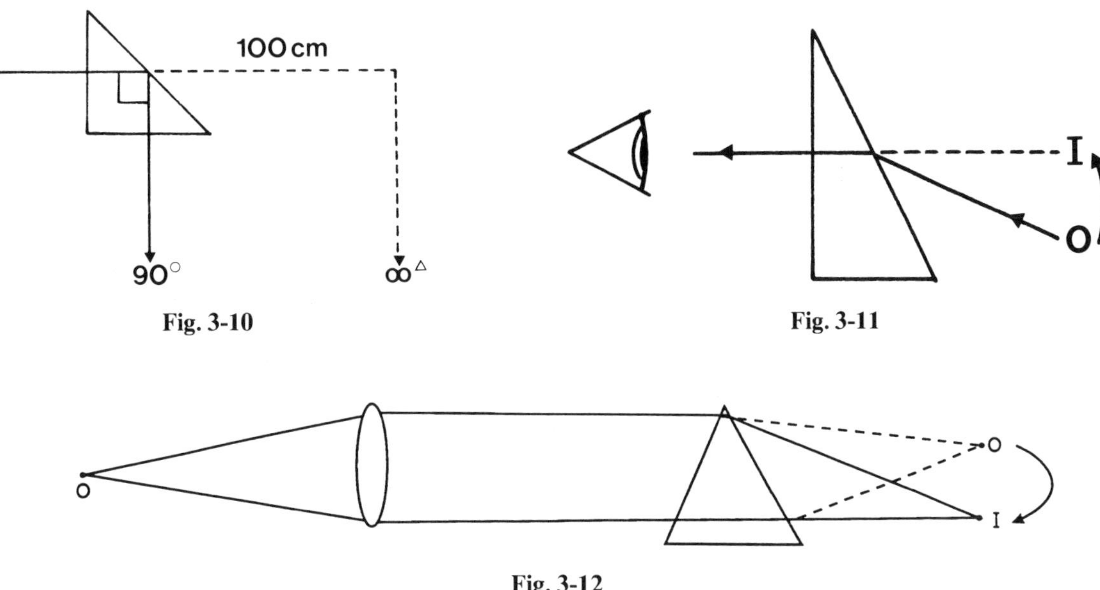

Fig. 3-10

Fig. 3-11

Fig. 3-12

prism, the image is virtual and *displaced toward the apex* (Fig. 3-11). (Note that the ray emergent from the object is reversed i.e., travelling right to left, and the object is virtual.)

If it is a real object in an optical system with a prism, it actually displaces the image toward the base of the prism (Fig. 3-12).

It is more important to remember that in visual imagery, as depicted in Fig. 3-11, the virtual nature of the object and the reversal of the usual direction of the light displace the image of the object to the apex of the prism. When one is looking at a patient with the prism in front of their eye, the eye will look displaced to the apex of the prism, i.e., both the patient and the examiner see their respective images displaced toward the apex of the prism.

A heterophoria or tropia is a latent or manifest deviation of the eye. This is an everyday clinical problem in which prisms are used to measure the deviation. An esotropia is an eye deviated toward the nose; an exotropia is a temporal deviation; a hypertropia or hypotropia is a vertical deviation.

Fig. 3-13 depicts an esotropic eye with a prism that is base out, deviating the ray to fall on the central fixing portion (fovea) of the deviated eye. As can be seen, the *prism apex of the correcting prism points in the direction of the deviation.*

Similarly, if a prism such as a pair of glasses is placed in front of a straight eye, a deviation will be produced. The direction of the induced deviation is again pointed out by the apex of the prism required to correct it. For example, 4 P.D. base out is accidentally placed in a patient's glasses. A deviation is noted on clinical testing, which is neutralized by 4 P.D. base in. The apex of the prism that neutralizes the deviation is out or lateral, so an exodeviation is present.

Prisms are not the only optical means of deviating light. If you think of any lens, all rays off the optical axis are bent toward or away from the axis depending on the vergence power of the lens (Fig. 3-14). This is known as the *prismatic effect of lenses.* In fact, lenses can be thought of as prisms of progressively increasing prismatic power outward from the optical center of the lens (which has no prism power).

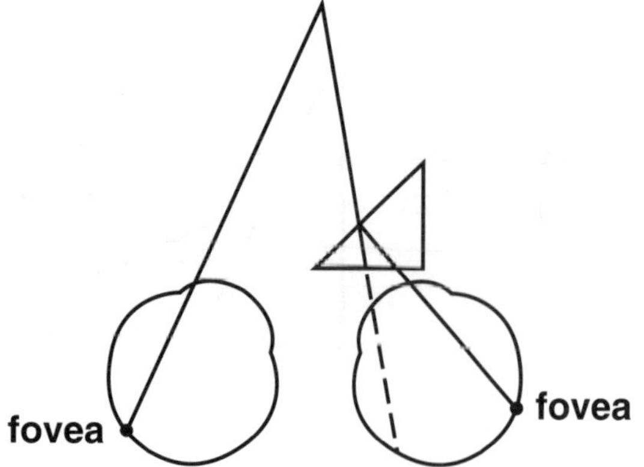

Fig. 3-13 Right esotropia neutralized by base out prism.

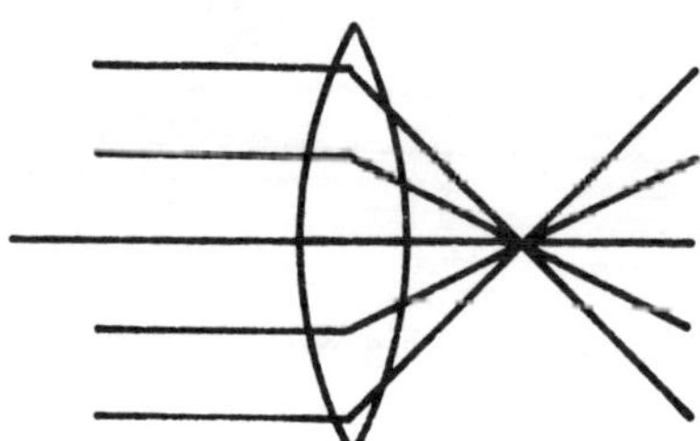

Fig. 3-14

PRENTICE'S RULE

As seen in Fig. 3-15(*a*), a plus lens can be thought of as an upper base down and lower base up prism, depending on which decentered portion of the lens one is viewing through. The reverse is true of a minus lens (Fig. 3-15*b*). Physiologically this is important, since the reading position carries the visual axes approximately 2 mm nasally and 8 mm down into a portion of the lens with prismatic effect. As expected, the induced prism depends on two factors: (1) the power of the lens in that meridian and (2) the distance decentered from the visual axis. This relationship is the basis of *Prentice's rule.* This simply states that the induced prismatic effect of a lens (P) is equal to its distance decentered from the optical center of the lens (h) (in centimeters) times the power of the lens (D) (in diopters) in that meridian (Fig. 3-16).

$$\text{Induced prism } P \text{ P.D.} = h \text{ (cm)} \times D \text{ (diopters)}$$

where: h = distance from the optical center in centimeters
D = power of the lens

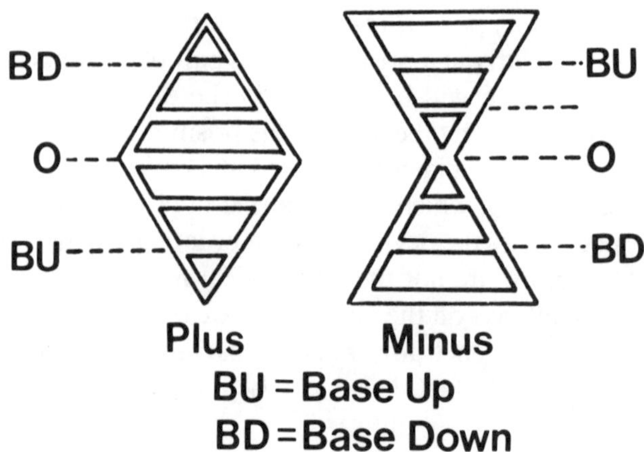

Fig. 3-15

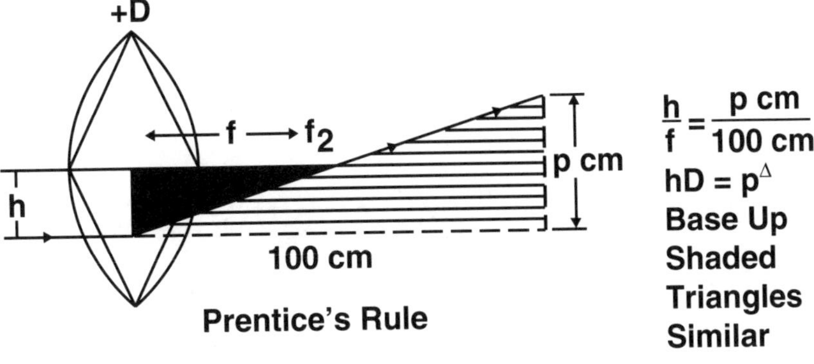

Fig. 3-16

In Fig. 3-16 the two shaded triangles are similar so that:

$$\frac{h}{f} = \frac{P}{100 \text{ cm}}$$

$$h \times \frac{1}{f} = \text{P P.D.}$$

$$h \times D = P \text{ P.D.}$$

This is an inevitable examination topic, so let us spend a little more time examining the intricacies (it's also important clinically, of course). As just discussed, with normal spherical lenses consideration must be given to the reading position. If one wears a +5.00 D lens over both eyes (Fig. 3-17), what will be the induced prismatic effects at the usual reading position (2 mm in, 8 mm down)?

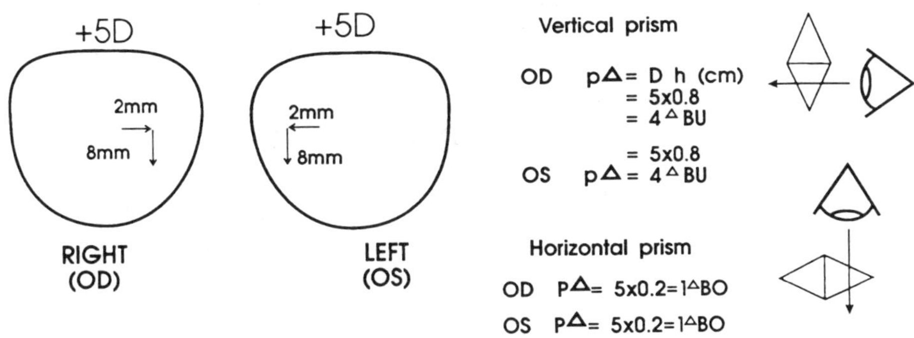

Fig. 3-17

ANISOMETROPIA AND INDUCED DEVIATIONS

If one considers the effect of prisms on the eye alignment, one will learn how to deal with these numbers. If, as in Fig. 3-18, a patient has a right hyperdeviation, normally he would fix the object of regard with his left eye. To neutralize this, a correcting prism base down, apex up (apex pointing to the type of deviation) would be placed over his right eye. If, on the other hand, his left eye is covered,

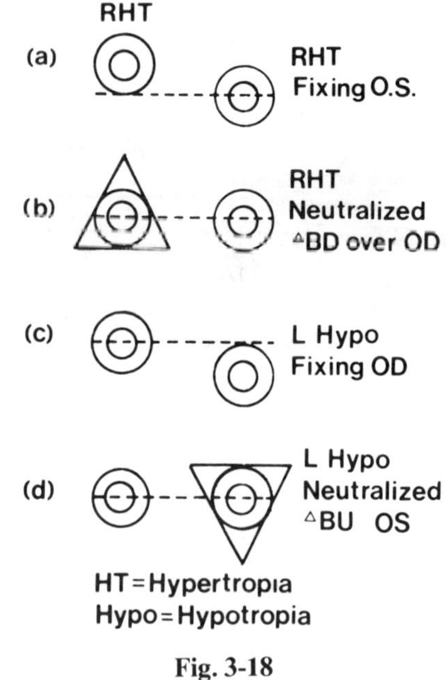

Fig. 3-18

his right eye would then fix and his left eye would be hypodeviated (left hypotropia). To neutralize this, a prism base up over his left eye is required. Thus, a hyperdeviation in one eye is equivalent to a hypodeviation in the opposite eye (excluding dissociated hyperdeviation). That is to say, placing a base down prism over the right eye is equivalent to placing a base up prism over the left eye. In Fig. 3-17 then, 4 P.D. base up over the right eye is equivalent to 4 P.D. base down over the left eye. The total or net effect is 4 P.D. base down + 4 P.D. base up = 0. Thus, although each image is displaced 4 cm at 1 m, it is done so in opposite directions but equally for both eyes, and no problems will arise unless there is a difference in power in the lenses—a condition called anisometropia. If the right eye is +5.00 D and the left eye is +1.00 D, what would happen to the vertical prismatic effect?

$$OD\ P\ \text{P.D.} = Dh = +5 \times 0.8 = 4\ \text{P.D. base up}$$

$$OS\ P\ \text{P.D.} = Dh = +1 \times 0.8 = 0.8\ \text{P.D. base up}$$

$$4\ \text{P.D. base up right eye} = 4\ \text{P.D. base down left eye}$$

$$\text{Net effect} = 4\ \text{P.D.} - 0.8\ \text{P.D.} = 3.2\ \text{P.D. base down left eye}$$

To neutralize this, a 3.2 P.D. base up whose apex points down would be required. Therefore a left hypodeviation is induced or a right hyperdeviation of 3.2 P.D. The implication is that the patient would now be required to exert 3.2 P.D. of vertical fusional movement to maintain single binocular vision. In a single vision lens this is no problem. One would simply avoid this reading portion, tilt the head or elevate the reading material and look through the optical centers of the lenses where no induced prism is found. In the presbyopic patient wearing bifocals to replace lost accommodative power, this region of the lens is necessary to see clearly. In this instance two alternatives are available: (1) single vision reading glasses or (2) ground-in prism or lens decentration of the appropriate amount (if of adequate power). An appropriate technique is to "slab off" some base down prism by decentered grinding (Fig. 3-19).

What effect on the eye deviation is achieved with induced horizontal prism? Consider a horizontal deviation, for example, the esotropia (ET) depicted in Fig. 3-20. With the right eye fixing, a left ET is seen that is neutralized with prism base out over the left eye. If one covers the right eye, the left eye picks up fixation and a right ET is seen, which again requires a base out prism to neutralize it. Thus if one has an esodeviation or exodeviation, the direction of the correcting prism for the deviation is in the same direction no matter which eye is covered. Placing a base out prism over the right eye is equivalent to placing a base out prism over the left eye. To neutralize this, a base in–apex out prism is required. An *exo*deviation is produced. Horizontal fusional movement is required to remain in single binocular vision. This is seldom a problem clinically. Most individuals have much greater horizontal fusional amplitudes than vertical fusional amplitudes. Just as often as creating problems, decentration of the optical centers of plus or minus lenses is often beneficial for an individual with an exodeviation or esodeviation to obtain an induced prismatic effect in the direction of an eso or exo shift. This lessens the requirements on the fusional amplitudes and increases comfort.

In summary then, the induced eye deviation is in the direction of the apex of the neutralizing or correcting prism. The magnitude of this decentration is the net difference between the eyes for similar vertical prisms and the sum of both eyes for dissimilar vertical and horizontal prisms.

If a problem with decentration arises, calculate the difference between the pupillary distance and the optical centers of the lenses and split the distance equally among both eyes (Fig. 3-21). For example, if the optical centers are 70 mm apart and the pupillary distance is 64 mm, the lenses are decentered 6 mm or decentered out 3 mm in each eye.

Another frequent variation is to have a spherocylindrical correction in a bifocal lens. Although cylinders have not yet been discussed, the power of the cylinder is in the meridian 90° to its axis. For example, a cylinder +2.00 × 180 has all its

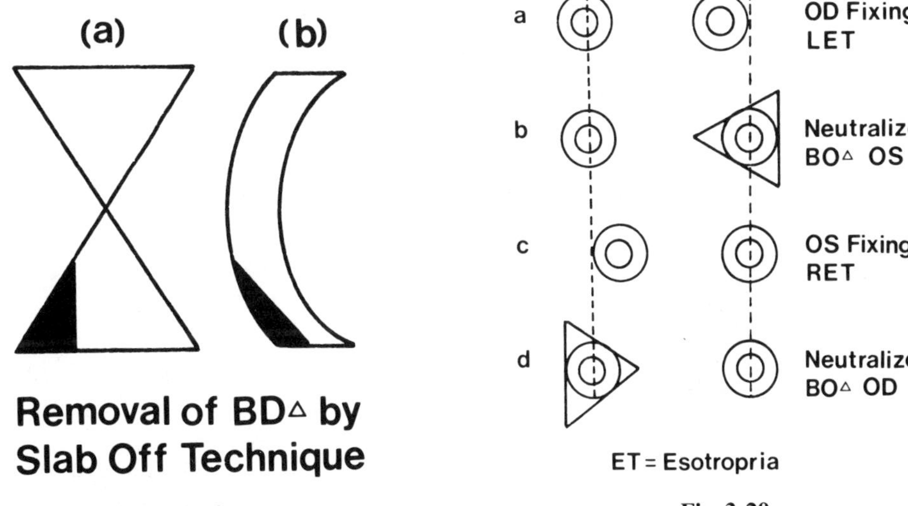

Fig. 3-19

Fig. 3-20

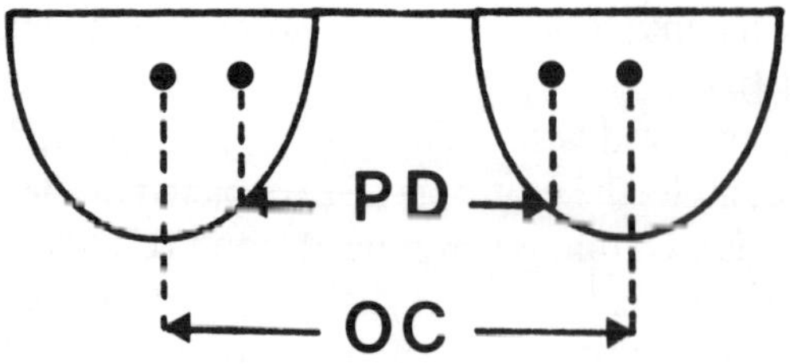

PD
OC

Fig. 3-21

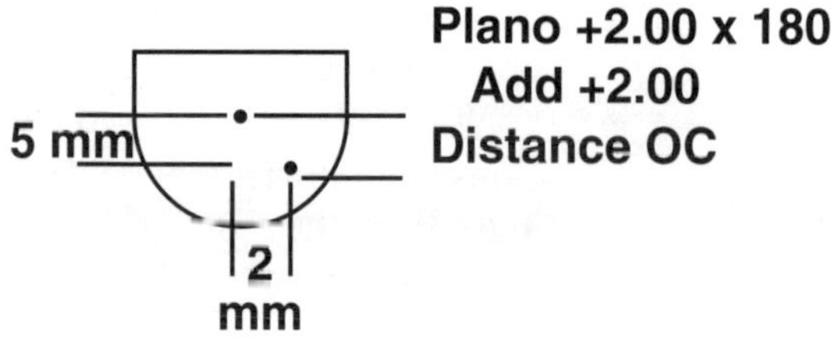

Right Lens
Distance
Plano +2.00 x 180
Add +2.00
Distance OC
5 mm
2 mm

Fig. 3-22

power acting at 90°. In Fig.3-22 the distance correction has all the power in the 90° vertical meridian. It also has, for near, an additional +2.00 D. The total power in the vertical meridian is therefore +4.00 D. To calculate the vertical prism induced, P P.D. = hD = 0.5 × 4 = 2 P.D. Since it is a plus lens, it is 2 P.D. base up. Similarly, the power in the horizontal meridian would be only the power of the bifocal, and the induced horizontal prism would be P P.D. = 0.2 × 2 = 0.4 P.D. base out. One can ignore the power of the add if it is equal in both eyes, set at the same height, and of the same style.

MEASUREMENT ERROR

If this were not enough, Scattergood and Guyton have called attention to the fact that beneath high plus or minus lenses the prismatic effect of the lenses can alter the amount of deviation measured for strabismic patients. Fig. 3-23 illustrates the principles involved. If the measuring prism is in the same direction as the induced

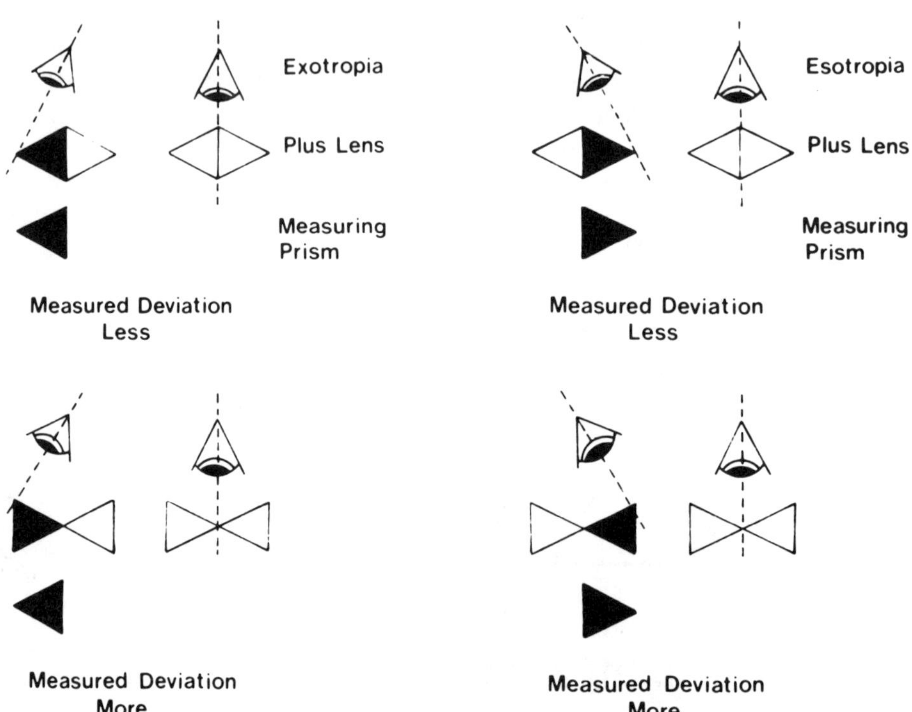

Fig. 3-23

prismatic effect of the spectacle correction, the amount of measuring prism will be less than the true deviation.

Similarly, if it is opposite to the induced prism, this additional prism must be neutralized before the deviation is measured; the measured deviation is therefore greater. This is, of course, related to the power of the lens and becomes significant if it is greater than ± 5.00 D. The amount of induced error in measurement is approximately $2.5 \times$ D%.

For example a $+20.00$ D aphakic patient with a measured esotropia of 40 P.D. would actually have an 60 P.D. esotropia! ($2.5 \times 20 = 50\%$, i.e., a plus lens decreases the measured deviation to 50% of the true value). As is readily appreciated, if one is to contemplate surgery according to the measured deviation, this error should be corrected for.

In summary, *plus* lenses *decrease* the measured deviation; *minus* lenses *increase* the measured deviation. A useful way to remember this is the 3M rule: *m*inus *m*easures *m*ore.

Another aspect of prism neutralization relates to measuring primary versus secondary deviations. If the patient has a left sixth paresis with a left esotropia, the patient fixes with the nonparetic right eye and a base out prism is placed over the paretic left eye to measure the deviation. Prism is increased until the primary deviation is neutralized. With the paretic left eye fixing, the prism is added to the right eye until neutralization. This is the secondary deviation. In this case it will measure more. The definition of the fixing eye then becomes the eye without the prism.

Measuring deviations automatically is now possible. Projecting prisms into free space is equivalent to projecting lenses into free space (Humphrey). (This latter assembly is used in automated refraction.) Combining a remote prism projection to an eye movement scanner allows the measurement of a deviation without placing a physical prism in front of a patient (Guyton). In adults, the position of two targets can be neutralized by prisms controlled by hand-operated, computer-assisted trackball or mouse arrangements. In children too young for subjective testing, the movement of the eyes to projected targets can be neutralized by the ghost prisms and the eye movement scanner. These techniques hold great promise for screening and measuring motility disorders.

For simple photography, holding the flash under the camera gives a beautiful Krimsky reflex, and increasing the pantoscopic tilt of the glasses reduces unwanted reflections (Guyton).

IMAGE JUMP AND DISPLACEMENT

Image jump is the sudden shift in the image position when the visual axis descends from the distance optical center to the bifocal segment. If the optical center is far from the top of the segment, the visual axis must first encounter the prismatic effects of the add before reaching the reading segment optical center. This prismatic effect causes the image to jump. Conversely, the flat top or executive style has optical centers in the segment that are very close to the top of the segment, so very little prismatic effect or jump is experienced. This is depicted in Fig. 3-24.

Image displacement is the displacement of the image by the total amount of prism effective in the bifocal portion, i.e., that contribution from the distance and near correction. From Fig. 3-24 one sees that for minus lenses an ideal situation exists. With the flat top or executive type bifocal both image jump and displace-

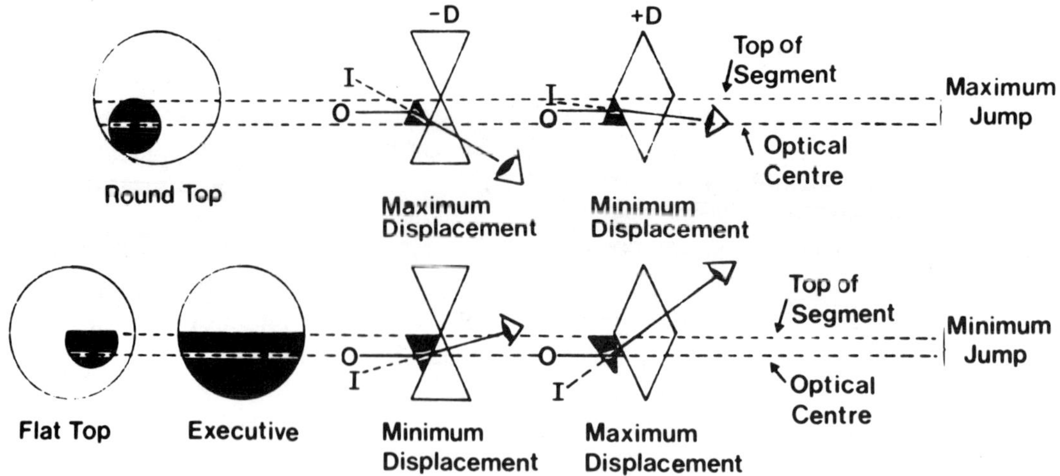

Fig. 3-24

ment are minimized. In a plus lens, however, one must decide between the best of two evils, since no single type minimizes both effects. Contrary to what the name implies, an executive with a plus executive bifocal would probably complain more of the displacement with this lens and might prefer to put up with the image jump of the round top to minimize this.

Conversely, a waiter would prefer the minimized jump with the executive or flat top type. In the anisometropic patient before slab-off bicentric grinding was popularized, a flat top was used in the more minus or less plus lens and a round top in the other. This is a cosmetically poor alternative. Don't forget that all of this can be avoided by single vision reading glasses. They are also easier on the neck and are encouraged for cervical disc disease sufferers!

SPECIAL PRISMS

The *biprism* is a useful device present in most trial sets, although its clinical use is not popular. It is, however, used in many ophthalmic instruments such as the keratometer and applanation tonometer as a doubling device. Fig. 3-25 depicts the imagery of doubling with this device. The beauty of doubling from a *single* source is that, if one image moves, so does the other. When attempting to take a measurement on a nonstationary object such as the eye, small movements shift both images, so an end point can still be obtained.

A *rotary prism* (Fig. 3-26) (e.g., Risley) is constructed of two prisms with back-

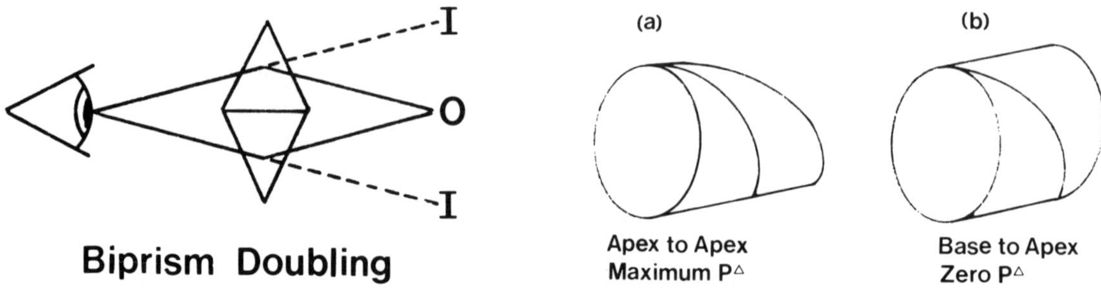

Fig. 3-25

Fig. 3-26

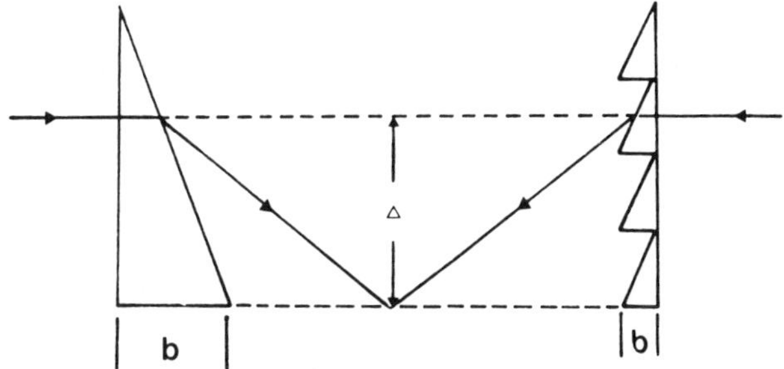

Fresnel Prism 'Stacking'
Same Power-Reduced Base (b)

Fig. 3-27

to-front juxtaposition and is capable of 360° rotation. This varies the power of the prism such that it is maximum in the apex-to-apex position and minimum when base-to-apex. Variable powers in between are calibrated. This handy device is used for the measurement of eye deviations.

Another special form of prism is the *Press-On Fresnel Prism* (Optical Sciences Group, Inc., California). In an attempt to reduce the base thickness of prisms, the fact that the prism power is related to the apex angle is employed. No matter how small the prism, as long as the apex angle is the same, the power of the prism is the same. The smaller the prism, the smaller the size of the base and the lighter the prism (Fig. 3-27).

The Press-On prism can be simply affixed to the surface of a regular spectacle lens in a reversible fashion. Its use in eye deviations that are unstable or in those in which a trial of prisms is indicated is obviously superior and cheaper than ground-in prisms. The disadvantages include reduced visual acuity from reflection and scatter at the interface, peeling, dirt, discoloration, and factors such as chromatic aberration, which are inherent in all ophthalmic prisms. Additional uses include correction of the induced deviation in anisometropic bifocals, static

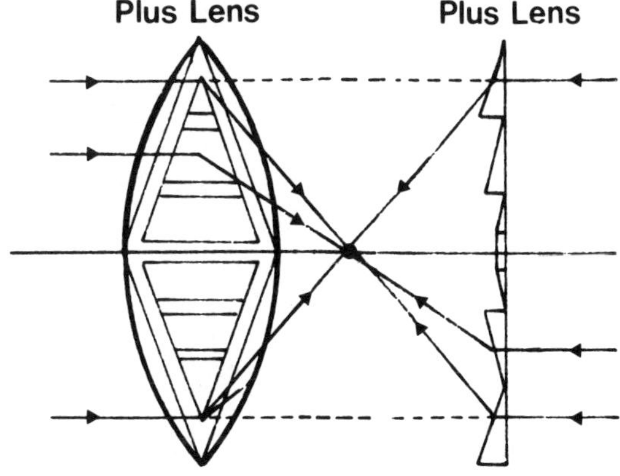

Fresnel Lens
Increasing Apex Angle
From Optical Centre

Fig. 3-28

incomitant deviations, nystagmus, visual field defects, and for temporarily bed-ridden patients (see prescribing prism guidelines).

The same principle can be applied to the construction of lenses. In the discussion on the prismatic effect of lenses it was said that lenses can be thought of as prisms of progressively increasing prismatic power as measured from the optical center of the lens. If prisms of increasing apex angle are stacked on top of each other, a situation equivalent to a spherical lens is derived Fig. 3-28. As with the prisms, they are lighter, can be cut to any size, and can be simply applied to any spectacle in a reversible fashion. Their uses include temporary aphakic lenses, occupational bifocal adds, low vision–high power segments, penalization devices, and temporary bifocal adjustments as well as medically induced refractive errors with anticipated variability. The same disadvantages exist as for the prism variety.

Please see Part II: Problems and Part III: Solutions for typical examination questions pertaining to the material in this chapter.

CHAPTER 4: VISUAL IMAGERY

Vision is a faculty, seeing an art—Anonymous

The discussion thus far has dealt with the effects of various devices on the vergence of light. This is a necessary prerequisite to the understanding of the formation of images by the eye that lead to the cortical perception of these images in the form of vision. It is easily appreciated that the eye is a multiple thick lens system with many refractive surfaces and many refractive media.

REFRACTIVE SURFACES

If we consider one surface at a time, some understanding as to the relative powers and hence the relative contribution of each surface to the overall dioptric power of the eye will be derived. Gullstrand has done this very eloquently using thick lens formulae that consider the thickness of each "lens" in the system. To perform this exercise, it is necessary to invoke our old friend the single smooth refracting surface, whose vergence relationships you will recall were

$$nU + \frac{n' - n}{r} = n'V$$

For the anterior surface of the cornea:

$$D_{SA} = \frac{n_C - n_{AIR}}{r_{CA}}$$

where: n_C = refractive index of the cornea
n_{AIR} = refractive index of air
r_{CA} = radius of curvature of the anterior air-tear-cornea interface as illustrated in Fig. 4-1

Substituting these values, it is found that the refracting power of the anterior air-tear-cornea interface is 48.80 D. Similarly, the posterior cornea-acqeous interface would have

$$D_{SP} = \frac{n_{AQ} - n_C}{r_{CP}} = \frac{1.336 - 1.376}{0.0068} = -5.90\text{D}$$

If one considers this a thin lens and ignores the separation between the two surfaces, $D_C = D_{SA} + D_{SP} = 48.8 - 5.9 = 42.90$ D.

The anterior air-tear-cornea interface is not only a refracting surface but also a reflecting surface with the amount of nearly normal incident light reflected (approximately 2% at this interface) as follows:

$$\left[\left(\frac{n' - n}{n' + n}\right)^2\right]$$

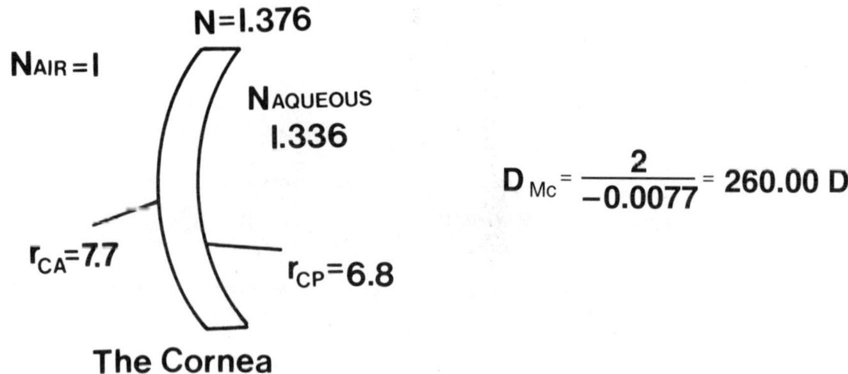

Fig. 4-1

The power as a mirror is as follows:

$$D_{Mc} = \frac{2}{-0.0077} = 260.00 \text{ D}$$

Thus the cornea is a much more potent reflecting surface than it is a refracting one. This is a useful property with advantages for keratometry. Using the front interface as a mirror, the image can be measured to derive the radius of curvature.

The image of an object at infinity would lie at the focal point of the mirror = $\frac{1}{D_{M_c}} = \frac{1}{-260} = -3.85$ mm. This is the first Purkinje-Sanson image, and since it is located posterior to the mirror (Fig. 4-2, *a*), it is virtual. It is also erect and minified, as seen in the illustration. The posterior corneal surface and the anterior lens

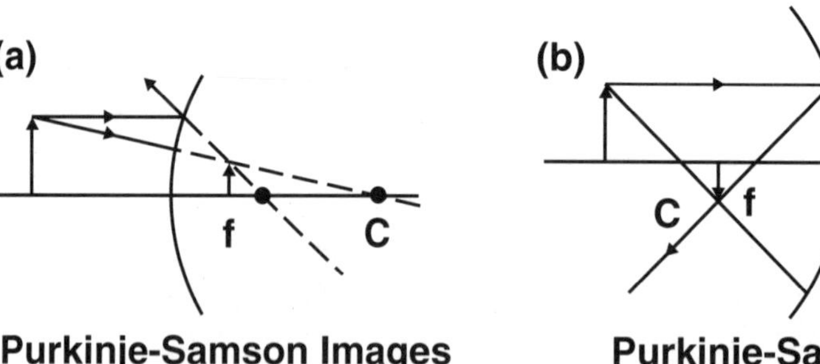

Fig. 4-2

surface are also convex (minus) mirrors whose consecutive images are *virtual, erect,* and *minified* (mnemonic vermin). The posterior lens surface is a concave (plus) mirror whose image is real, inverted, and smaller (Fig. 4-2, *b*). These details are in themselves not very important but somehow always manage to sneak onto examinations.

When we consider the two lens surfaces, the refracting powers become:

$$D_{LA} = \frac{n_L - n_{AQ}}{(+)r_{LA}} = \frac{1.42 - 1.336}{0.0102 \text{ m}} = 8.24 \text{ D}$$

$$D_{LP} = \frac{n_v - n_L}{(-)r_{LP}} = \frac{1.336 - 1.42}{-0.006 \text{ m}} = 14.00 \text{ D}$$

where: n_{AQ}, n_L, n_V = indices of refraction for aqueous, lens, and vitreous, respectively

r_{LA}, r_{LP} = radii of curvature of the lens anteriorly and posteriorly in the unaccommodated eye

The total lens power as a thin lens $D_L = D_{LA} + D_{LP} = 8.24 + 14.0 = +22.24$ D. The total eye power would then equal $D_E = D_C + D_L = 22.24 + 42.9 = 65.14$ D, but corrected for the distance between the cornea and lens (4.5 mm) it becomes 60.82 D. A schematic eye can thus be created using a simple combined eye power at the corneal surface of approximately 60.00 D. The usefulness of this will become apparent.

Fig. 4-3 shows a schematic eye with a power of +60.00 D and an average index of refraction of all the ocular media at $n' = 1.333$. The anterior focal point is $\frac{1}{-D} = 17$ mm (actually $\frac{100}{60} = 16.67$ but rounded off to 17), and the posterior focal point if the reduced distance $\frac{n'}{D} = 1.333 \times 17 = 22.6$ mm from the principal point at the front surface of the cornea. The nodal point is thus located at 22.6 − 5.6, or 17, mm from the posterior focal point, which in the emmetropic (no refractive error) eye is on the retina.

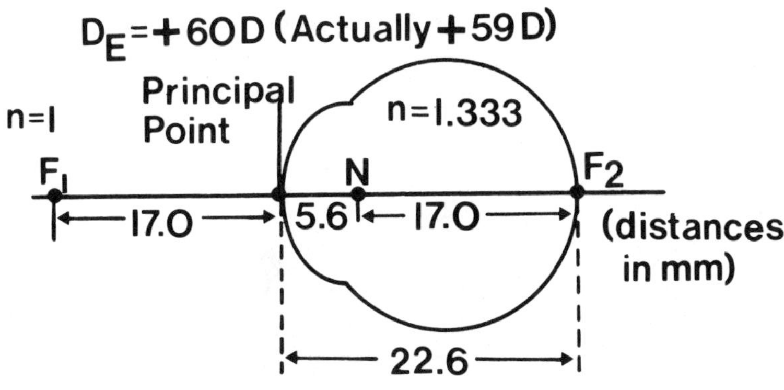

Fig. 4-3

REFRACTIVE AND AXIAL MYOPIA

The schematic eye is a useful tool for the calculation of image size on the retina for a known object at a known distance. Fig. 4-4 depicts the same two similar triangles through the nodal point of the eye from which linear magnification was determined.

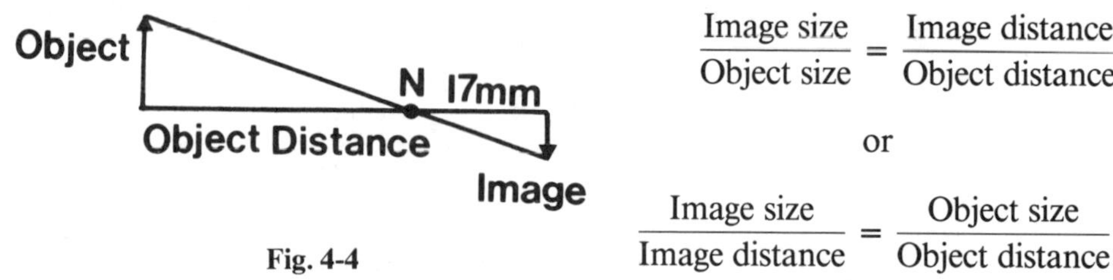

Fig. 4-4

$$\frac{\text{Image size}}{\text{Object size}} = \frac{\text{Image distance}}{\text{Object distance}}$$

or

$$\frac{\text{Image size}}{\text{Image distance}} = \frac{\text{Object size}}{\text{Object distance}}$$

For example, a nonseeing area, or a scotoma, is found to measure 20 mm on a Goldmann perimeter (330 mm). What is the corresponding size of the retinal lesion?

$$\frac{I}{17\text{ mm}} = \frac{20\text{ mm}}{330\text{ mm}}$$

$$I = \frac{20 \times 17}{330} = 1.03\text{ mm}$$

What would happen if the power of the eye were greater than that of the schematic eye? In Fig. 4-5 the eye depicted is +5.00 D stronger than the emmetropic schematic eye. Parallel rays would come to focus 2.1 mm anterior to the retina. This is the condition known as *myopia,* or nearsightedness,and since it is based solely on the fact that the refractive power of the eye is too strong, it is referred to as *refractive myopia.*

If the eye in question has normal refractive power (+60.00 D) but is 5 mm too long, how would this affect the posterior focal point? From Fig.4-6 one sees that the posterior focal point is still at 22.6 mm where it was for the normal sized eye, but the normal refractive power in this instance is too much. This is known as *axial myopia.*

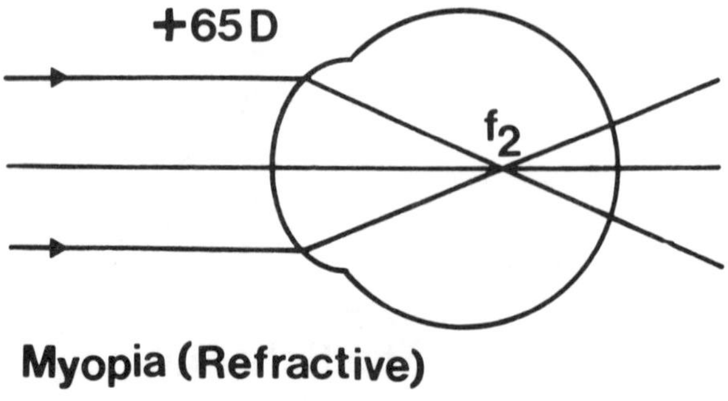

Fig. 4-5

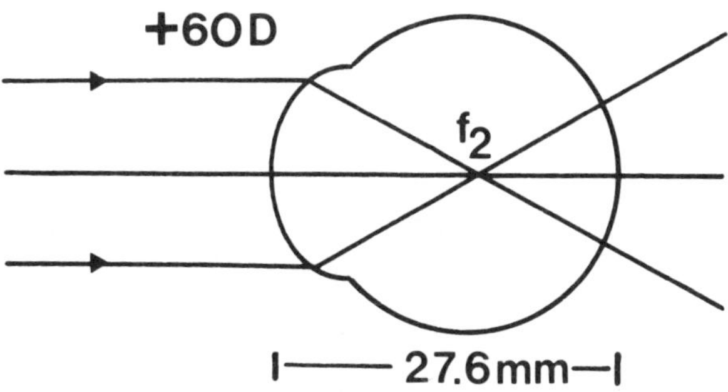

Myopia (Axial)

Fig. 4-6

REFRACTIVE AND AXIAL HYPEROPIA

In a similar fashion it can be determined that, if the power of the eye is insufficient to focus rays on the retina, the posterior focal point will be behind the retina (Fig. 4-7). This is known as *refractive hyperopia.* If the power is normal but the length of the eye is short,the retina will lie in front of the posterior focal point—a condition known as *axial hyperopia.*

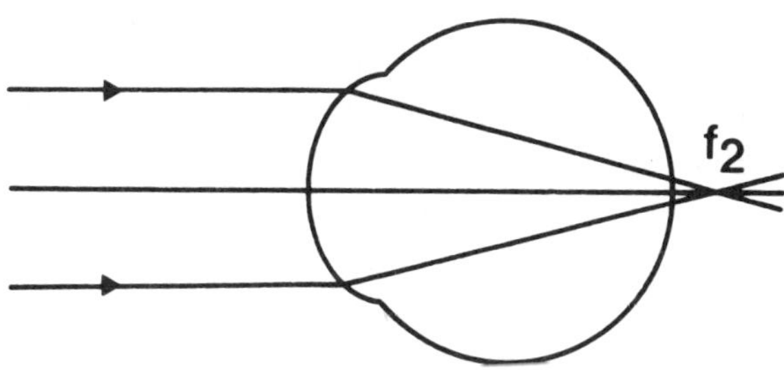

Hyperopia

Fig. 4-7

A curious phenomenon occurs in all optical systems. As an object is moved along the optical axis, the image moves in the same direction. This can be predicted from the simple vergence formula $U + D = V$. If D remains the same, a change in object position will always result in a change in image distance in the same direction relative to the light: $\frac{1}{u} + D = \frac{1}{v}$. As u decreases (e.g., from 100 cm to 50 cm), so must v increase from 50 cm to 100 cm if D remains the same (Fig. 4-8).

In this example the object moves away from the light but so does the image,

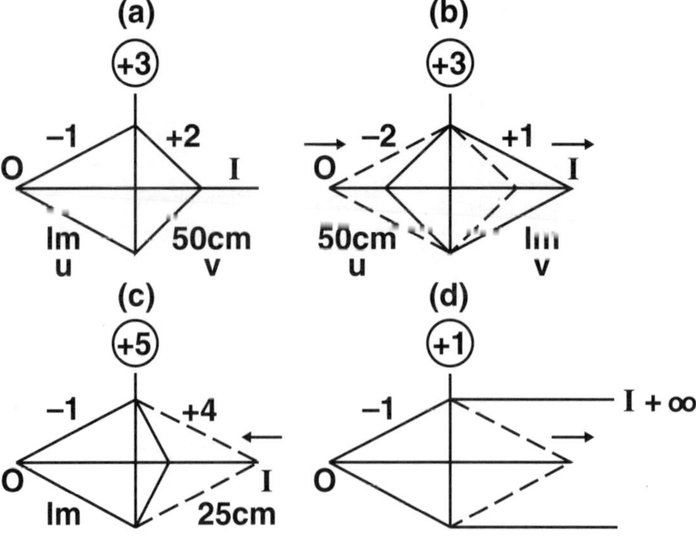

Fig. 4-8

In this example the object moves away from the light but so does the image, i.e., in the same direction. The rate that the image moves is dioptrically and not linearly related to object movement (although in the example it is both!). Similarly, if the power of the lens is changed in the plus direction, the image is pulled against the light (Fig. 4-8, *c*) and if it is made less plus or more minus, the image moves with the light.

If one considers the myopic eye again for a moment, it becomes obvious that to place the image on the retina one has two alternatives: (1) moving the object closer to the eye, pushing the image in the same direction, onto the retina; or (2) placing a minus lens, which will also push the image with the light and onto the retina (Fig. 4-9).

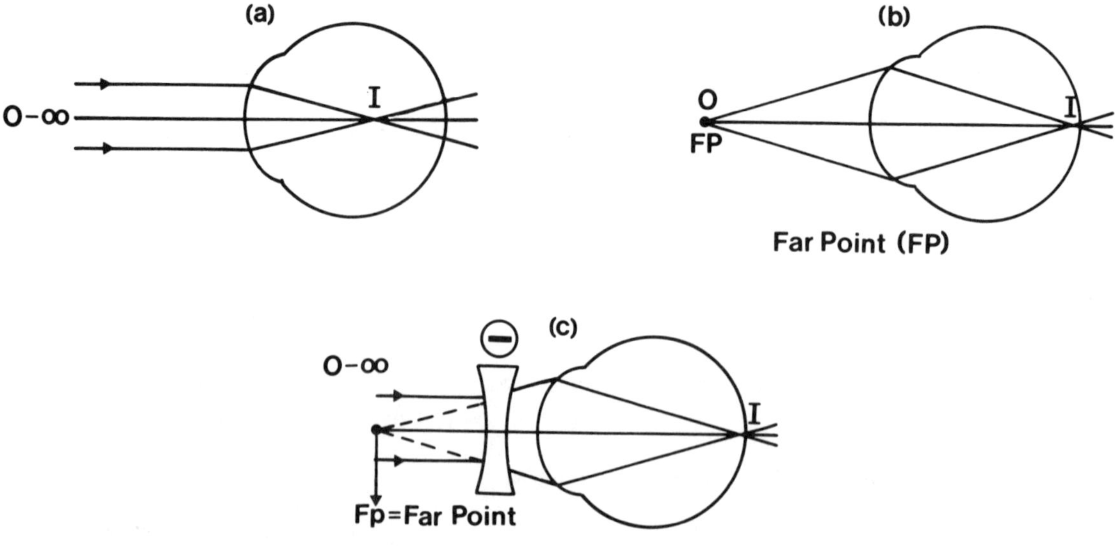

Fig. 4-9

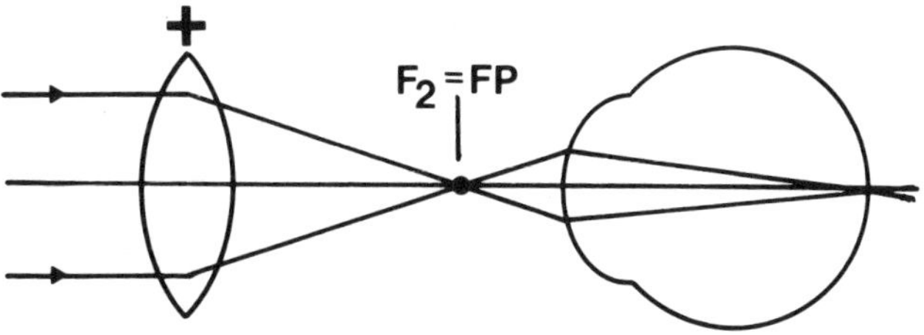

Fig. 4-10

FAR POINT

In the unaccommodated myopic eye the point imaged by the eye onto the retina is called the *far point.* (This is an extremely important concept to understand the correction of all ametropias and will again be used in the objective technique of retinoscopy to be discussed later.) At this point the object and the image can be reversed and the light changed in direction, and an image of the retina can be obtained at the far point. Fig. 4-9, *c*, is the second alternative described above. The minus lens causes the image to move with the light and onto the retina. If one looks closely, however, one will notice that the anterior or secondary focal point of the minus lens falls on the far point. This is a vital concept as well: *the corrective lens has its secondary focal point coinciding with the far point.* No matter what power of lens is used, as long as it is positioned such that this condition exists, it will image the object on the retina. Thus the secondary focal point is coincident with the far point, which in turn is conjugate to the retina.

Even a plus lens, if placed a long distance from the eye on the left side of the far point, meets these criteria and would theoretically (but not practically) correct the myopia (Fig. 4-10). In the hyperopic eye it has been seen that in the unaccommodated state the far point lies behind the retina. If one brings the object closer, the image location moves in the same direction and thus makes the situation worse. The only way would be to bring the object back through infinity and come from behind the eye. Unfortunately the rest of the head gets in the way with this manoeuvre. Alternatively, a corrective lens could be placed in such a position that its secondary focal point is coincident with the far point (Fig. 4-11). It's this latter

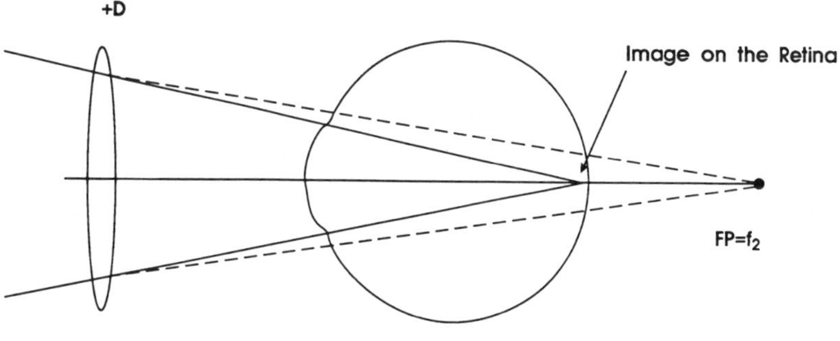

Fig. 4-11

modality that characterizes the clinical correction of hyperopia. The plus lens converges light to a focal point coincident with the far point. The combination of the lens plus the eye will image the object on the retina.

NEAR POINT

This situation, however, is complicated by the act of accommodation. In the myopic patient, accommodation adds more plus power to an already overplussed eye. This results in an image that is even more out of focus than before. The stimulus for accommodation is therefore not present until the image comes to focus behind the retina. After this point, accommodation is required to maintain the image focused on the retina. There is, however, a limit to the accommodative power of a lens that is age dependent. This is the basis of presbyopia with advancing age. It also is the basis of the measurable amplitude of accommodation, which shall be discussed later under the presbyopia section. Suffice it to say that using maximum accommodation, a near point is found, inside which a clear image cannot be maintained on the retina. This is appropriately called the *near point* and in the case of a myopic person would be represented dioptrically by the *amount of myopia plus the accommodative amplitude.* This describes an interval of clear vision between the far point and near point through which a myopic person without correction has clear imagery on the retina. Distal to the far point and proximal to the near point a crisp stigmatic focus is not achieved, and a *blur circle* is seen instead. Proximal to the near point the chromatic interval would be similar to that of the unaccommodated hyperopic person with the blue side in better focus than the red. This may be one of many central mechanisms differentiating a hyperopic blur circle from a myope past their far point, whose interval would be focused more clearly on the red side.

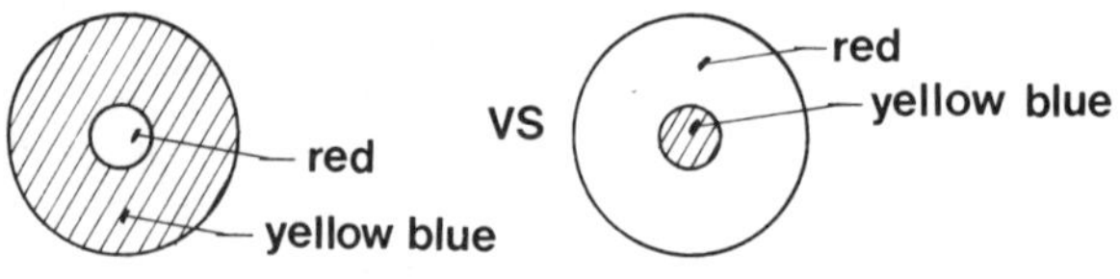

Fig. 4-12

The hyperopic patient has an image behind the retina. If there is any accommodative amplitude left, some or all will be exerted to bring the image onto the retina. Since this uses up some accommodation, he cannot focus on as near a point as his emmetropic or myopic counterpart. His near point is thus dioptrically represented by the difference between the amplitude of accommodation and the amount of hyperopia. For example:

1. What is the interval of clear vision for an uncorrected 4.00 D myope with 8.00 D of accommodative amplitude?

$$\text{Far point} = 100/4 = 25 \text{ cm}$$

$$\text{Near point} = 100/(8 + 4) = 8.33 \text{ cm}$$

$$\text{Interval of clear vision } 8.33 - 25 \text{ cm}$$

2. What is the interval of clear vision for an uncorrected 2.00 D hyerope with 4.00 D of accommodative amplitude?

Far point 50 cm behind the eye

With +2.00 D accommodation far point at $-\infty$

$$\text{Near point} = 100/(4 - 2) = 50 \text{ cm}$$

Interval of clear vision 50 cm to infinity

The emmetropic patient of course has their far point located at infinity, and their near point is simply related dioptrically to the amplitude of accommodation.

Please see Part II: Problems and Part III: Solutions for typical examination questions pertaining to the material in this chapter.

CHAPTER 5: ASTIGMATISM

Unfortunately not all eyes have purely spherical errors. In some eyes the power in one meridian is stronger. This is because two meridians, 90° apart, have different radii of curvature (which is called a *toric* surface). In the eye this can occur either in the cornea or the lens. It gives rise to the clinical entity of *astigmatism,* named after the imagery of this type of surface, which is not pointlike. To understand this entity and its correction, the optics of cylinders must first be clearly understood.

CYLINDER OPTICS

A cylinder is the simplest form of spherocylindrical lens because it has maximum power only in one meridian and no power at 90° to this meridian. Fig. 5-1, *a,* depicts a plus cylindrical form and *b* a minus cylindrical form. If a cross section is taken at 90° to the axis, as in Fig. 5-1, *c* and *d,* it becomes apparent that in this meridian the power is maximum. This is the *power meridian* and is *always* 90° to the axis. If for example this is a +5.00 D cylinder, it would have its power at 90° to its axis. If the axis is 45°, its power is at 135°. In notation form this is written +5.00 @ 135°.

A longitudinal section through the plus cylinder along its axis is shown in Fig. 5-1, *e.* It can be seen that this is no more than a plane parallel plate, which has no power. Similarly, in *f* a longitudinal section along the axis of a minus cylinder reveals the same situation. The power along the axis is thus written plano (zero) @ axis°. For the same example above this is written plano @ 45°. This is of course very confusing but so well entrenched in the nomenclature that it will never change.

A pictorial representation of this situation is the *power cross,* which depicts the power of a cylindrical or spherocylindrical lens along the appropriate power meridians. For the example above, + 5.00 @ 135°/plano @ 45° (Fig. 5-2). The notation for cylinders is *not* according to the power meridian but conventionally according to the *axis* of the cylinder. This above cylinder is thus specified as +5.00 × 45, where a times sign is followed by the axis. The degree sign is usually dropped so that when writing prescriptions confusion does not arise (e.g., 18 and 180). In this form the power cross can still be formed, but axis notation must be switched to power meridians.

$$+5.00 \times 45 = +5.00 \text{ @ } 135/\text{plano @ } 45$$

The axis is also guided by a convention illustrated in Fig. 5-3. Note that the axis is the *same for both eyes* and starts at zero with reference to the left ear. Since axis 90 = 270 with cylinders, from zero to 180° only is used on the scale. Since zero is the same as 180, the latter is always used in standard notation.

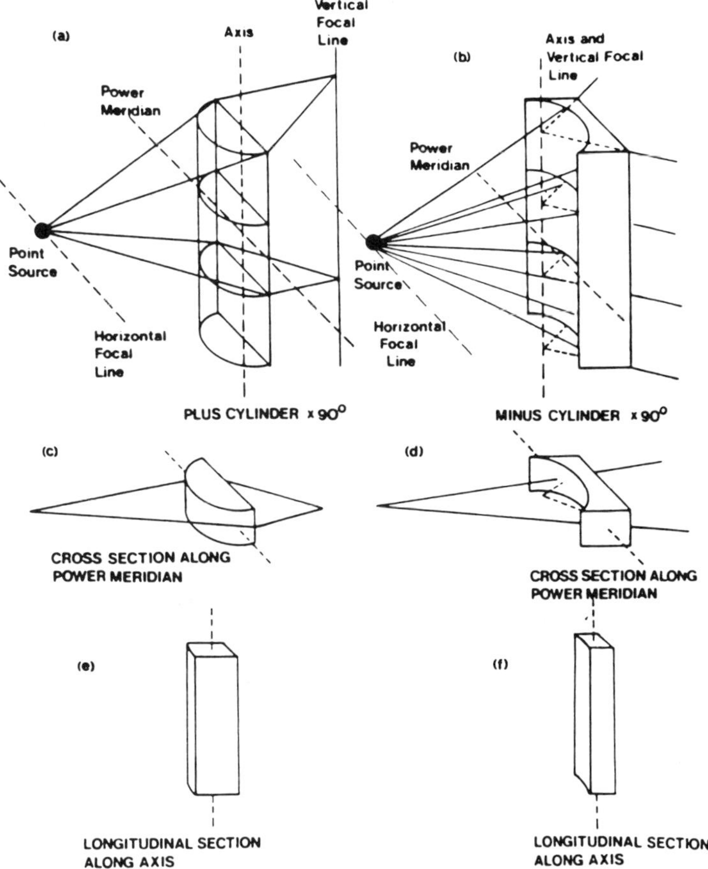

Fig. 5-1

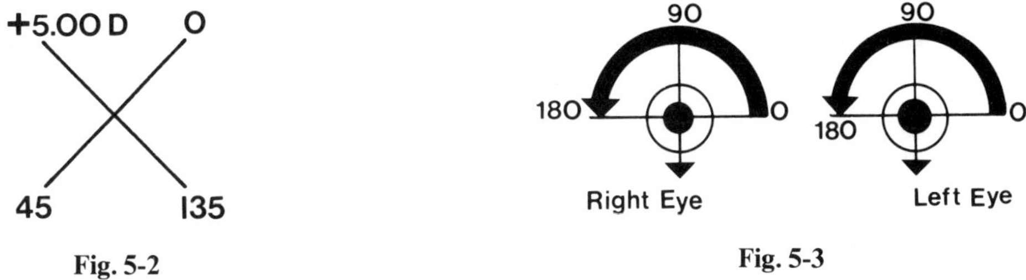

Fig. 5-2

Fig. 5-3

The power of the cylinder has been seen in action in Fig. 5-1, but how are the images formed and where are they located? From the illustration, if multiple little cross sections are taken, each will come to a point focus. The sum total, however, transcribes a *focal line*. In the power meridian each cross section will have a power D, the power of the cylinder. The image will be formed according to $U + D = V$. Take the example of the high plus cylinder in Fig. 5-4.

If a light source is held at ⅓ m:

$$U + D = V$$

$$-3 + 203 = +200$$

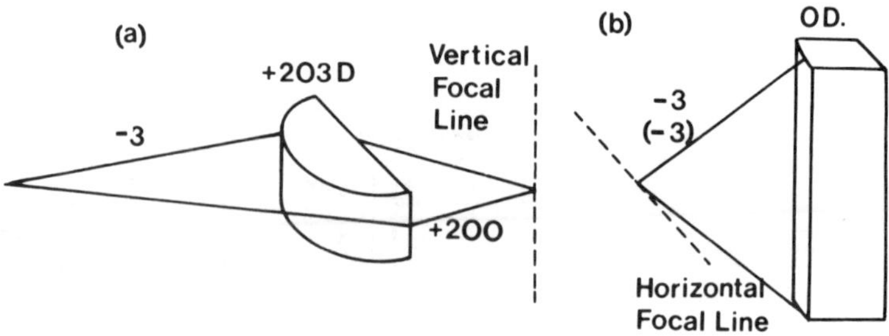

Fig. 5-4

The image will be located at 100/200 = 0.5 cm or 5 mm, and since it is to the right of the cylinder, it will be real and linear in the same direction as the axis. In the axis meridian the power is zero: $-3 + 0 = -3$. The image is virtual, linear, and in exactly the same spot as the object. This is the basis of the *Maddox rod,* a device used clinically for the measurement of eye deviations. A high plus cylinder of red or white plastic is held before one eye and a light source is held such that it is visible before both eyes. The eye with the Maddox rod is presented with two focal lines. The one at 5 mm is so close that it is not visible. The virtual image, which is horizontal and perpendicular to the axis, is seen. The uncovered eye sees a spot image of the source. Since a red line and a white spot are not "fusible material," the two eyes are dissociated and the deviation can be measured by placing prisms in the appropriate direction to place the "light spot on the line."

In summary:

1. A cylinder is specified by its axis.
2. The power of a cylinder in its axis meridian is zero.
3. Maximum power is at 90° to its axis, in the power meridian.
4. The image formed by the power meridian is a focal line parallel to the axis.
5. The image formed by the axis meridian is a focal line perpendicular to the axis at the object.

A *spherocylinder* has a toric surface with two principal meridians at 90° to each other with a different radius of curvature in each meridian. Fig. 5-5 depicts such a lens and its imagery. Each principal meridian can be thought of as a simple cylinder with a focal line parallel to its axis. The combination of two cylinders at opposite (normal) meridians transcribes a complex conical image space called the *conoid of Sturm,* which is bound by the two focal lines of the spherocylinder. The position of the focal lines depends on the power meridian of each cylindrical component and is in the direction of its axis. The distance between the two focal lines is called the *interval of Sturm.*

Dioptrically midway between the two focal lines is where the horizontal and vertical dimensions of the blurred image are approximately equal. This forms the *circle of least confusion,* at which point the image is least blurred. This would be the focal point, if the average power of the lens over all meridians were combined to form a spherical lens. The circle of least confusion is therefore described by the *spherical equivalent* of the spherocylindrical lens. Its shape is determined by the shape of the lens and the aperture.

The spherical equivalent can be calculated from any spherocylinder by the following formula:

$$\text{Spherical equivalent} = \text{Sphere} + \frac{\text{Cylinder}}{2}$$

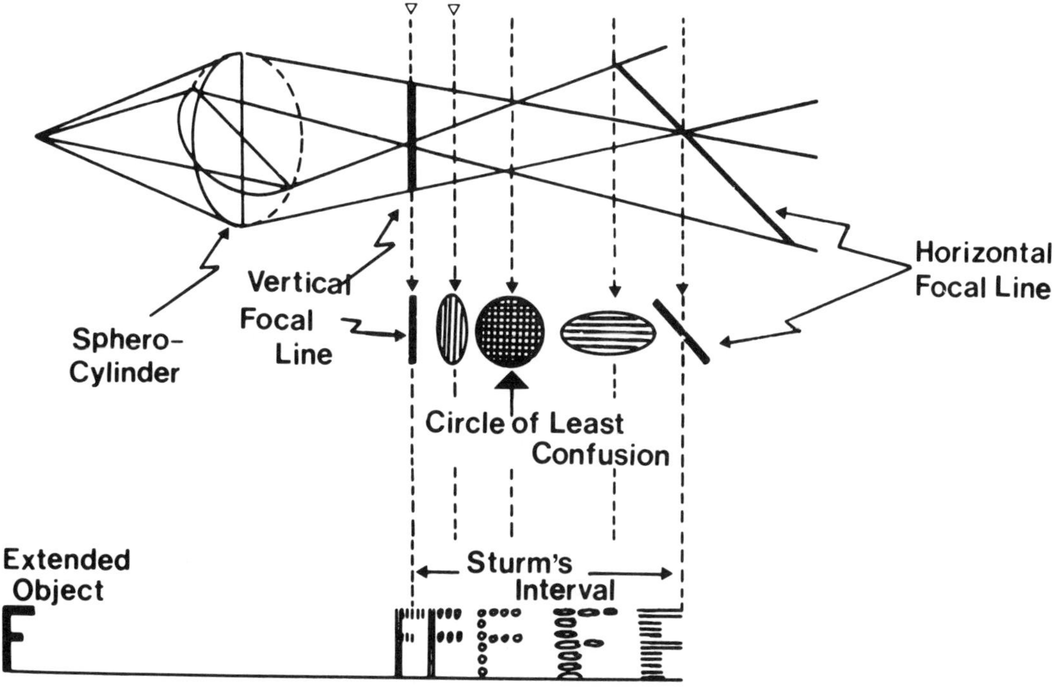

THE SPHEROCYLINDER AND ITS IMAGERY

Fig. 5-5

For any combination of sphere and cylinder with the same spherical equivalent, the circle of least confusion will be in the same location, but the *size* of the blur circle will depend on the interval size. The smaller the interval, the smaller the circle of least confusion. Spherocylinders can be thought of as a combination of two cylinders of different powers in two principal meridians at 90° to each other. The power cross can be used to visualize this, just as was done for simple cylinders. Consider first a +2.00 D sphere (Fig. 5-6). This can be thought of as a combination of two +2.00 D cylinders acting at right angles to one another. If a power cross emerges with the same power at two meridians 90° to each other, it is by definition a sphere.

As can be seen, all three notation forms are equivalent ways of expressing the same lens. As such, they are freely interconvertible and each practitioner should be capable of doing so with facility. When dealing with spectacles, either the plus or minus cylinder form is acceptable, but contact lenses are always dealt with in minus cylinder form. The following methods of interconversion are useful as bypass methods to avoid the often cumbersome power cross.

To convert from *plus to minus or minus to plus cylinder form*:

1. Add the sphere to the cylinder to yield a new sphere.
2. Change the sign of the cylinder.
3. Change the axis by 90.

For example:

$$+2.00 = +1.00 \times 90 \text{ to minus cylinder form}$$

$$\text{Sum of sphere} + \text{cylinder} = +2 + (+1) = +3$$

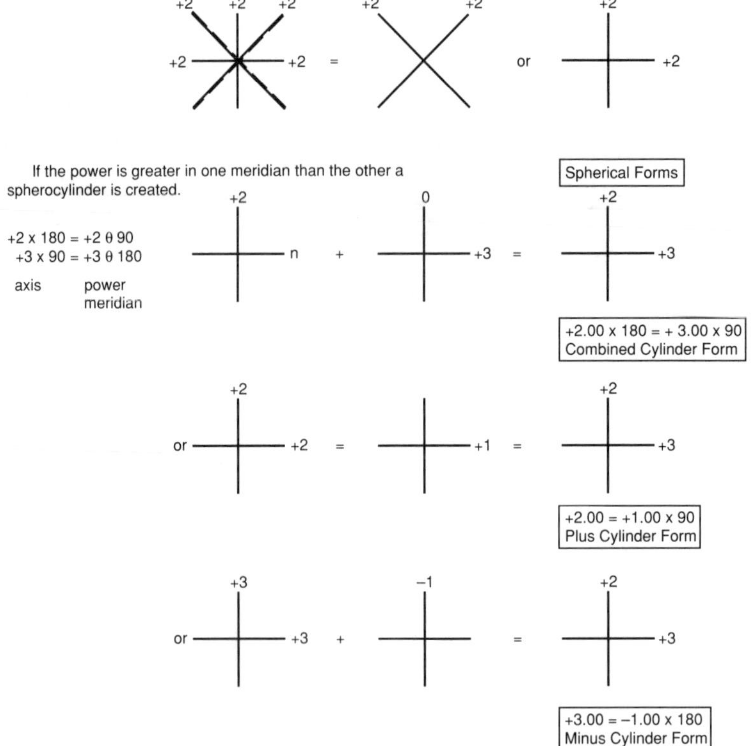

Fig. 5-6

$$\text{Change sign of cylinder} = +1 \rightarrow -1$$

$$\text{Change axis by } 90^\circ = 90 \rightarrow 180$$

$$\text{Minus cylinder form} = +3.00 = -1.00 \times 180$$

The conversion (Fig. 5-6) of a combined cylinder to a spherocylinder is easily done with the power cross but can be also easily performed with a little mathematic "sleight of hand." Add an equal cylinder at 90° to one of the cylinders in the combination form such that the sum in that meridian is now a sphere. If a cylinder of equal magnitude but opposite sign is placed in the same meridian, the net effect is zero. The resultant sum is the spherocylinder form.

For example:

$$\begin{array}{rcl|c|rcl|l}
+2.00 \times 180 & = & +3.00 \times 90 & & +2.00 \times 180 & = & +3.00 \times 90 & \text{combined cylinder} \\
\underline{+2.00 \times 90} & = & \underline{-2.00 \times 90} & \text{or} & \underline{-3.00 \times 180} & = & \underline{+3.00 \times 180} & \text{net zero cylinder} \\
+2.00 & = & +1.00 \times 90 & & -1.00 \times 180 & = & +3.00 & \text{spherocylinder} \\
\multicolumn{3}{r|}{\text{Plus cylinder form}} & \text{or} & \multicolumn{3}{l|}{\text{Minus cylinder form}} &
\end{array}$$

It is equally simple to convert spherocylinders into two combined cylinders. The sphere, by definition, has equal cylinders at all meridians. Any combined cylinder with equal cylinders at 90° meridians will be determined to be a sphere. The sphere component in the spherocylinder can be divided into an equivalent combination of spherocylinders at 90° to each other.

$+2.00$	$= +400 \times 45$	original spherocylinder
$+200 \times 135$	$= +200 \times 45$	$+2.00$ sphere equivalent
Add $\quad 0$	$= +400 \times 45$	remaining cylinder
$+200 \times 135$	$= +600 \times 45$	combined cylinder form

The advantage to these mathematic methods of interconversion is not only their speed but also the elimination of one step in power crossing. Each power cross requires conversion from axis to meridional power and back again. This is just one more step where an easy error can be made. From the combined cylinder form it is easier to conceptualize the two focal lines and to determine their position. For the first combined cylinder above and an object at infinity: $+2.00 \times 180 = -3.00 \times 90$.

$$+2.00 \times 180 = +2.00 \text{ @ } 90 \qquad U + D = V \qquad 0 + 2 = +2 \qquad 100/2 = 50 \text{ cm}$$

$$+3.00 \times 90 = +3.00 \text{ @ } 180 \qquad U + D = V \qquad 0 + 3 = +3 \qquad 100/3 = 33 \text{ cm}$$

Thus the interval of Sturm is between 33 & 50 cm; the horizontal focal line (parallel to the $+2.00$ cylinder axis 180) is at 50 cm; the vertical focal line is at 33 cm; the circle of least confusion is dioptrically midway: $(+3 + 2)/2 = +2.50$ D, $100/2.5 = 40$ cm (note 40 cm is not linearly midway between 33 and 50 cm).

For example, where is the circle of least confusion and the interval of Sturm with the combined cylinder $+3.00 \times 90 = -1.00 \times 180$ and an object at infinity?

$+3.00 \times 90$: $U + D = V$
$0 + 3 = +3$
$100/3 = 33$ cm
Vertical focal line 33 cm to the right of the lens

-1.00×180: $U + D = V$
$0 - 1 = -1$
$100/-1 = -100$ cm
Horizontal focal line 1 m to the left of the lens

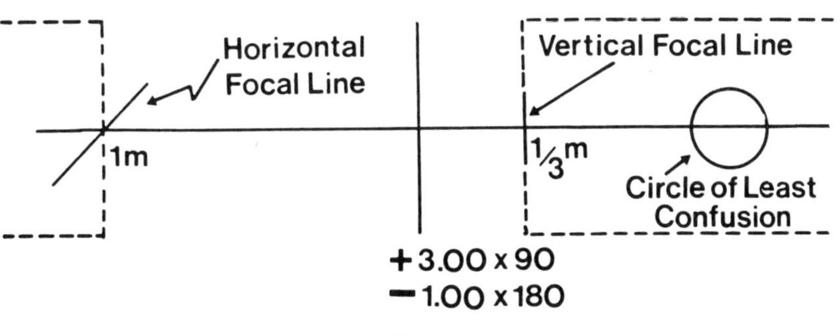

Fig. 5-7

The circle of least confusion is $\frac{+3 - 1}{2} = \frac{+2}{2} = +1$ m to the right of the lens!

This indicates that the interval of Sturm is not between the lines but actually extends from the vertical line behind the lens through infinity and emerges from the left to reach the horizontal focal line. The interval thus "bridges infinity," and its length is infinite (∞), but its bounds are the two focal lines.

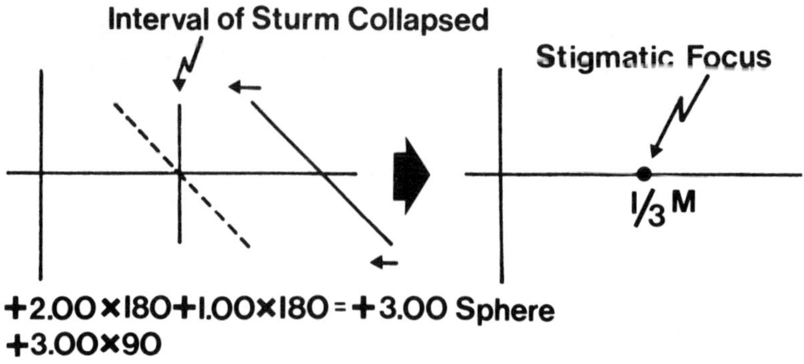

Fig. 5-8

For example, what is the effect of adding a cylinder of +1.00 × 180 to the combined cylinder +2.00 × 180 = +3.00 × 90? This is the same combined cylinder as used in the first example. The horizontal focal line is at 50 cm and the vertical focal line is at 33 cm. Adding plus cylinder axis 180 will move the horizontal line toward the light (Fig. 5-8). In this case the resultant combined cylinder is +3.00 × 180 = +3.00 × 90, which is of course a sphere. In this fashion the interval of Sturm has been collapsed. Instead of a two focal line astigmatic focus, a new stigmatic or point focus is formed at the focal point of the sphere, i.e. ⅓ m.

TYPES OF ASTIGMATISM

In dealing with the clinical entity ocular astigmatism, it has already been mentioned that either the cornea or the lens can be responsible for the toricity of the refracting surfaces. One can think of this in the same fashion used to deal with spherical refractive errors. If this approach is taken, it is observed that there are two focal lines that lie somewhere in relation to the retina. Fig. 5-9 defines these entities according to the position of the focal lines and the deviation from the power of the schematic eye.

As seen in Fig. 5-9, depending on the power in each meridian, the eye error can be expressed in combined cylinder form. If placed at the corneal plane, the corrective combined cylinder lens will be equal in magnitude but of opposite sign to the eye error. The nature of the astigmatism is still readily identifiable from this form. The corresponding spherocylinder depends on whether plus or minus cylinders are used. The nature of the astigmatism can be determined by which is larger—the sphere or the cylinder or if both are equal in magnitude. This is considerably more difficult than with the combined form, but once one is familiar with the spherocylindrical form it can easily be performed.

When sphere is added, both lines move an equal amount dioptrically, but linearly the interval of Sturm changes slightly or dramatically depending on the power added.

To selectively move one line, a cylinder with its axis parallel to the line is used. If it is desired to move the focal line towards the light, a plus cylinder is used. Plus

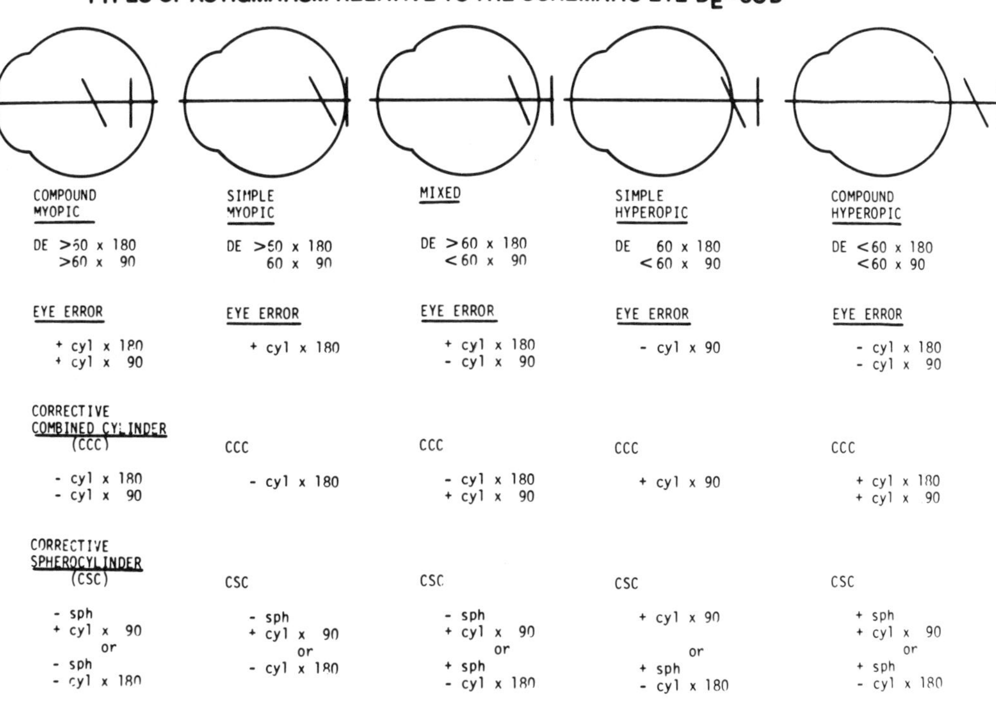

Fig. 5-9

cylinder refracting techniques may be thought of as converting all forms of astigmatism to simple hyperopic astigmatism by adjusting the sphere such that the anterior focal line is on the retina. A plus cylinder then moves the posterior focal line toward the light and onto the retina, collapsing the astigmatic interval into a point focus (Fig. 5-10). Similarly in minus cylinder technique, sphere is adjusted to obtain simple myopic astigmatism, and the anterior focal line is pushed away from the light with minus cylinders.

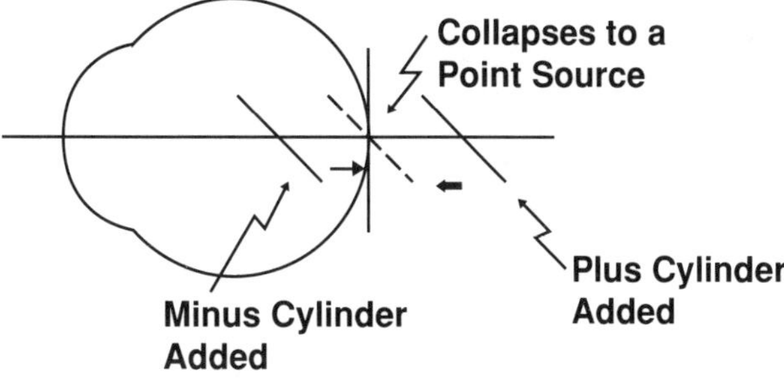

Fig. 5-10

For example, what type of astigmatism is corrected by a $+3.00 = -2.00 \times 90$ spherocylindrical lens at the corneal plane? Since it is not readily apparent from this spherocylindrical form, the lens is converted to combined form.

$$
\begin{array}{lcrcr}
+3.00 \text{ D sphere} & = & +3.00 \times 180 & = & +3.00 \times 90 \\
-2.00 \times 90 & & & & -2.00 \times 90 \\
\hline
 & & +3.00 \times 180 & = & +1.00 \times 90
\end{array}
$$

This corrects an eye error: $-3.00 \times 180 = -1.00 \times 90$. This is compound hyperopic astigmatism.

Of course it is not always practical to correct astigmatism in the corneal plane, and the spectacle plane at a specified vertex distance must be selected. In this situation it is useful to invoke the far point concept just as was used for spherical lenses. In an astigmatic eye there is not a single far point or far point plane but rather two far point planes corresponding to the eye error in the two principal meridians. Just as in spherical lenses, the spherocylindrical lens can be placed anywhere as long as the secondary focal lines of the correcting lens are coincident with the far point planes of the eye. Once this is achieved, by definition conjugacy between distant objects and the retina is achieved. For example, what power of spectacle lens at vertex distance 10 mm is required to correct an eye error of $+8.00 \times 180 = +6.00 \times 90$?

In the corneal plane a $-8.00 \times 180/-6.00 \times 90$ is required.

$$\text{Horizontal far line plane} = 100/-8 = -12.5 \text{ cm}$$

$$\text{Vertical far line plane} = 100/-6 = -16.6 \text{ cm}$$

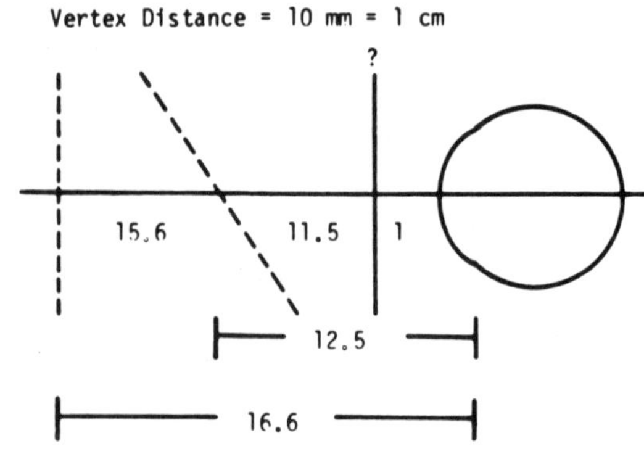

$$\text{D Horizontal} = \frac{100}{12.5-1} = \frac{100}{11.5} = -8.7 \times 180$$

$$\text{D Vertical} = \frac{100}{16.6-1} = \frac{100}{15.6} = -6.4 \times 90$$

Combined Cylinder Form	-8.7 x 180	= -6.4 x 90
	-8.7 x 90	= +8.7 x 90
Plus Cylinder Form	-8.7	= +2.3 x 90
Minus Cylinder Form	-6.4	= -2.3 x 180

These three forms are the same expression for the required spectacle lens

Fig. 5-11

Astigmatism also has other clinical nomenclature associated with it. *Symmetrical astigmatism* is said to exist when the axes of the two eyes are mirror images of each other and whose sum is thus 180° (Fig. 5-12, *a*). *Asymmetrical astigmatism* exists when the two axes do not summate to 180° (Fig. 5-12, *b*).

Regular astigmatism exists when the toricity of the cornea in the visual axis has a uniform refractive surface and the amount of astigmatism is repeatedly consistent. The retinoscopic reflex is crisp and reliable for the axis of astigmatism.

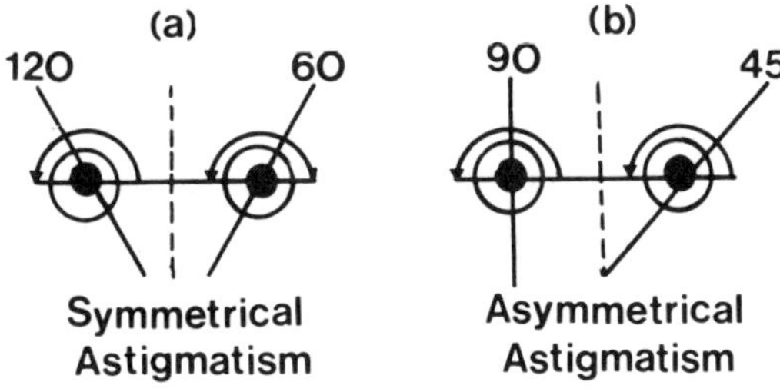

Fig. 5-12

Irregular astigmatism is when a different astigmatic error is obtained with only small excursions from the very central portion of the visual axis. The radii of curvature are thus highly variable and give rise to abnormal scissor type reflexes at retinoscopy. A single spherocylindrical correction will correct only one minute portion of the pupillary aperture, often difficult for the lens wearer to find. If the problem arises from the corneal surface, a contact lens may smooth out the surface, yielding regular astigmatism.

A clinical example of this is keratoconus, where a degenerative process affecting the corneal thickness results in out-bowing of the central or paracentral cornea in an irregular fashion. If the lens is the cause by means of abnormal configuration such as lenticonus, lentiglobus, or spherophakia (conical, globular, or spherical distortion of the lens), a contact lens will not correct the irregular astigmatism.

A common misconception is prevalent about irregular astigmatism. Many people feel that it is present when the two principal meridians are *not* at 90° to each other. This is *wrong*. Mathematically this is *impossible*. Any toric surface, no matter how irregular, always has two principal meridians normal to each other. If keratometry or refraction suggests otherwise, two different areas or zones of the cornea or pupillary aperture are being tested. Another common clinical classification is *with the rule* and *against the rule* astigmatism. As far as I can determine, this serves no real use in the optical world but it is another vestige of the past entrenched and engrained in clinical practice.

With the rule astigmatism is present when the axis of the *correcting* cylinder is at 90° when using plus cylinders and at 180° when using minus cylinders. It does not have to be exactly in these axes, but within 20° usually qualifies. *Against the rule* would have the correcting plus cylinder at axis 180° or minus at 90°. Newborns and very young children start with against the rule, but with the rule astigmatism is more common in older children, and a gradual tendency with age is to drift into against the rule astigmatism again. This is such a common examination question that it may be helpful to consider the various permutations and combinations.

If given any eye error, combined corrective cylinders, or spherocylindrical correction, by converting this to the plus cylinder spherocylindrical form the type of astigmatism is easily determined. For example, given an eye error of $-3.00 \times 90 = -5.00 \times 180$, is this with or against the rule astigmatism?

$$
\begin{array}{rl}
\text{Eye error} & -3.00 \times 90 = -5.00 \times 180 \\
\text{Corrective lens} & +3.00 \times 90 = +5.00 \times 180 \\
\text{Spherocylindrical form} & +3.00 \times 90 = +5.00 \times 180 \\
 & \underline{+3.00} \times \underline{180} = \underline{-3.00} \times \underline{180} \\
 & +3.00 \qquad\quad\; = +2.00 \times 180
\end{array}
$$

This is against the rule astigmatism.

If given keratometry readings, the powers in the two principal meridians of the cornea are already known. By converting these to the appropriate amount of eye error, the type of correcting cylinder can be determined.

For example, keratometry yields *K* readings of 42.00 D horizontally and 48.00 D vertically. Is this with or against the rule astigmatism?

$$42.00 \text{ D horizontally} = 42.00 \text{ D @ } 180 = 42 \times 90$$

$$48.00 \text{ D vertically} = 48.00 \text{ D @ } 90 = 48 \times 180$$

$$\text{Eye error} = +6.00 \times 180$$

$$\text{Corrective cylinder} = -6.00 \times 180$$

$$\text{Plus cylinder form} = +6.00 \times 90$$

This is with the rule astigmatism.

If given any type of astigmatism, such as compound hyperopic, simply convert to simple hyperopic and check the direction of the focal line that is corrected with the plus cylinder. For example (Fig. 5-13), once the anterior focal line is on the retina, plus cylinder axis 180 will bring the posterior focal line toward the light onto the retina. Since +cyl × 180 is against the rule, that is the type of astigmatism.

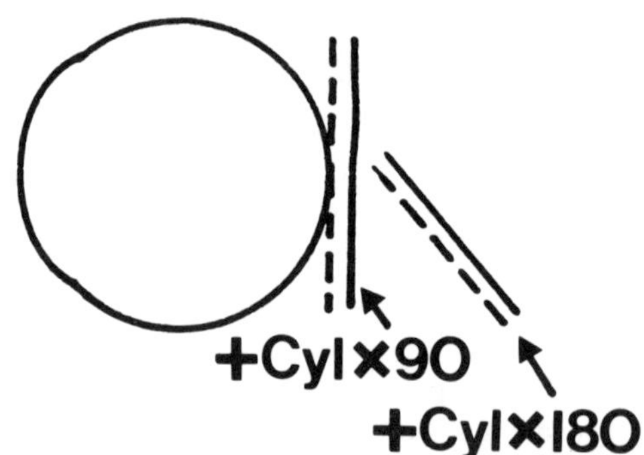

Fig. 5-13

PANTOSCOPIC TILT

Tilting a lens induces spherical and cylindrical power due to astigmatism of oblique incidence. The *pantoscopic tilt* is a measure of the tilt of a spectacle lens in the spectacle plane. Whenever a lens is tilted, the amount of induced sphere and cylinder is proportional to the power of the lens and the amount of tilt. All that need be remembered is that tilting a minus lens induces a small amount of minus sphere and a larger amount of minus cylinder at axis 180. Similarly, tilting a plus lens induces a small amount of plus sphere and a larger amount of plus cylinder at 180. If a plus lens is tilted, plus cylinder at 180° or minus cylinder at

90° is produced, which is with the rule astigmatism—it requires plus cylinder at 90° to correct it.

Effect of tilting a +10.00 D sphere:

$$10° + 10.10 = +0.31 \times 180$$

$$20° + 10.39 = +1.32 \times 180$$

$$30° + 10.83 = +3.33 \times 180$$

Similarly, an intraocular lens implant can be tilted. This can be measured approximately by orienting the positions of the third and fourth Purkinje—Sanson images. When the implant is tilted, these images are separated. By having the patient follow the examiner's finger while keeping the hand light fixed, the two images can be aligned and the angle between the light and finger estimated as the degree of tilt (DL Guyton).

Astigmatism can be divided into *corneal* and *lenticular* as outlined above in the discussion on irregular astigmatism. For example, a patient is wearing a spectacle correction +3.00 = +4.00 × 90. Keratometry reveals *K* readings of 42.00 D horizontally by 44.00 D vertically. Although the total astigmatic error is +4.00 D, only +2.00 D can be attributed to the cornea (a little more if vertex distance is corrected for). The remaining +2.00 D is said to be the amount of lenticular or lens-induced astigmatism. The implication of this is that a contact lens which reduces corneal astigmatism (such as a hard contact lens) will leave a residual astigmatic error of +2.00 D. A specially constructed soft toric or bitoric rigid contact lens could conceivably correct both components.

SUTURE TENSION

In Fig. 5-14 the effects of suture tension on the cornea are considered. A suture placed too tight decreases the chord diameter vertically, reducing the radius of curvature in the same meridian. This, in effect, gives more power to this meridian. Conversely, a suture that is too loose weakens the power of this meridian. How might this be recognized clinically? Look at the following example. A pseudophakic patient (with an intraocular lens implant) complains of poor vision 2

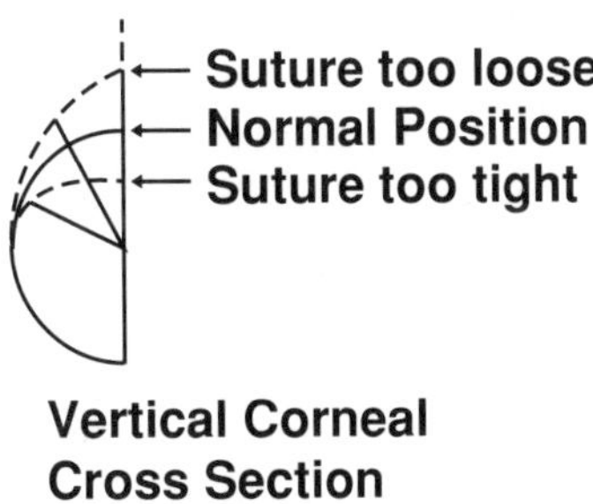

Fig. 5-14

months postoperatively. 10.0 interrupted nylon sutures were used for closure and the wound is well healed. K readings are 40.00 D horizontally and 50.00 D vertically. What type of astigmatism exists, and what would be the appropriate management?

$$40.00 \text{ D horizontally} = 40 @ 180 = 40 \times 90$$

$$50.00 \text{ D vertically} = 50 @ 90 = 50 \times 180$$

$$\text{Eye error} = +10.00 \times 180$$

$$\text{Correcting cylinder} = -10.00 \times 180$$

$$\text{Transpose to plus cylinder form} = +10.00 \times 90$$

This is with the rule astigmatism induced by sutures that are too tight at the 12 o'clock meridian (Fig. 5-15). Cutting these sutures is indicated. If, after cutting the sutures, the K readings are 45×45, what would be the anticipated change in spherical correction? This would be equal to the spherical equivalent of the lost astigmatism $= \dfrac{10.00 \text{ D}}{2} = 5.00$ D in the plus direction.

The general rule is: *A tight suture will cause plus cylinder astigmatism in the axis of the offending suture.* Similarly, absorbable sutures may prematurely absorb or trauma to the wound may cause the wound to gape. Sutures placed too loose will also exert the same effect. Under these circumstances the power in this meridian is weakened by the lengthened chord diameter and increased radius of curvature (see Fig. 5-14). The power in this meridian is reflected by a lower K in the gaping area. If the gape was present vertically, against the rule astigmatism would result. *A loose suture will cause plus cylinder astigmatism at 90° to the axis of the offending suture.*

Work through another example. The postoperative K readings on a patient are 44.00 D in the 120° meridian by 36.00 D in the 30° meridian. What is the implication?

$$44 @ 120 = 44 \times 30$$

$$36 @ 30 = 36 \times 120$$

$$\text{Eye error} = +8.00 \times 30$$

$$\text{Correcting cylinder} = -8.00 \times 30$$

$$\text{Plus cylinder form} = +8.00 \times 120$$

This implies that the suture is loose or the wound is gaping at 90° to the offending plus cylinder or at 30°. If all the sutures have been removed and the wound is healed or gaping, this same rationale can be used in repair. Plus cylinder can be relieved by a relaxing incision in that meridian. The gaping wound can be tightened maximally in the meridian 90° to the plus cylinder, with sutures or a wedge resection at the gape.

Some centers in Europe are contrarian. In pseudophakic patients they are trying to induce astigmatism. In simple myopic astigmatism (Fig. 5-16) one focal line is conjugate with infinity and the other with the corresponding far point plane,

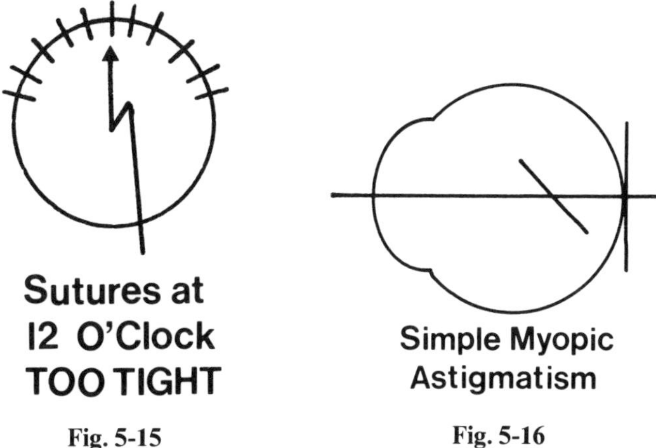

Fig. 5-15

Fig. 5-16

hopefully close to the reading position. In this way without any spectacle correction, some vision is obtained at both distance and near. As seen later, a problem may arise with spectacle correction of this error because of the induction of distortion.

CYLINDERS AT OBLIQUE AXES

To deal with eye errors, the correcting cylinder has been placed in the corneal or spectacle plane at exactly the same axis as the error lies. If the axis of astigmatism is different from the correcting cylinder, a complex situation arises where there are two cylinders at oblique axes. Consider first the situation of a $+1.00 \times 180$ cylinder taken at an oblique axis. The shaded area in Fig. 5-17, *a*, would represent such a section. It no longer has the same radius of curvature as the basic cylinder and secondarily has a different power. There exists an approximation formula

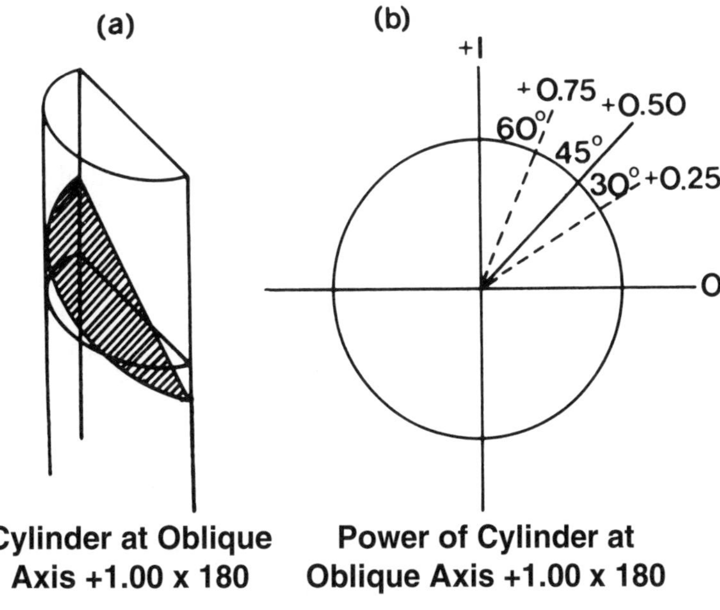

Fig. 5-17

based on $\sin^2\theta$ where θ is the number of degrees off axis. Using this, Fig. 5-17, *b*, can be derived and is probably more useful to remember.

Now it can be imagined that the trigonometric relationship between two cylinders at oblique axes is quite complex. Not only a new power but a new axis is obtained as well as some induced sphere. Suffice it to say that when obliquely crossed cylinders of equal power and different sign (as when dealing with corrective cylinders and eye error) are crossed, the new axis is 45° away from the axis of the eye error. This can be shown by vector addition (Ogle). The power can be read by the simulated system in a lensmeter or calculated by trigonometry or matrices.

CROSS CYLINDER

In the last example the lens used is a special entity called a *cross cylinder.*

$+1.00 \times 90 = -1.00 \times 180$	combined cylinder form
$+1.00 \times 180 = -1.00 \times 180$	transpose with net zero cylinder
$+1.00 = -2.00 \times 180$	minus cylinder form
or $-1.00 = +2.00 \times 90$	plus cylinder form
$-1 + +2/2 = 0$	spherical equivalent

A cross cylinder can be recognized by any of its forms. In the combined cylinder form, the two cylinders are of equal magnitude, opposite sign, and 90° apart. In the spherocylindrical form a quick check always reveals that the *spherical equivalent equals zero.* The implication of having a zero spherical equivalent is that when the cylinder is placed in front of any eye the position of the circle of least confusion remains undisturbed. This is the basis of its clinical use in the form of the *Jackson cross cylinder,* named after the man who described it. This extremely useful test is used in the refinement of the cylinder power and axis in any patient capable of *subjective refraction.* It has already been stated that the circle of least confusion is not changed, but what other effects are invoked and how is this device most efficiently employed?

Consider first the refinement of the cylinder power, since it is the easiest to understand, but it is performed *after* refinement of the axis. To perform this test, objective or subjective refraction techniques must have the circle of least confusion already on the retina. This by definition is either mixed astigmatism or emmetropia. In emmetropia there is no astigmatic interval except the one created by the cross cylinder, which also happens to be the mixed form. Keep in mind that the figures for the cross cylinders are not power crosses but representative of where the axes are located and therefore which focal lines they will affect (i.e., those parallel).

In Fig. 5-18, *a*, the plus axis is aligned with the posterior focal line and moves it toward the light. Similarly, the minus axis moves the horizontal line away from the light. This decreases the interval of Sturm, decreases the diameter of the circle of least confusion, and improves vision. In Fig. 5-18, *b*, the minus cylinder is now oriented with the posterior focal line but pushes it with the light. The plus cylinder

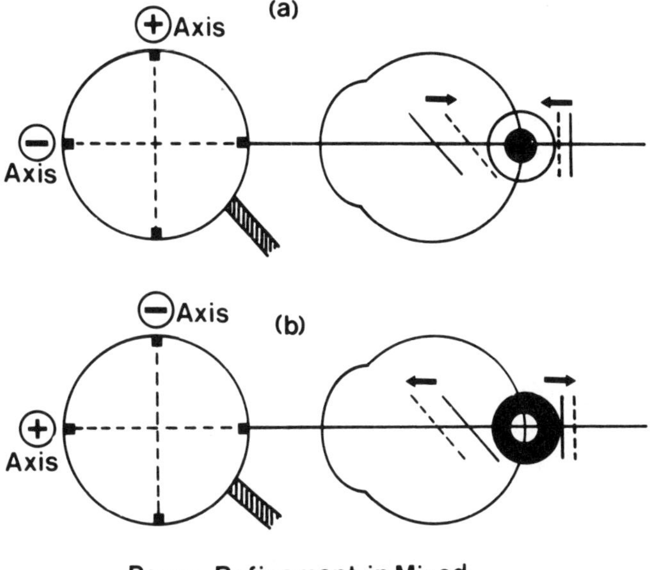

Power Refinement in Mixed Astigmatism

Fig. 5-18

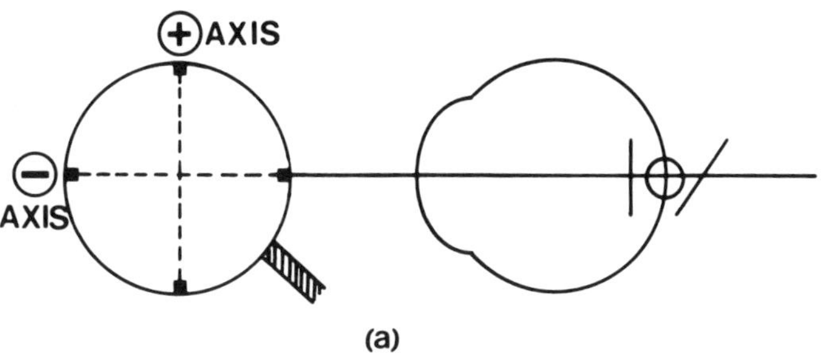

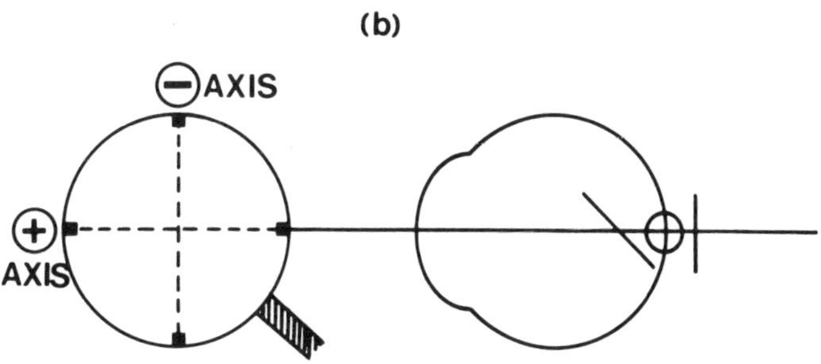

Fig. 5-19

draws the horizontal line even further into the vitreous. The interval of Sturm increases, the circle of least confusion enlarges and the vision diminishes. (Q: Which is better A or B? A: A.)

Plus cylinder at 90° or minus cylinder at 180° is added (in this instance) and the procedure is repeated until no difference is noted between the two positions. This is the end point and is illustrated in Fig. 5-19. At the end point, as seen in Fig. 5-

19, there is no residual astigmatism except that induced by the cross cylinder itself. The vertical plus axis draws the vertical focal line anterior to the retina, and the horizontal minus cylinder pushes its focal line further away. When the lens is flipped, the focal lines are reversed. The circle of least confusion stays on the retina and does not change in size, and the interval of Sturm remains the same length. The vision is the same for both alternatives. (Q: Which is better, A or B, or are they both the same? A: The same.)

The power refinement rests on the premise that the circle of least confusion is always maintained on the retina. If, in the first part of the test, 0.50 D of plus cylinder is added, the circle will be shifted by an amount equal to the spherical equivalent. If plus cylinders are used, the circle has been drawn into the vitreous and for each +0.50 D of cylinder added, −0.25 D of sphere must be used to compensate for the shift. Similarly, in minus cylinder technique for each −0.50 D of cylinder +0.25 D of sphere must be added.

The power of the cross cylinder used depends on the visual acuity of the patient. The better the vision, the lower the power of the cross cylinder and the more subtle and exact the refinement. The test hinges on the difference between two alternatives, which must be made different enough for the patient to appreciate (Table 5-1).

Table 5-1

Visual Acuity	Power of Cross Cylinder
$> \frac{20}{30}$	±0.25 D
$\frac{20}{40}$ to $\frac{20}{70}$	±0.50 D
$\frac{20}{70}$ to $\frac{20}{100}$	±1.00 D
$< \frac{20}{100}$	No benefit

To refine the axis with the cross cylinder is a much easier task to perform than it is to understand. Look first at the situation where the axis is already correct with just the cross cylinder before it. There are three cylinders to consider: (1) the eye error, (2) the correcting cylinder, and (3) the cross cylinder. Since the axis of the correcting cylinder is correct, there are no oblique cylinders to consider. The cross cylinder is placed so that the two axes straddle the correcting cylinder equally (Fig. 5-20). The vision will be equally blurred by the astigmatic interval and stay blurred with reversal flip of the cross cylinder axis. This is, in fact, the end point of axis refinement with the eye error axis coincident with the axis of the correcting cylinder.

If you recall, when first introduced to cross cylinders the discussion was about the effect of two obliquely crossed cylinders. The new axis created is at 45° to the eye error axis if the cylinders are of equal magnitude but opposite sign (Fig. 5-21).

If the correcting cylinder is not at the correct axis relative to the eye error, two oblique cylinders exist. Their new axis is 45° to the eye error axis, which falls close to one of the axes of the cross cylinder. If the plus axis position corresponds to the induced minus axis, the resultant cylinder is less. If the minus position is there, the resultant cylinder increases. When using plus cylinders, the correcting cylinder

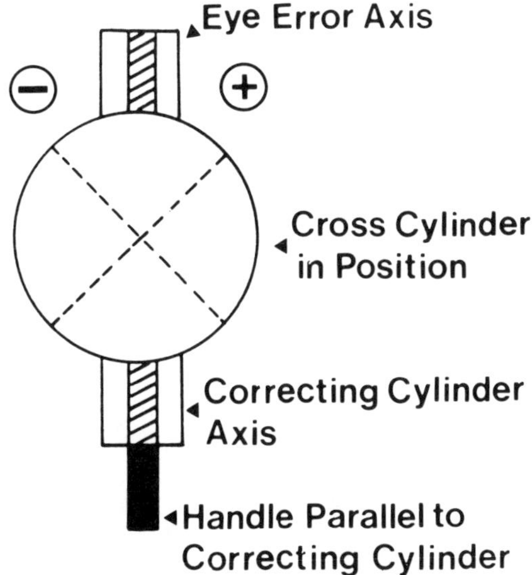

Fig. 5-20

is rotated toward the plus axis of the cross cylinder and the lens flipped again. The rotation is continued until the correcting cylinder is in the correct axis and no oblique cylinders are present (Fig. 5-21, the endpoint). If minus cylinders are used, the correcting minus cylinder is rotated toward the minus cylinder on the cross cylinder. (An alternative explanation can be found in Rubin M: *Optics for clinicians,* Triad Publishers, 1974, pp. 181-185.)

The patient is asked which position is better or worse, and the cylinder is rotated a few degrees toward the plus axis if the correcting cylinder is a plus cylinder. The endpoint is when both alternatives are equal. The number of degrees

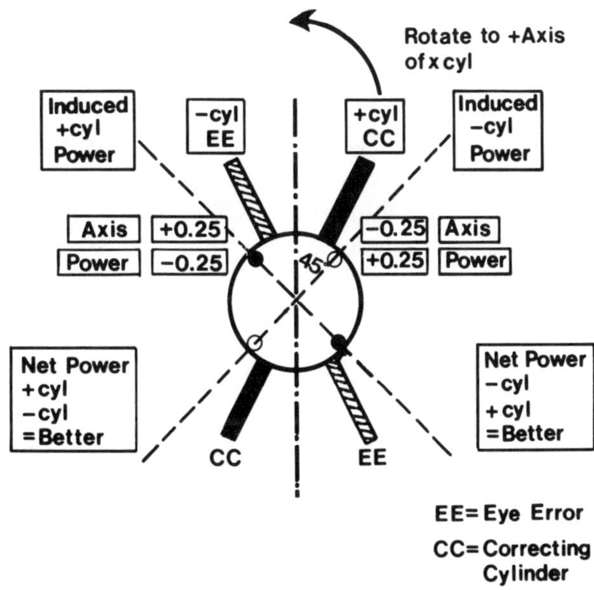

Fig. 5-21

Position "B" Cross Cylinder

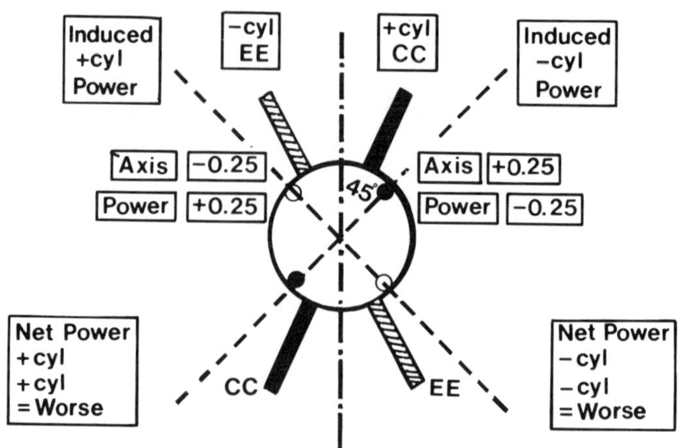

Fig. 5-21, cont'd.

rotated depends on the amount of the correcting cylinder and the strength of the cross cylinder. To produce the equivalent of a +0.25 D astigmatic blur, the correcting cylinder should be rotated as in Table 5-2.

Table 5-2

0 to 1.00 D	10°
1.00 to 1.75 D	5°
1.00 to 1.75 D	3°
>3.00 D	2°

It should be reinforced that the axis is refined first and then the power. If the reverse is done, the power refinement only minimizes the power of the resultant induced cylinder of the obliquely crossed cylinders. This gives you the best power for the cylinder in the incorrect axis! In skilled hands this is a very accurate refinement technique. Recent developments in the art *simultaneously* present both alternatives to the patient, allowing direct comparison and hopefully better refinement. The Simulantest (Zeiss of West Germany) and Simulcross (American Optical) are two such devices.

ASTIGMATIC CLOCK

Another useful test in dealing with astigmatism is the astigmatic clock or dial. This test is based on the imagery of the extended object (see Fig. 5-5). In the interval of Sturm, when the vertical focal line is on the retina, the vertical aspects of an extended object are in focus; conversely, when the horizontal focal line is on the retina, the horizontal aspects are better imaged. If an astigmatic patient were to

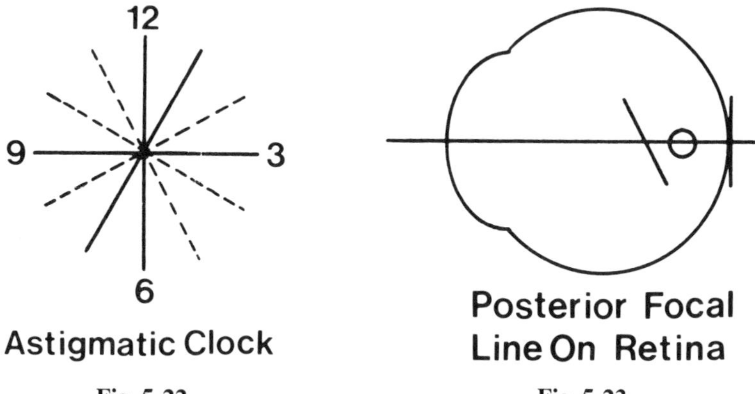

Fig. 5-22

Fig. 5-23

look at six equally dark lines in the configuration of a clock, the sharpest line would correspond to the axis of the focal line nearest the retina (Fig. 5-22).

Under normal seeing circumstances the examiner would have no idea whether this is the anterior or the posterior focal line. This is easily controlled if one converts all types of astigmatism to compound myopic with just enough plus sphere to bring both focal lines into the vitreous. This achieves two objectives. First, one knows that as the plus sphere is lessened or minus sphere is added, the line that is clearest now corresponds to the posterior focal line. Second, it controls any stimulus to accommodation, which would now only further blur the image. This technique is known as *fogging.* As one "unfogs," the posterior focal line now lies on the retina, and that line on the clock is very sharp. The patient viewing Fig. 5-23 would respond that the 1 o'clock meridian is sharpest.

At this point one now wants to move the anterior focal line with the light and onto the retina. This requires minus cylinder in the axis of the anterior line. This is where it becomes obvious that this technique is very useful for those practitioners employing minus cylinders. The addition of minus cylinder moves the anterior focal line posteriorly, collapses the interval of Sturm, and creates a situation where all lines achieve equal clarity.

The axis of the correcting cylinder is guided by the clearest line appreciated by the patient. In the above example, the 1 o'clock meridian was selected by the patient. This response implies the posterior focal line is in the axis corresponding to the 1 o'clock meridian and is hence in best focus. The anterior focal line is naturally oriented 90° to the posterior focal line and is somewhere in the vitreous, as in Fig. 5-23. But how can the axis of the correcting cylinder be determined by the patient's response?

If the line best seen by the patient is projected onto the patient's face as the *examiner* sees it, it becomes apparent that it is a mirror image (Fig. 5-24, *a*). To the examiner the 1 o'clock meridian in fact corresponds to 11 o'clock on the patient's face. This corresponds to the location of the posterior line. The anterior focal line is 90° to it. As viewed by the examiner, this lies at the 30° axis in conventional axis notation (Fig. 5-24, *b*). To move this anterior focal line against the light, minus cylinder is added at this axis. The general dictum that evolves is that for *each* clock hour between 1 and 6 o'clock, 30° of correcting minus cylinder are added. For example, if the 4 o'clock line is sharpest, $4 \times 30 = 120°$ is the axis of the correcting minus cylinder.

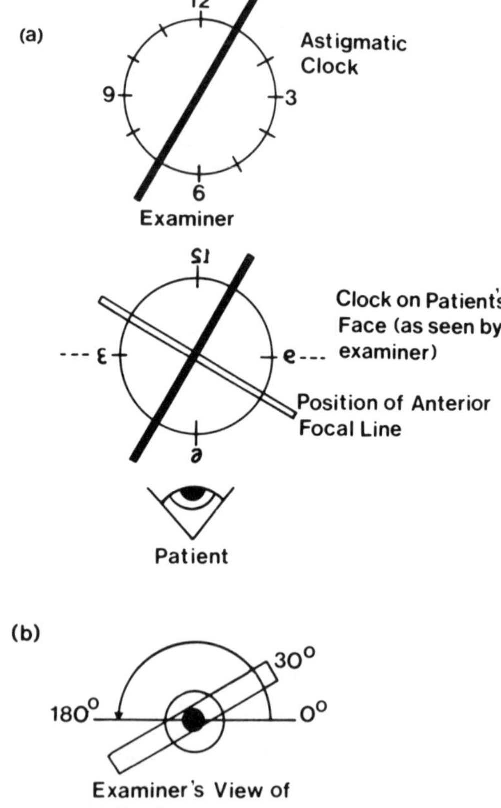

Fig. 5-24

DOUBLE CLICK METHOD

If plus cylinders are used, the *double click* method must be employed. In the above example, to move the anterior focal line, minus cylinder at a specific axis was used. Consider the minus cylinder plano = −0.25 × 90. Transposing to plus cylinder form, this becomes −0.25 = +0.25 × 180. In other words, adding −0.25 D of sphere with +0.25 D cylinder at 90° to the original minus cylinder axis has exactly the same effect as adding the original minus cylinder. In this fashion the anterior focal line can be moved posteriorly just as with minus cylinder. The double click of −0.25 D sphere and +0.25 D cylinder at the (*clock hour* × *30) plus 90°* can thus be used. This added click, however, has been enough to dissuade most plus cylinder refractionists from using this method.

It should be mentioned that the posterior focal line should be kept slightly in front of the retina at all times or accommodation will be stimulated. The standard method is to maintain the fog at about the 20/40 level, which ensures that the posterior focal line will still be slightly in front of the retina. When this method is employed, the desired endpoint is when all the lines of the clock or dial become equally blurred. If doubt about the maintenance of the fog exists, the visual acuity chart can be introduced as verification. The results from the dial or clock methods are then refined according to the cross cylinder technique outlined already.

The prescription is given to the patient, and when he first puts the glasses on, he curses and swears, threatens litigation, and claims that their only use would be as an alternative to a house of mirrors. What went wrong? Inherent in the spectacle correction of astigmatism is the distortion it produces. To understand this well, the basics of magnification must first be understood.

Please see Part II: Problems and Part III: Solutions for typical examination questions pertaining to the material in this chapter.

CHAPTER 6: MAGNIFICATION

An object has height, width, and depth.An image of the object can thus appear taller or wider (meridional magnification), larger (magnification), smaller (minification), deeper, or more elevated (axial magnification). Whether the image of an object appears larger or smaller is related to the *linear or lateral magnification* that was considered earlier in the discussion of the uses of the schematic eye. At that time it was determined that by similar triangles:

$$\text{Linear magnification} = \frac{\text{Image size}}{\text{Object size}} = \frac{\text{Image distance}}{\text{Object distance}}$$

MERIDIONAL, AXIAL, AND ANGULAR MAGNIFICATION

If the image appears taller or wider than the object, magnification in one meridian is greater than in the other. For example, if a square appears as a rectangle, either the height or the width is selectively magnified or minified. This is often referred to as *meridional magnification or minification.* This can occur when different powers are applied to different portions of an extended object. This is commonly seen with spherocylinders and is the basis of distortion. The recognition, causes, and treatment of this will be dealt with later.

If the image appears to be more elevated or depressed than the object, it is said to have undergone *axial magnification.* If it is less elevated or depressed, this is axial minification. Thinking in terms of measurement, linear magnification is measured relative to the distance *away* from the optical axis, whereas axial magnification is related to the distance *along* the optical axis (Fig. 6-1).

x = Axial magnification along the optical axis

y = lateral magnification away from the optical axis

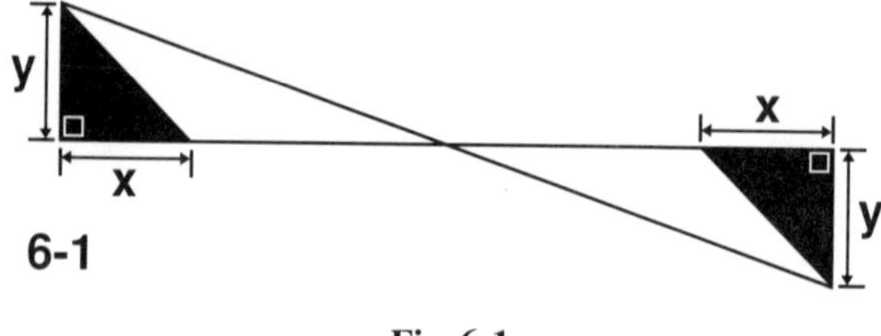

Fig. 6-1

The axial magnification is related to the linear magnification not linearly but exponentially: Axial magnification = (linear magnification).[2] After simple magnification has been detailed, the application of this to indirect ophthalmoscopy will become apparent.

When the distance or size of an object cannot be measured, one is not able to derive the above relationships. This is the problem when dealing with the eye as an optical system. What can be done is to compare the size of the image without the optical system to the size of the image with the optical system.

In Fig. 6-2, *a*, the object subtends an angle α at the nodal point of the eye. If angle α is small, $\tan \alpha = \frac{\text{Opposite}}{\text{Adjacent}} = \frac{\text{Object size}}{\text{x}}$ (1). The size of the image without the optical system is therefore related to the angle α subtended at the nodal point without the optical system.

If an optical system is introduced such as the plus lens as in Fig. 6-2, *b*, the angle subtended with the object at the anterior focal point of the lens is angle α'. The size of the image is therefore related to the angle α' subtended at the nodal point with the optical system. Thus:

$$\text{Angular magnification} = \frac{\text{Angle subtended with the system}}{\text{Angle subtended without the system}}$$

But if α' is small, $\alpha' = \tan \alpha' = \frac{\text{Opposite}}{\text{Adjacent}} = \frac{\text{Object size}}{\text{f}} = \text{Object size} \times \frac{1}{f} =$ object size $\times$ D (2)

$$M_A = \frac{\alpha'}{\alpha} = \frac{\text{Object size} \times \text{D (2)}}{\frac{\text{Object size (1)}}{x}} = \frac{\text{Object size} \times xD}{\text{Object size}}$$

$$M_A = xD$$

where: x = distance in meters from the object to the nodal point

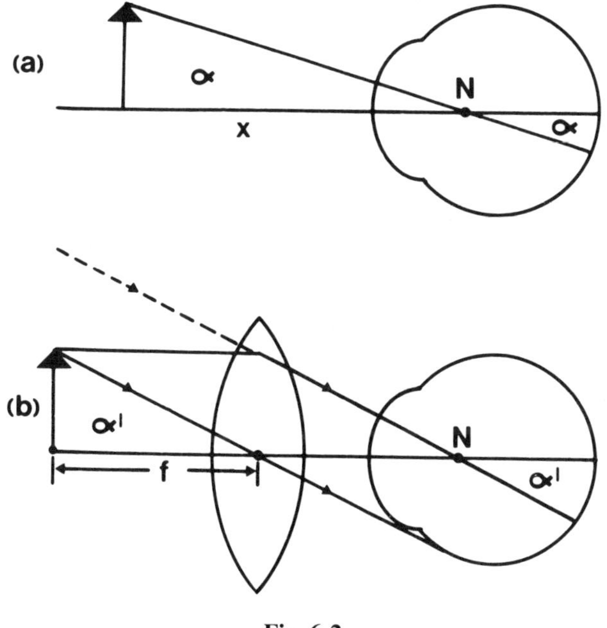

Fig. 6-2

This relationship tells us that the angular magnification is related not only to the angular subtense at the nodal point but also to the power of the magnifier and some reference distance x. This has been standardised with few exceptions to 25 cm or ¼ m. Thus:

$$M_A = \frac{D}{4} \quad \text{Angular magnification of a simple magnifier}$$

Having chosen this standard, what has really been done? The size of the image of any system is compared to its size at the reference distance of 25 cm without the system. Several very common examples are used extensively on examinations. For example, what is the magnification (1) of the fundus as visualized with the direct ophthalmoscope and (2) of the aphakic eye with an anterior focal point of 25 mm using the direct ophthalmoscope?

Solutions:

(1) The power of an emmetropic eye is found from the reduced schematic eye to be +60.00 D. The magnification is then $D_{eye}/4 = +60/4 = 15\times$.

(2) An aphakic eye with an anterior focal point of 25 mm or 2.5 cm is equivalent to an eye of 100/2.5 or +40.00 D.

$$M_A = \frac{+40}{4} = 10\times$$

Occasionally a question will appear altering the viewing distance, e.g., from 25 to 40 cm. The magnification is calculated the same, but consideration is given to viewing at 40 cm rather than 25 cm. The image would appear smaller at the further distance by 25/40.

$$M_2 = \frac{25}{40} \times M_1$$

GALILEAN TELESCOPE

Telescopes are common devices that use angular magnification, since their objects and images are large and distant. There are two common forms of telescopes, Galilean and astronomical, which vary according to their eyepiece and imagery.

The Galilean telescope has a plus objective lens and a minus eyepiece (closest to the eye) lens. These lenses are placed such that the secondary focal point of the first plus objective lens coincides with the primary focal point of the second (minus eyepiece) lens. The real image of the first lens becomes the virtual object for the second, and the rays emergent from the eyepiece are parallel. These subtend a greater angle α' than the incident parallel rays (angle α) (Fig. 6-3, *a*). The image on the retina is thus larger and inverted (but perceived upright). But how much larger? Inspection of Fig. 6-3, *b*, shows two triangles bounded by a base, y, which is the image formed by $+D_O$ in the focal plane of both lenses. If α and α' are small:

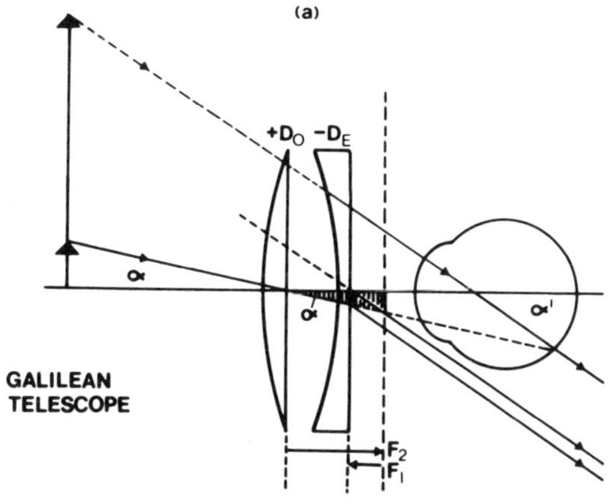

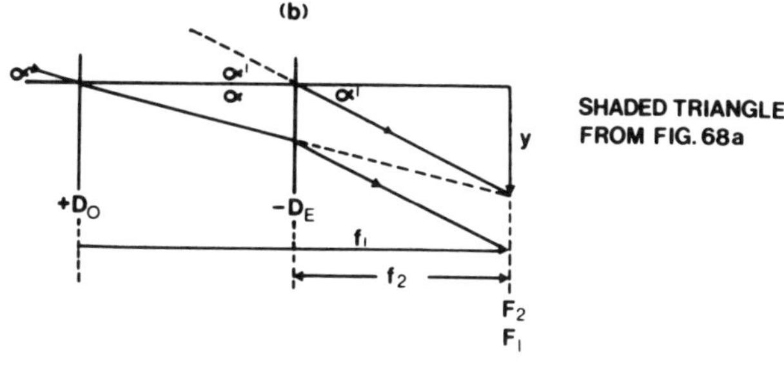

Fig. 6-3

$$\alpha = \tan \alpha = \frac{\text{Opposite}}{\text{Adjacent}} = \frac{y}{f_1} \quad \text{and} \quad \alpha' = \tan \alpha' = \frac{y}{-f_2}$$

$$\text{The } M_A = \frac{\alpha'}{\alpha} = \frac{\frac{y}{-f_2}}{\frac{y}{f_1}} = \frac{y}{-f_2} \times \frac{f_1}{y} = \frac{f_1}{-f_2} = \frac{-D_{\text{EYEPIECE}}}{D_{\text{OBJECTIVE}}}$$

$$M_A = \frac{-D_E}{D_O}$$

where: M_A = angular magnification
D_E = power of the eyepiece lens
D_O = power of the objective lens

This is a very important relationship because it represents not only the magnification of telescopes but also any combination of lenses whose secondary focal point of the first lens is coincident with the primary focal point of the second. The correction of ametropia is one such combination.

Consider first a telescope with D_O + 20.00 D and D_E − 40.00 D. The magnification $M_A = \frac{-D_E}{D_O} = \frac{-(-40)}{20} = 2\times$. The separation of a Galilean telescope is the difference between their focal lengths 100/20 − 100/40 = 2.5 cm or 25 mm (Fig. 6-3, *b*). If the M_A is positive, the *perceived* image is upright and if negative it will be inverted.

If D_E is plus instead of minus, what is the result? $M_A = \frac{-D_E}{D_O}$ so the image is inverted when perceived. This is the situation with the astronomical telescope, which for this very reason is used much less than the Galilean in ophthalmic optics. This is illustrated in Fig. 6-4, and again it can be seen that f_2 of the objective lens coincides with f_1 of the eyepiece. This ensures emergence of parallel rays. The separation will thus be the sum of the focal lengths.

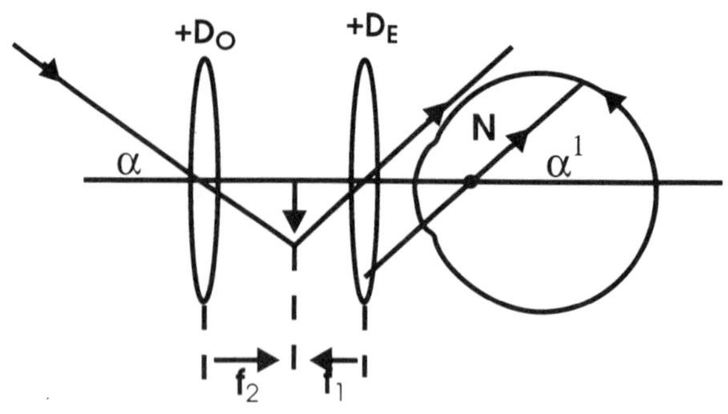

Fig. 6-4

As the object is brought closer for near viewing, the object vergence is naturally more divergent. It is easy to focus solely on accommodation and forget about the convergence demands of near viewing. Loupes and other systems may magnify not only the accommodative demands but also those of convergence. Similarly, if accommodation is invoked, accommodative convergence may also occur, inappropriately turning the eyes in. Measures can be taken to manipulate these factors to reduce these problems.

Consider first the accommodative demands of an object at near when viewed through a telescopic device. This requires not only the normal accommodation for this distance but also more accommodation to overcome the increased demand by the telescope. The approximation formula below is instructive.

$$\text{Accommodation through a telescope} = \text{Normal accommodation} \times M_A^2$$

$$\text{or} \quad A_T = A_N \times M_A^2$$

Suppose an object at 50 cm is viewed through a 3× Galilean telescope $A_T = 2 \times 3^2 = 18.00$ D! If the telescope was to be used at this distance, a +2.00 D lens positioned in *front* of the objective lens would collimate or make parallel the light entering the telescope. This would eliminate the accommodative demand. The new magnification of the telescope would be $M_A = \frac{-D_E}{D_O} = \frac{-D_E}{D_O + 2.00\text{ D}}$. This principle is applied when dealing with telescopic low vision aids or surgical operating loupes. Consider a 3× magnifier with a desired working distance of 25 cm. As described above, a +4.00 D lens is added to, or incorporated into, the objective lens. To achieve the same 3× magnification, a simple magnifier would be required to be $\frac{D}{4} = 3\times = +12.00$ D. A +12.00 D lens, however, has a focal length of 100/12 or 8.3 cm. The obvious advantage of the telescopic system is the further working distance it affords. Practically, however, they are more cumbersome and cosmetically displeasing.

What would happen if this telescope inadvertently had the +4.00 D lens incorporated into the eyepiece lens? The telescope, when the near object is viewed, has already exerted its diverging effect by the time it encountered the + 4.00 D lens. The accommodative requirement would then be $A_T - 4.00\text{ D} = (4 \times 3^2) - 4 =$ 32.00 D.

When dealing with multiple systems, the total magnification of the system is the product of each component magnifier.

$$\text{Total magnification } M_1 \times M_2 \ldots\ldots \times M_n$$

When one considers the correction of ametropia, one is dealing with two lenses of different powers—the correcting lens (D_O) and the eye error (D_E). Since the correcting lens is coincident with the far point of the eye, one again has a situation where the secondary focal point of the first lens is coincident with the primary focal point of the second (far point). This is therefore a telescope.

Consider first the example of extreme hyperopia—aphakia. What is the magnification of a +12.00 D spectacle-corrected aphake at a vertex distance 10 mm (Fig. 6-5)? The +12.00 D spectacle images objects at the far point $f_2 = \frac{100}{12} =$ 8.33 cm. The spectacle vertex distance is 10 mm, but to this must be added the distance to the removed crystalline lens (approximately 5 mm) = 15 mm = 1.5 cm. The eye error is:

$$D_E = \frac{-100}{8.33 - 1.5} = \frac{-100}{6.8} = -14.7$$

$$M_A = \frac{-D_E}{D_O} = \frac{-(-14.7)}{12} = 1.22\times \text{ or } 22\%$$

From this relationship it is easily appreciated that, as the vertex distance decreases, D_E approximates D_O and the magnification approaches 1. This fortifies the clinical fact that in the optical correction of aphakia, as one goes from a spec-

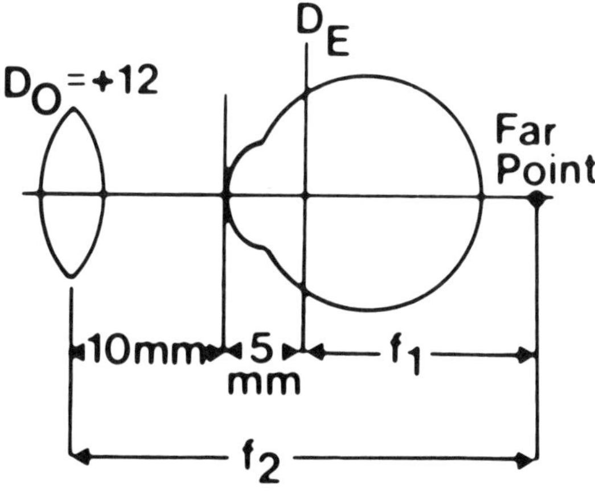

Fig. 6-5

tacle to a contact lens to an intraocular lens, the magnification becomes insignificant. Similarly a myopic patient would have a minus D_O and a plus D_E.

$$M_A = \frac{-(-D_E)}{(D_O)} = \frac{D_E}{D_O}.$$

If $D_O > D_E$ (as it is with spectacles), $\frac{D_E}{D_O} < 1$ or *minification* occurs. This is like looking through a Galilean telescope backward, and the world is minified. Again, as the vertex distance approaches zero, the minification approaches unity.

As mentioned previously, an astigmatic patient gets meridional magnification. Consider a $+6.00 \times 45$ astigmat. The far point plane is located at $100/6 = 16.6$ cm. With a vertex distance of 10 mm or 1 cm, the $-D_E = \frac{100}{16.6 - 1} = \frac{100}{15.6} = -6.40$ D. $M_A = -\left(\frac{-6.4}{6}\right) = 1.06$ or 6%. Since the power of the cylinder is at 90° to its axis, the $45 + 90 = 135$ meridian is magnified. A square might look as depicted in Fig. 6-6.

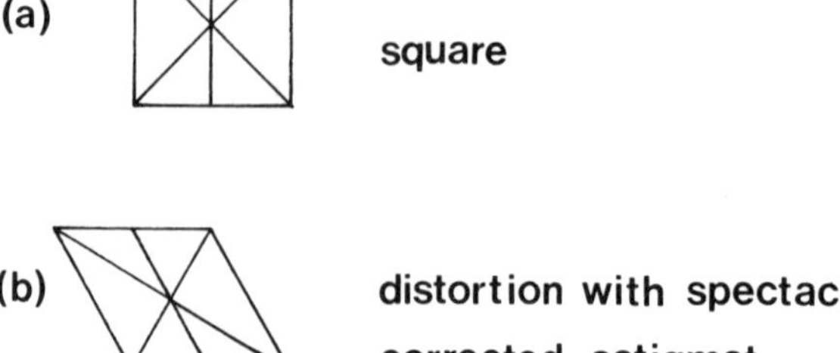

Fig. 6-6

ANISEIKONIA

In aphakia, anisometropia, and astigmatism this image magnification is the basis of *aniseikonia*—the perception of an image size disparity between the two eyes or when compared to normal seeing.

Under normal seeing circumstances an object of regard falls on corresponding retinal elements and is fused centrally into single binocular vision. If, under the above mentioned circumstances, magnification of the image in one eye or the meridian of one aspect of the image in one eye occurs, the image no longer falls on corresponding retinal points. In this case diplopia and visual confusion will occur. In diplopia the object of regard projects an image that falls on noncorresponding retinal points. In visual confusion different objects of regard fall on corresponding retinal points (Fig. 6-7). In young children visual adaption can occur by readjustment of the cortical value of corresponding retinal points (abnormal retinal correspondence). This usually occurs when an eye deviation or strabismus is present.

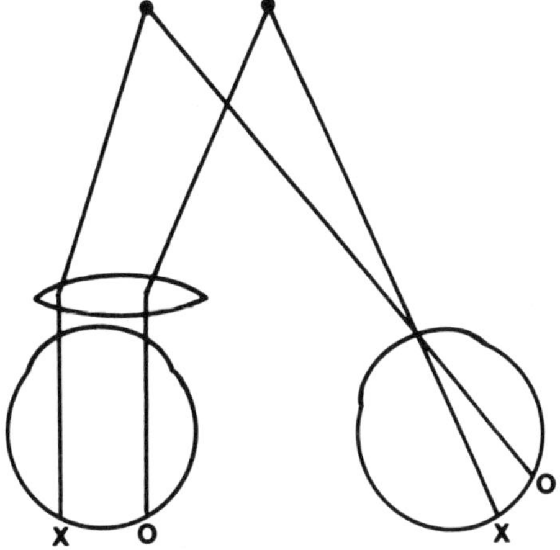

XX Different Object of Regard on Corresponding Retinal Points = Visual Confusion

XO Non-Corresponding Retinal Points With Same Object of Regard = Diplopia

Fig. 6-7

If the amount of image disparity and aniseikonia is small, the plasticity of the occipital cortex will allow adjustment. If the amount is large and the patient is a visually mature adult (a 70-year-old uniocular aphakic patient, for instance), the difference cannot be compensated for and the patient will see double. This can be eliminated by (1) a balance lens over the phakic eye to sufficiently blur the image to facilitate ignoring it, or (2) correction with an optical device whose magnification is reduced, such as a contact lens or intraocular lens. If the image size disparity is small but still bothersome, size, or iseikonic, lenses can be used. These are constructed as Galilean or reverse Galilean telescopes by virtue of different front and back surface powers that magnify or minify but maintain the same power. Some practitioners (Enoch) routinely overplus aphakic contact lens patients and overcorrect with minus spectacles to obtain the reverse Galilean telescopic effect. This reduces some of the 5% to 7% image disparity. In the days of the now defunct Dartmouth Eye Institute, image size and disparity were measured with a device called the eikonometer, which is seldom used today. Hand cards with sized semicircles and red-green glasses can be used instead (Awaya, et al. Handaya Corp., Japan).

KNAPP'S RULE

Another theoretical way of dealing with image magnification is illustrated in Fig. 6-8. By definition any rays incident at the primary focal point of a lens will emerge from the lens as parallel rays. Consider a myopic eye that has too much plus power ($+D_E$). If, as in Fig. 6-8, *a*, the incident rays are passed through F_A, they will emerge parallel. If the correcting minus lens is positioned at F_A, the rays will

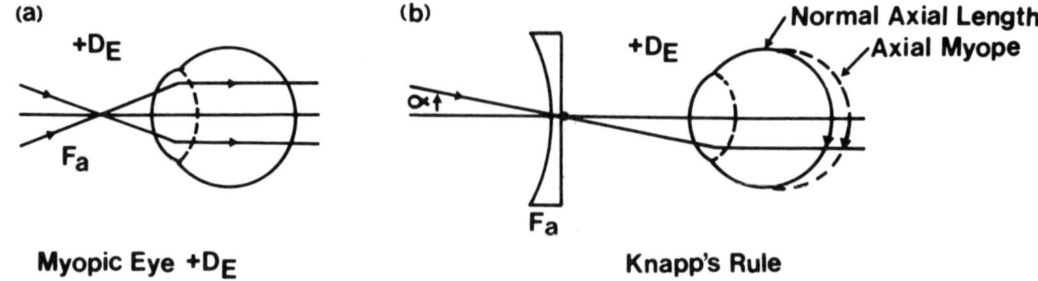

Fig. 6-8

still, by definition, emerge parallel. The retinal image thus subtended will remain the *same size* no matter what the axial length of the eye. This is *Knapp's rule.* Unfortunately, in a clinical setting one seldom knows how much of a refractive error is attributable to refractive versus axial components, nor the exact position of the anterior focal point. Even if known, it may not be practical to use this vertex distance. This may be true of some anisometropic patients whom one would *expect* to be symptomatic but are not.

When one deals with contact lens wearers, one not only has to consider the magnification factors in changing from spectacles to contacts but also the demands on accommodation. Consider the example of an 8.00 D spectacle-corrected hyperopic and myopic patients and the accommodative demands on each for an object at 25 cm (Fig. 6-9).

+8.00 Hyperopia

$$FP = \frac{100}{8} = 12.5 \text{ cm}$$

$$-D_E = \frac{100}{12.5 - 1} = \frac{100}{11.5} = -8.7 \text{ D}$$

$$M_A = \frac{-8.7}{-8} = 1.09\times$$

$$\text{Normal accommodation } A_N = \frac{100}{25} = 4.00 \text{ D}$$

$$A_T = A_N \times M_A^2 = 4 \times 1.09^2 = 4.75 \text{ D}$$

$$\frac{4.75 - 4.00}{4.00} = \frac{0.75}{4} \times 100 = 18.75\% \text{ more}$$

−8.00 Myopia

$$FP = \frac{100}{-8} = -12.5 \text{ cm}$$

$$+D_E = \frac{100}{12.5 + 1} = \frac{100}{13.5} = +7.4$$

$$M_A = \frac{-(+7.4)}{-8} = 0.925\times$$

$$A_N = 4.00 \text{ D}$$

$$A_T = 4 \times 0.925^2 = 3.40 \text{ D}$$

$$\frac{4.00 - 3.40}{4.00} = \frac{0.6}{4} \times 100 = 15\% \text{ less}$$

From these examples one can see that spectacle-corrected hyperopia of +8.00 D requires 18.75% more accommodation than contact lens–corrected hyperopia and 18.75 + 15 = 33.75% more than −8.00 D spectacle-corrected myopia. Thus, if this hyperopic patient converted to contact lenses, he would require 18.75% less accommodation than with spectacles. If he was prepresbyopic, this would delay his entry into bifocals. Similarly, the myopic patient who converts to contacts from spectacles must now exert 15% more accommodation. If prepresbyopic, his entry into bifocals may be precipitated.

The spectacle-corrected myopic patient also learns very early that he can remove his spectacles and see very clearly at his far point with *no* accommodation

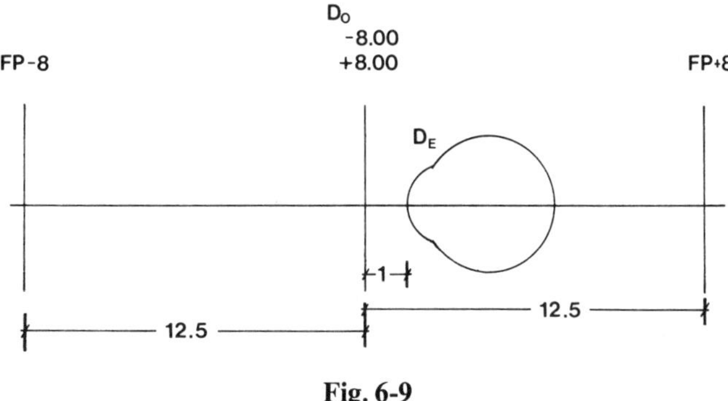

Fig. 6-9

(since the far point is conjugate to the retina). It is considerably more difficult to remove one's contacts to achieve this. This also eliminates the minification, since there is no longer a reverse Galilean telescopic effect.

This raises the interesting point that magnification, minification, and distortion are phenomena related to the *correcting lens* and not the ametropia itself. An astigmatic person who is uncorrected experiences no distortion (or very little) until he is spectacle corrected (see Guyton DL: Prescribing cylinders: the problem of distortion, *Surv Ophthalmol* 22(3):177-188, 1977.). Vision is blurred but not distorted. Although the amount of distortion monocularly may be small, the binocular appreciation is manifest multifold. This is especially true for stereoscopically perceived phenomena such as tilt or inclination, where small retinal image disparity is responsible for the perception of depth. A 0.4° monocular tilt that is opposite in the two eyes is perceived as a 35° forward or aft binocular tilt. This article proposes that distortion can be reduced by using minus cylinder (posterior toric) lenses and minimal vertex distances, which can be easily understood from the principles already learned. Since horizontal and vertical distortion are better tolerated, rotation of the offending cylinder toward 90° or 180° will convert oblique distortion to more acceptable forms. The clinical application of this will be dealt with when considering the prescription of lenses.

Please see Part II: Problems and Part III: Solutions for typical examination questions pertaining to the material in this chapter.

CHAPTER 7: RETINOSCOPY

Dealings with ametropia have so far been limited to subjective refining techniques and the power and position of the correcting lens. Since subjective testing depends on patient participation, it is often time consuming and not rewarding. An objective method that deals with light reflexes and shadows as they emerge from the eye gives us the "ballpark figure" from which to start our refinement. This is called *streak retinoscopy (or skiascopy)* and was popularized in North America by the late Jack Copeland, whose teaching of retinoscopy was almost evangelical in its fervor. Much of the following can be found and expanded on in his manual *Streak Retinoscopy,* available from Stereo Optical Co., Inc., 3539 North Kenton Ave. Chicago IL 60641.

To understand retinoscopy, the concept of the far point is crucial. Recall that in the unaccommodated myopic eye the far point is somewhere in front of the eye, its position varying with the amount of myopia. Similarly, in hyperopia the far point is behind the eye, and in emmetropia it is at infinity. In astigmatism two far lines exist whose positions depend on the type of astigmatism (e.g., compound myopic). If the retina is illuminated with a light source (such as the retinoscope), it then becomes an object whose image will be formed at the point conjugate to it, i.e., the far point. One can simulate eye errors and ametropia by placing plus or minus spheres in front of an emmetropic eye. It is instructive to see the movement of the far point as this is performed.

In Fig. 7-1 it is seen that, by the addition of plus or minus sphere, one can move the far point wherever desired in a controlled fashion. The next crucial aspect is how does one *identify* this change clinically? Fortunately, the direction of movement of the light reflexes changes with the different far point positions. The detection of these movements is the basis of retinoscopy. As shall be seen momentarily, the movement of the light reflex has a point where its direction reverses; unfortunately this position is at infinity, i.e., when the far point for emmetropia is reached. Since it is impractical to work at an infinite distance from the patient (although in some cases this might be desirable!), it is necessary to manipulate the point of reversal to a point that is more accessible: ⅔ m is a convenient distance at which to work. From Fig. 7-1 one sees that a +1.50 D lens moves the emmetropic far point to ⅔ m, which is desired. This is therefore called the *working lens.* This lens affects not only the emmetropic far point but also *all* far points. In essence it is redefining emmetropia for retinoscopy purposes as −1.50 D of myopia.

Fig. 7-2 depicts this difficult concept. From the diagram one sees that those eyes with a myopic error less than 1.50 D now behave during retinoscopy in a way that low hyperopic eyes would be expected to behave, i.e., they yield a "with" response. Being less myopic than the new "emmetropia", their far points are behind the examiner as a low hyperopic eye would be. This will be clarified when considering the origin of the with and against movements seen at retinoscopy.

Fig. 7-3, *a*, depicts a hyperopic patient with the working lens in place. The far point plane of the patient remains behind the retina. As the streak from the retinoscope descends, the retina is illuminated and becomes an object imaged at its

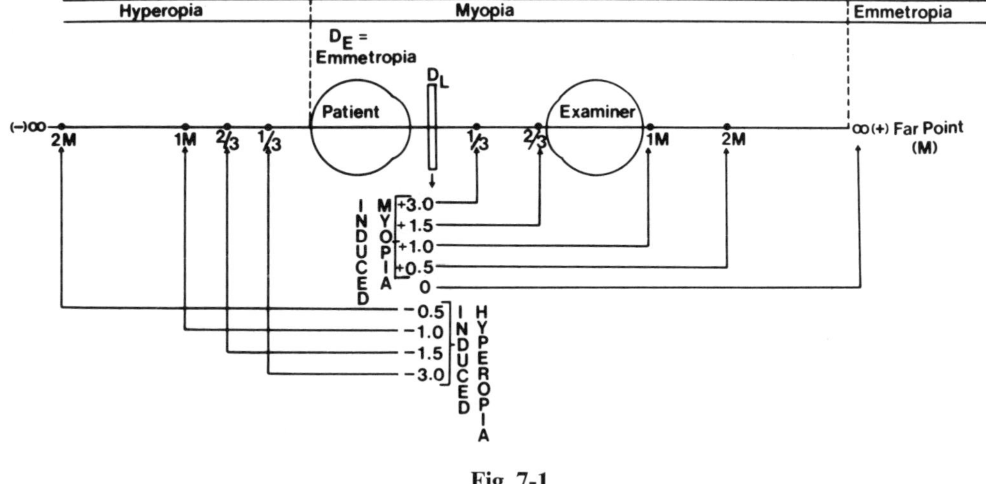

Fig. 7-1

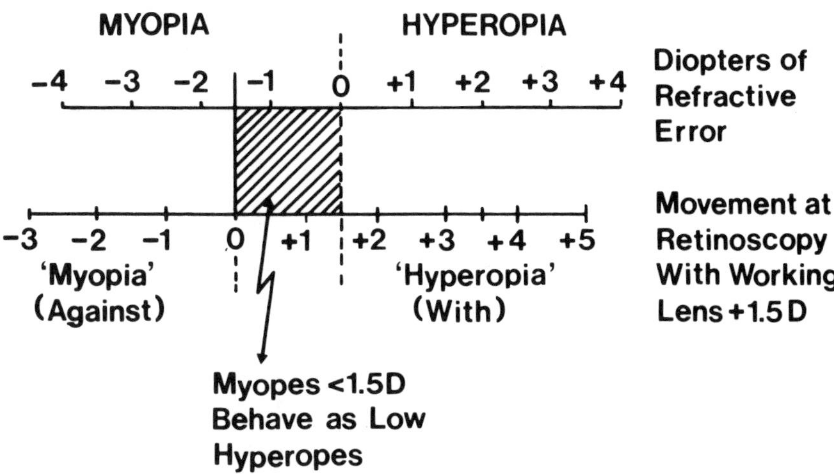

Fig. 7-2

conjugate point, the far point plane. This streak image is now an object for the examiner to follow. As she moves the retinoscope down, the new object or streak moves down in the far point plane. The image of this in the examiner's eye, however, is moving up. This is *perceived* by the cortical processing of retinal imagery as down. Thus the intercept on the face and rest of the eye (which indicates the direction the retinoscope is moving) and the streak (which is the perceived image) are both travelling in the same direction and represent a *with* motion. Similarly, the weak myopic eye whose refractive error is less than −1.50 D has a far point plane that lies behind the examiner. The intercept and streak both travel in the same direction, yielding a with motion (Fig. 7-3, *b*). In the myopic eye greater than −1.50 D, the far point plane lies between the examiner and the patient. The image of the streak again becomes the object for the examiner, but this time is transcribed to an inverted image on the retina. This means that as the intercept goes down, the perceived movement of the streak is up. This is the basis of the *against* movement. When the far point is at the peephole of the retinoscope, as in Fig. 7-3, *d*, the image of the light *fills* the examiner's pupil and no movement is seen. This corresponds to the far point of the emmetrope as newly defined.

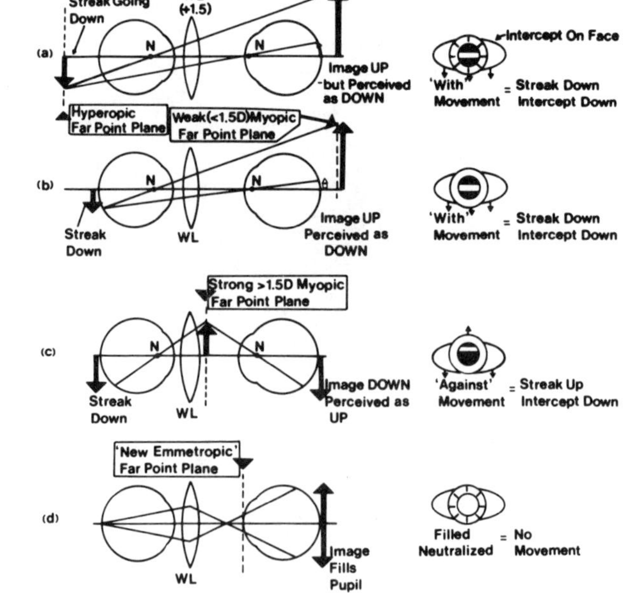

Fig. 7-3

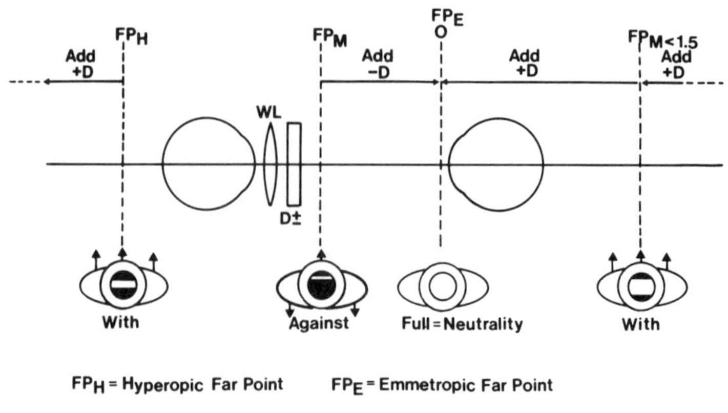

Fig. 7-4

Now that one can identify where the far point plane lies by the direction of the movement it transcribes at various positions, one can utilize the system of altering its position with the various lenses to advantage. Fig. 7-4 shows how this might be done. If an against movement is seen, one knows that the far point is between the patient and the examiner. If one neutralizes the eye error with minus lenses (−D), the far point will recede and the reflex will fill when no against movement is seen. In a similar fashion plus lenses can be added to weak myopic and hyperopic eyes to neutralize the with movements until neutrality is achieved.

The point of neutrality is often difficult to judge precisely and is more of a neutral zone than a sharply defined point. One way to verify this is seen in Fig. 7-5. If one has achieved neutrality, by changing the position of the examiner relative to the far point the movement of the reflex can be changed. If the examiner moves forward, the far point is behind her, and a with movement is seen. Rather than

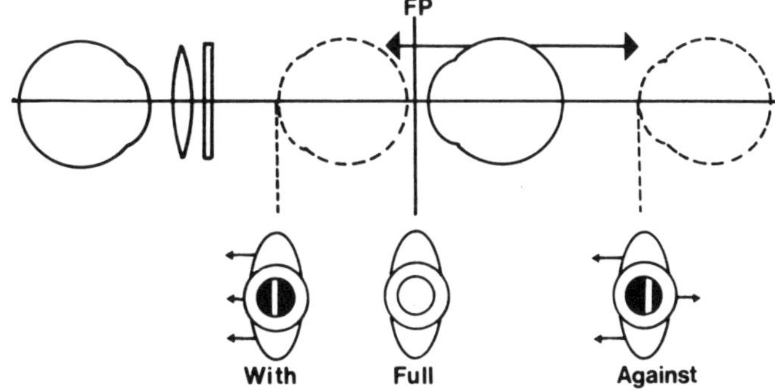

Fig. 7-5

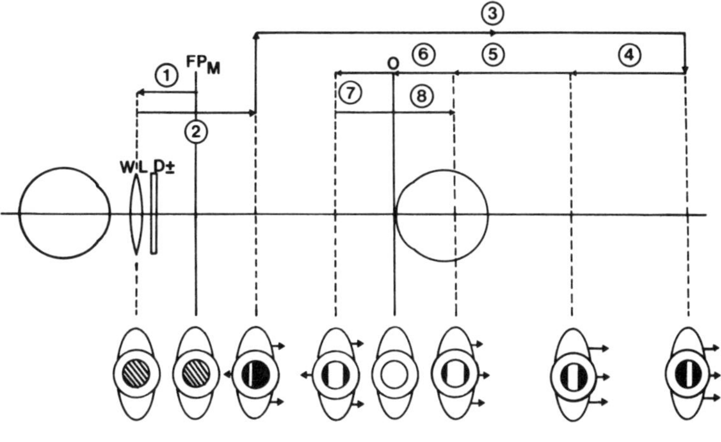

Fig. 7-6

moving, adding −0.50 D will achieve the same far point effects. Clinically, with motion is more easily appreciated than against movement. This is why many refractionists leave "just a touch" of with motion at neutrality so that it is more easily recognized. It is also the reason myopic patients are not treated by neutralizing the against movement. It is much easier to add a lot of minus sphere to convert all high myopia to low myopia or hyperopia and neutralize the with motion.

Consider for a moment the neutralization of high myopia and high hyperopia to illustrate these principles. High myopia is shown in Fig. 7-6: (*1*), With the sleeve of the retinoscope all the way up (or down depending on the make of the retinoscope), a poor light reflex is seen, which resembles a blob. It might be mistaken for neutrality, but moving in and out has no effect. Some plus sphere is added, but no improvement is seen. (*2*), Minus sphere is added and a definite against reflex is seen. (*3*), Minus is added until a strong with is seen. (*4*) to (*6*), Plus sphere is added until neutrality is seen. Minus is added until a "tough of plus" remains. Two interesting points are made here. A blob reflex could be either high myopia or high hyperopia, which are often separable by the addition of ±3.00 D. (This may also be due to poor clarity of the refractive media, in which case nothing will improve it.) In very high refractive errors, steps of ±3.00 D may be required to over ±20.00 D before a clear reflex one way or another is seen and identified.

Also note that, as neutrality is approached, the reflex becomes broader and picks up speed. In hyperopia the far point begins behind the eye and with more

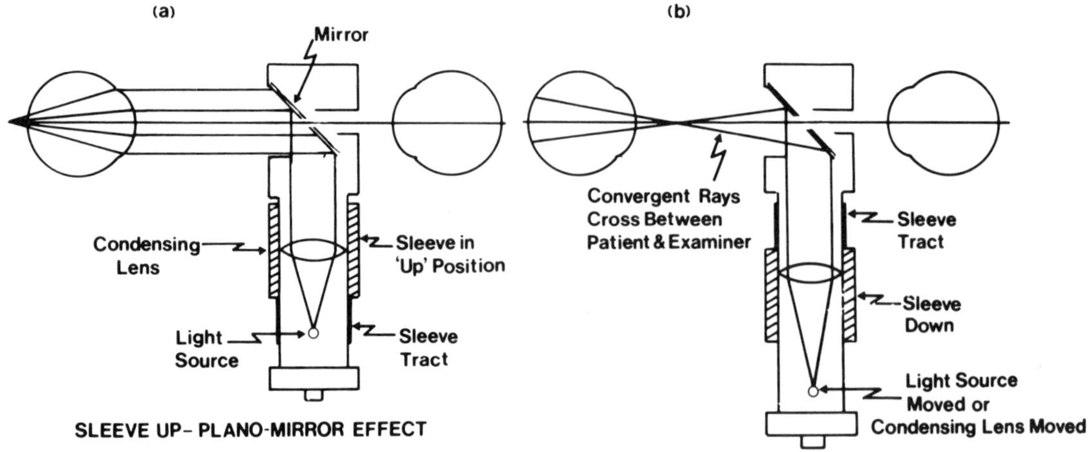

Fig. 7-7

plus sphere comes through infinity, and approaches the neutrality point. From this point on it is the same as myopia.

There are other ways of enhancing the reflex if high hyperopia or myopia is suspected from a blob image. To understand these, the construction of a retinoscope is briefly required. (The following discussion applies to a streak retinoscope used in the sleeve-up position. If a sleeve-down style is employed, reverse everything.)

In the sleeve-up position the emergent light is divergent. In the sleeve-down position the light source or the condensing lens position is varied such that the emergent light is convergent to a point of focus between the patient and examiner. This has the effect of reversing the traditional motion so that against becomes with motion. In the sleeve-down position, with a highly myopic patient, it is often possible to obtain a with motion where an against was difficult to discern with the sleeve up. For a blob reflex this is a useful manoeuvre. In a hyperopic patient, dropping the sleeve may sometimes enhance the image about midway between the up and down positions. Just as the band width is useful in estimating the proximity to neutrality, the enhanced band width is also useful in estimating the proximity to neutrality. If the enhanced reflex is narrow and is about the same size as the intercept, approximately +5.00 D of hyperopia exists. If the band is wide and not enhanced well, it is only about +1.00 D.

If the eye is astigmatic, instead of a single far point one has two far line planes in meridians 90° to each other. Inspection of all meridians is performed with a rotation sweep of the retinoscope. Two bands of unequal (or perhaps opposite) motion can be identified. This portends no real difficulty but requires slightly different approaches depending on whether the refractionist is dealing with spheres only or plus or minus cylinders.

Plus cylinders are probably best suited to streak retinoscopy, and consideration to plus cylinder technique will be dealt with first. Two far line planes exist irrespective of the type of astigmatism. With the addition of enough minus sphere, all types of astigmatism are converted to compound hyperopic astigmatism, which will yield *with* motions of different streak widths and speeds, normal to each other. One band will be approaching neutrality faster than the other. This is illustrated in Fig. 7-8.

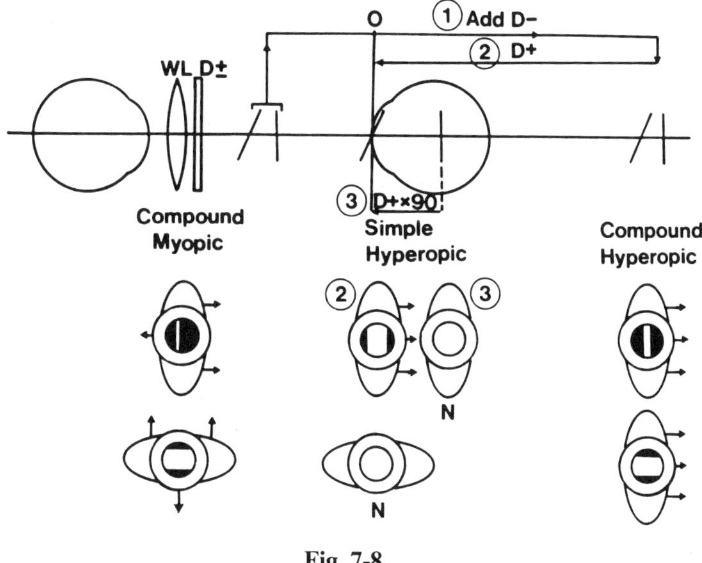

Fig. 7-8

The band that neutralizes first corresponds to the spherical correction. The remaining band in Fig. 7-8 remains at 90°. The axis of the plus cylinder is aligned with the streak, and plus cylinder axis 90° is added until neutrality is achieved in both meridians.

It is not always that easy to be certain about the axis of the correcting cylinder. Five descriptive phenomena aid in the refinement of the cylinder axis (Fig. 7-9). These are self-explanatory and are used by the seasoned practitioner at a subconscious level.

The *minus cylinder technique* can be performed in several ways. One method is to use the double click method previously described under transposition. Recall that $+0.25 = -0.25 \times 90$ is equivalent to plano $+0.25 \times 180$. Using exactly the same technique as plus cylinders, i.e., neutralizing with motion in both directions, minus cylinder at 90° to the streak is added with an equal amount of plus sphere. When refining the axis by straddling, always remember to go toward the wider instead of the finer band.

The second minus cylinder technique is to proceed with sphere addition until neutralization of the first meridian. At this point the first, far point plane is passed through and the *second* meridian is neutralized to become the sphere. This con-

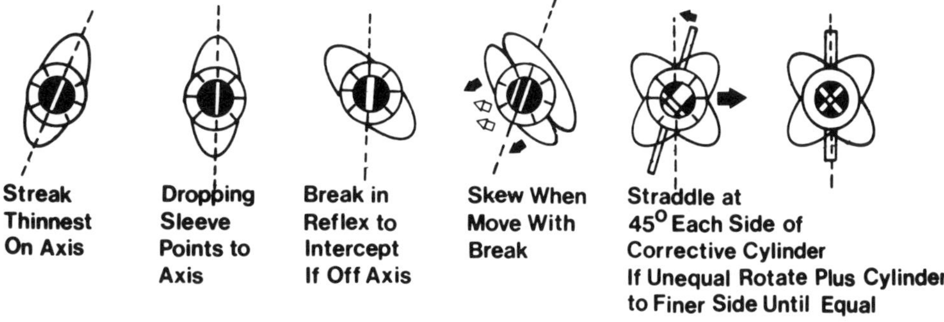

Fig. 7-9 Axis refinement during retinoscopy.

verts everything to simple myopic astigmatism, and the anterior far point plane can be pushed back with minus cylinder in the meridian of the against motion. (One can also neutralize the against motion in both meridians or drop the sleeve for the concave mirror effect to reverse the against to with motion. Both of these are inferior methods to those cited above.)

If so inclined, the use of spheres only to neutralize the two principal meridians is also feasible. In so doing, the recording is in *meridional power* and forms a power cross, which must be converted to axis notation in the usual way. Refinement of the cylinder axis is the major deficiency as well as the two-step recording required.

Two major problems that arise during the course of retinoscopy can detract from its accuracy: (1) loss of accommodative control and (2) irregular reflexes. When performing retinoscopy only one eye is scoped at a time. The other eye should be fogged with +1.00 or +1.50 D fixing a distant, nonaccommodative target such as a fixation light. Many practitioners use their working lens as a fogging lens. The problem with a working lens is that an extra lens causes an extra reflection. It is just as easy to add plus to the sphere. One of the great attributes of cycloplegia is that fogging and accommodative problems are relatively controlled. If the pupil is constricting or the values are shifting during retinoscopy, recheck fixation and fog and consider using cycloplegia.

The irregular reflexes the retinoscopist sees are most common in younger individuals with widely dilated pupils, and they occur especially prominently approaching neutrality. The etiology is presumed to be spherical aberration which, as you will recall, is the increased refraction of peripheral rays. At neutrality, this leads to a central filled zone but a peripheral against zone representative of the peripheral myopic rays. This is best ignored while confining your findings to the central few millimeters.

Irregular astigmatism can give rise to a related phenomenon. In this entity either corneal or lenticular radii of curvature change from one point to another across the pupillary aperture. This gives rise to irregular intervals of myopia and hyperopia, which wreaks havoc with the retinoscopic reflex. The most common form is the scissors reflex. Cycloplegic refraction of the central visual axis while the patient is fixing the light of the retinoscope is most accurate, although over-refraction with an appropriate contact lens may help (if the irregularity is in the cornea). If all else fails, perform a completely subjective refraction.

Please see Part II: Problems and Part III: Solutions for typical examination questions pertaining to the material in this chapter.

CHAPTER 8: REFRACTION

Virtually all of the skills and understanding necessary to perform a refraction to the final refinement stage have been covered. After a brief review of this latter entity, the sequence that should logically be followed will be summarized.

Assume for a moment that the cylinder correction has been objectively refined by retinoscopy and subjectively further refined with the Jackson cross cylinder. The fog and working lenses have been removed and now one wishes to refine the sphere. This can be achieved by two means, one of which has already been discussed. The ultimate goal is to determine the most amount of plus or least amount of minus sphere that affords the best visual acuity. If this is not performed, overminusing may result in excessive accommodative demands, or overplusing may compromise visual acuity. Consider giving minus away the same as giving money away.

The first method is simply adding +0.25 D sphere in a monocular fashion and asking the patient if the vision is better or worse. If better, continue adding plus until no further improvement is achieved. If the patient is accommodating, he will say it is worse. If he can relax the accommodation it will stay the same. At this point, change the question to "Is this worse or about the same?" Adding plus makes things bigger, introducing a bias. Checking the acuity is useful to rule out this bias. Recheck the visual acuity to verify that acuity has remained maximal. If the patient responds that vision is worse, remove +0.25 or prepare to add −0.25 D of sphere; ask if the letters are sharper and clearer or just smaller and darker. This will detect the reverse Galilean telescopic effect of induced accommodation with a corrective minus lens. The end point is when vision no longer improves or minification is reached.

The second method is the *duochrome or bichrome test,* which has been mentioned previously. Chromatic aberration by the crystalline lens results in blue and green being refracted more than red. The dispersion of white light into its spectral components in this way transcribes a chromatic interval, which bridges the retina for 1.50 to 2.00 D (up to 3.00 D). Clinically, during this test a red-green split filter is added to the visual acuity chart projector so that only these colors are used. Since a paucity of blue-sensitive receptors are present centrally (although the interval would be expanded by the use of blue), vision is preferentially reduced for this wavelength. By employing green-red, an interval of only 0.75 D exists, with yellow holding the emmetropic position on the retina midway between the myopic green waves and the hyperopic red waves (0.37 D on each side). Since this is due to the physical characteristics of the incoming white light and the aberration of the lens, color perception and hence color deficiency will not present a barrier to administration. In aphakic and pseudophakic patients the test is of little value because the green appears so much brighter after removal of the normal crystalline lens with its natural blue-green filter. The patient must be able to discriminate 0.37 D changes to appreciate the difference in acuity on each side of the chart. This precludes its use in those patients with less than 0.5 (20/40) vision. To perform the test, the preferred method is to fog the patient to the 0.67 (20/30) level with approximately +0.50 D sphere. This ensures that accommodation is con-

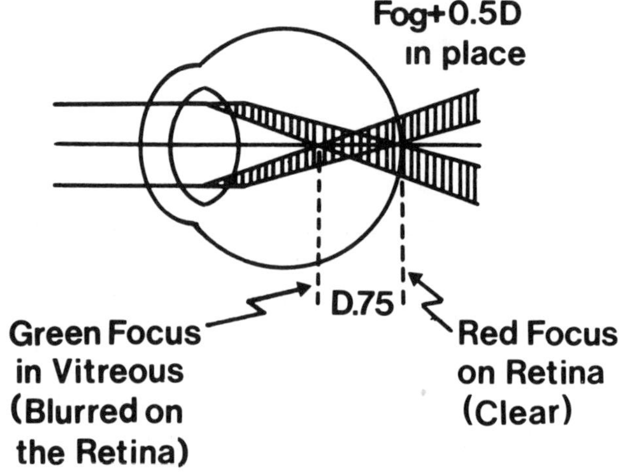

Fig. 8-1

trolled and that a predictable red interval should be closer to the retina and should therefore be the clearer side (Fig. 8-1). Once the patient has confirmed this, minus sphere is added until equality of the two sides exists and no further. Once carried onto the green side, accommodation can maintain equality and too much minus will be given. If the patient responds initially "in the green," plus is added again until the red side is clearer and brought back to equality with minus sphere. To the observant patient this is a very precise end point. To the less observant, it tends to be confusing and the examiner is wiser to stay with "better or worse."

The final step in the refinement process is to ensure that both eyes are equally controlled with respect to accommodation. If a cycloplegic refraction has been performed and there has been no evidence during testing that the cycloplegia is inadequate, I usually bypass this test, although the purists would consider this heretical. The technique is called *binocular balancing* and is more easily performed with a refractor than loose lenses. The one prerequisite is that visual acuity be equal in both eyes. If this is not so, the end point is tenuous and may be inaccurate. Two currently practised methods are prism dissociation and balanced fogging. Polarizing lenses with vectorgraphic slides can dissociate the eyes and be used in a similar fashion to the prism technique.

Prism dissociation requires that the patient be binocularly fogged to the 0.5(20/40) or so level with +1.00 D spheres. A 3 P.D. base up is placed over one eye and 3 P.D. base down over the other. In so doing the prism-induced decrease in vision is equal in both eyes. Others ignore this fact and place a vertical prism over one eye. A single line (20/40) is presented, which is now vertically diplopic so that simultaneous comparison of both eyes can be achieved. Plus sphere is added to one eye at a time to ensure that the two images are equally blurred or balanced. The prisms are removed and sphere refinement is performed binocularly by the "better or worse" method or the duochrome test again.

Similarly, without the prisms both eyes can be equally fogged, and an alternate cover test can be performed to compare the two. If a vision disparity exists, the fog is weaker on the side with the better vision. Plus sphere is added to equal blur and binocular sphere refinement performed as for the prism dissociation test.

All the necessary components have now been reviewed but not in their chronologically appropriate sequence. The following is presented as a guide to accurately obtaining the distance spectacle correction. The final prescription requires more knowledge of the art of prescribing, such as the amount of sphere or cylinder or reducing or changing cylinder axis. This is forthcoming.

Please see Part II: Problems and Part III: Solutions for typical examination questions pertaining to the material in this chapter.

SUMMARY OF REFRACTING SEQUENCE

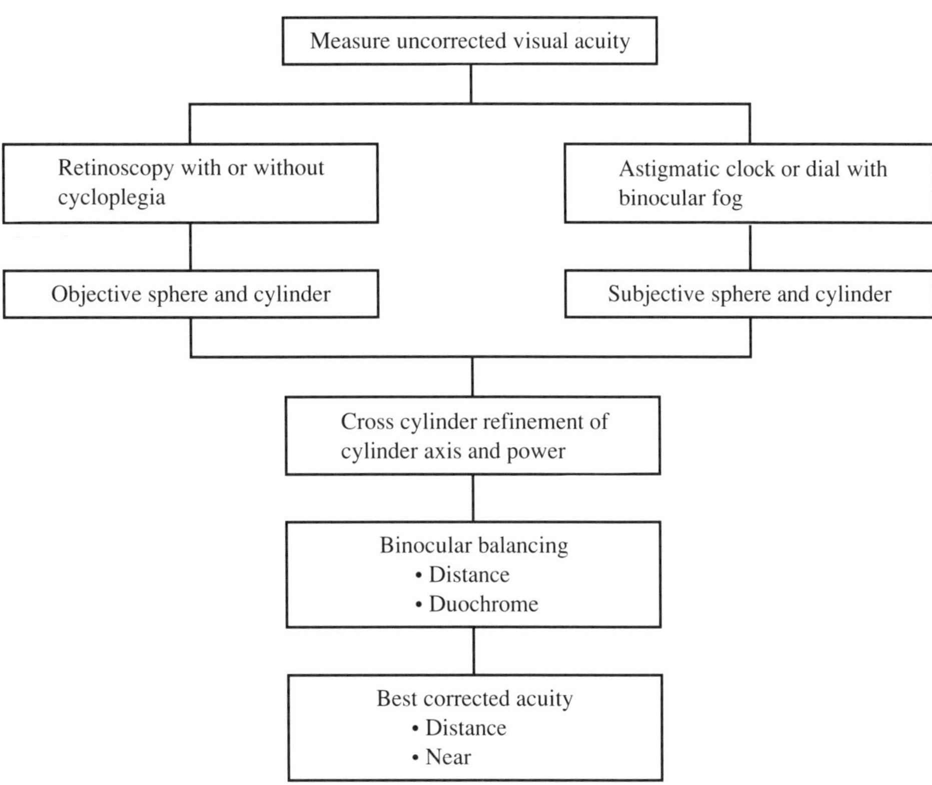

RECORD
(1) Uncorrected acuity
(2) Manifest refraction
(3) Present R_x
(4) Acuity with (2), (3) Distance and Near
(5) Cycloplegic refraction
(6) Cycloplegic agent
(7) Prescription given
(8) Vision with prescription

Fig. 8-2

CHAPTER 9: VISION TESTING

In the refraction sequence the initial and final steps both involve determining *visual acuity*. The measurement of visual acuity is influenced by many physiologic, psychophysical, and optical factors. Factors such as illumination, contrast, retinal area and illumination, state of adaption, pupil size, and diffraction all contribute to what is known as visual acuity. Some of these factors will be dealt with later and others will only be mentioned in passing. Complete treatment of these factors can be found in other texts.

SNELLEN FRACTION

To the ophthalmic practitioner, vision testing usually revolves around central visual acuity, peripheral visual fields, color vision, and steroacuity. These nonlaboratory office tests provide a plethora of data which cumulatively express the concept of the visual status of a patient. It is on these criteria that decision-making is performed and surgery undertaken. The optical aspects of central visual acuity are synonymous with the Snellen fraction. Other tests and measurements such as the minimum discernible and Vernier acuity all are important but not as useful on a day-to-day basis.

The 20/20 Snellen letter or optotype is so designed that at a distance of 20 feet the letter measures 8.9 mm and subtends, at the nodal point of the eye, 5 minutes of arc. Each stroke width and gap represent 1′. To identify the letter, the eye must be able to resolve this minimum separable or visual angle of 1′. The Landolt C and Allen picture cards are based on the same visual angles but are more suited to children and illiterate patients (Fig. 9-1).

The clinical entity that is called visual acuity is measured by having the patient read the smallest letter possible on a graduated chart at 20 feet or 6 m. The result is expressed as a fraction, e.g., 20/40 or 6/12. (A projector with an adjustable magnification tube can be used to calibrate the chart to accommodate lanes other than 20 feet or 6 m.) This (20/40) means that the smallest letter read, *when held at 40 feet,* subtends the same visual angle (5′ total or 1′ minimum separable) as the standard Snellen letter at 20 feet. Thus to know the Snellen fraction, the visual angle has to be known first, so one can decide where to put the letter so that it subtends 1 minute of minimum separable angle. This is the reason there has been so much confusion and controversy over what the best notation for visual acuity should be.

Consider first the visual angle as depicted in Fig. 9-2. This is the standard Snellen E held at 20 feet and subtending a minimum visual angle or minimum separable of 1′. If *E(1)* is moved toward the eye as *E(3)*, the angle subtended is an angle α which is obviously greater than 1′. If *E(3)* was the first position that the E was *identified as an E,* it can be said that this is the distance that 1′ of minimum separable angle could be discriminated by the patient. This occurs at a distance x feet. Since these angles are small, one can say:

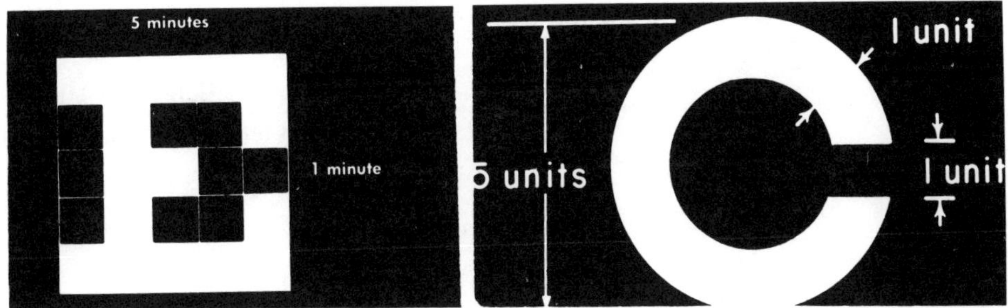

Fig. 9-1 Construction of the Snellen letter to subtend an angle of 5 minutes, with each part subtending an angle of 1 minute (1 minute equals $\frac{1}{60}$ degree). The 20/20 "E" measures 8.9 mm at 20 feet.

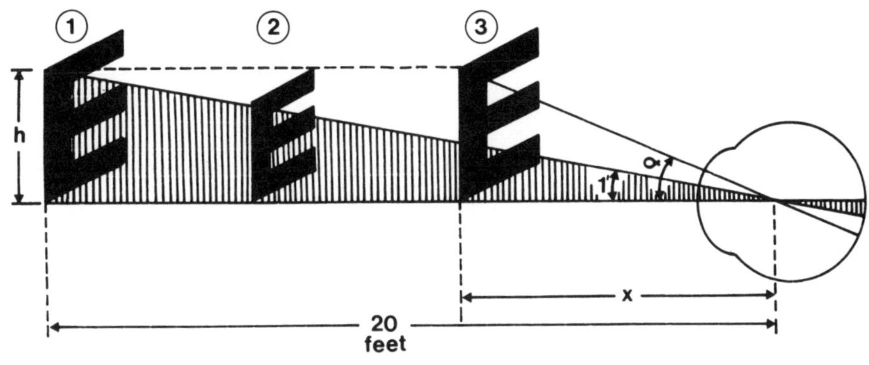

Fig. 9-2

$$\text{Visual angle} = \frac{\alpha}{1'} = \frac{\tan \alpha}{\tan 1'} = \frac{h/x}{h/20'} = \frac{h}{x} \times \frac{20}{h} = \frac{20}{x}$$

In other words:

$$\text{Minimum visual angle} = \frac{\text{Distance the Snellen letter subtends } 1' \ (+20 \text{ feet})}{\text{Distance } 1' \text{ of minimum separable angle is discriminated by the patient}}$$

For example, say the *E(3)* had to be brought to 10 feet before being identified as an E:

$$\text{Minimum visual angle} = \frac{20 \text{ feet}}{10 \text{ feet/minute}} = 2'$$

Thus, if the visual angle is 2′ it must be held twice as far (40 feet) as the standard Snellen E to subtend only 1′ at the nodal point. This is the same as saying that with 20/40 acuity, the patient can resolve at 20 feet what the normal patient with 20/20 acuity can resolve standing back at 40 feet.

Rather than moving the patient to 10 feet, the letter construction doubles the size and hence the angle. The Snellen chart contains the range from 20/10 to 20/800 optotypes.

Since the Snellen fraction is:

$$\text{Visual acuity} = \frac{\text{Test distance Snellen letter subtends } 1'}{\text{Distance identified letter must be held to subtend } 1'}$$

$$\text{In our example} = \frac{20}{40}$$

$$= \frac{1}{2} \times \frac{20}{20}$$

$$\text{Visual acuity} = \frac{1}{\text{Minimum visual angle}} \times \left(\frac{20}{20}\right)$$

Conversely:

$$\text{Minimum visual angle} = \frac{1}{\text{visual acuity}}$$

Similarly, if the Snellen fraction is 20/100, the visual angle would be 5′ and automatically it could be said that this must be held five times as far as the standard E to subtend 1′. In this way it doesn't matter if the notation used is in meters (referable to 6 or 5 or 4 m) as some use (and others desire) or in terms of fractions (e.g., 20/40 = 0.5) as in decimal acuity. Scientifically, to use the visual angle rather than the Snellen fraction makes the most sense, but it would require everyone to change their concept of what visual acuity is. The Snellen fraction, whether in feet or meters, is here to stay but at least you know from whence it came.

JAEGER NOTATION

The situation for near vision testing is even worse. Again it would make sense to note the visual angle at a certain distance or even the equivalent Snellen fraction. The fact is, this is seldom done. Instead, the Jaeger notation is commonly used. Jaeger himself never specified how it was derived or at what distance it should be administered. Usually the smallest Jaeger print (e.g., Jaeger 2) is noted at the position it is read best (e.g., 20 cm). There are so many variables (e.g., strength of bifocals) that this is really more of a description than a measurement and should be accepted as such. The point print system is equally arbitrary. There exists no known way to convert from one system to the other. As David Michaels, M.D., says about these problems "[It] . . . is a historic enigma whose abolition appears to have diplomatic immunity."

GLARE TESTING AND CONTRAST SENSITIVITY

Visual acuity testing has legal implications, such as driving standards, occupational standards, registration as blind, and so forth. Practically, it also gives the surgeon some objective measurement on which to assess indications for ocular surgery. It does not always correlate with patient complaints. This has led to other methods of acuity testing such as glare testing and contrast sensitivity testing.

Patients with media opacities, especially central ones such as corneal stromal scarring or posterior subcapsular cataracts, are very sensitive to bright lights and reflected light. Not only do the opacities degrade the axial and immediate paraxial rays, but in bright photopic conditions the pupil is smaller and the impairment is worse. Light can wash out the contrast, like opening the curtains while watching television on a bright afternoon. Scattering of the light may be simulated by commercial glare testers or testing the acuity with an acuity chart in a bright room rather than with a projector in a dark room. The consensual pupillary response is useful to constrict the pupil by shining light on the nonfixing eye. This unfortunately dazzles the eye with the light.

A similar phenomenon is contrast sensitivity. This is the ability to detect slight changes in luminance in regions without sharp contours. Clinically it is a measure of the difference of luminance from object to background (dL) divided by the background luminance (L) such that values define a sensitivity (and threshold) over varying spacial frequencies from 1.5 to 18 or more cycles per degree. Although it is as nonspecific for disease as is the Snellen acuity, it is more sensitive. Early optic neuropathy to corneal edema can affect the contrast sensitivity. Testing can be either in projected, oscilloscope, or printed chart form. Clinically the chart forms are easiest to administer, although the hardest to control for lighting, distance, etc. As with glare, reduced contrast can be a significant patient complaint with excellent Snellen acuity. This has been a concern with bifocal intraocular lens implants.

The diffractive implant (J. Futhey, 3M) employs multislope concentric diffractive rings on the back of a conventional implant. These rings are specially designed to establish only two orders of diffraction, presenting two foci where the visible spectrum is in phase. This is different from two focal points with a Fresnel or annular design. The question that arises with all of the refractive and diffractive bifocal lenses is whether the light that is defocused by the part of the lens to which one is inattentive degrades the contrast of the one focused on the object of regard. If the contrast sensitivity is reduced, is it outweighed by the advantages of the bifocal? These are questions to which I have no answer.

STEREOACUITY

Another important aspect of visual acuity is the ability of the visual system to appreciate depth. Aside from monocular cues and clues, stereopsis in terms of *stereoacuity* is a binocular phenomenon. For fine stereopsis to be perceived, an axial or horizontal object of regard within Panum's fusional space (the sum total of all fusible material) must be appreciated. This is stereopsis within the confines of single binocular vision. Gross stereopsis, on the other hand, can occur outside Panum's space in the sense that depth is implied by the bitemporal retinal disparity of close objects and the binasal disparity of far objects. When stereoacuity is spoken of, fine stereopsis is a function of the slightly different and disparate images of an object presented to each eye. This perspective difference is related to the distance the eyes are apart or the interpupillary distance (PD).

Consider Fig. 9-3. An object with a depth of x is located a distance d away from the eye. The horizontal retinal disparity induced by x subtends an angle θ at the nodal point. As long as x falls within Panum's space, the image disparity gener-

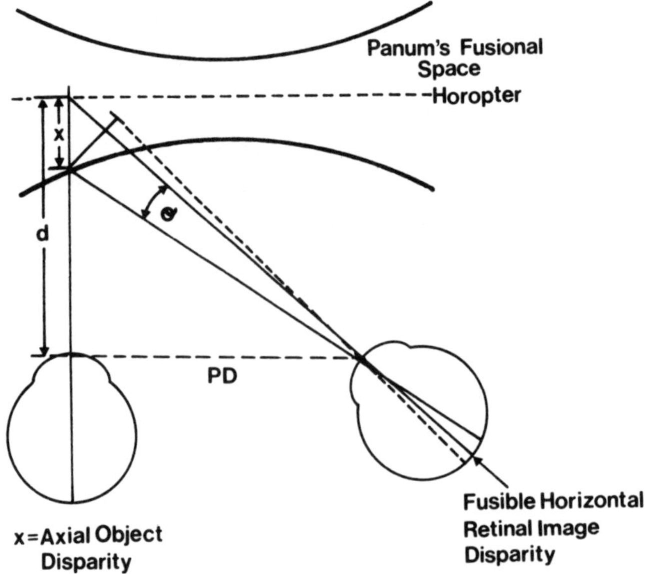

Fig. 9-3

ated by angle θ still falls on corresponding retinal points and can be fused. Trigonometrically it is easily derived that:

$$\theta = \frac{PD \times x}{d^2}$$

This confirms what one suspects intuitively, i.e., as the distance away from the eye increases, a marked decrease in stereoacuity is experienced. Similarly, as the depth (x) increases, the greater the angle it subtends and the easier it is appreciated as having depth. Perhaps unexpectedly, the wider apart one's eyes, the better the stereoacuity. This angle θ can therefore be used as a measure of stereoacuity if one considers how small angle θ can be for a patient to still be able to perceive depth. This is the *angle of stereoacuity* that is tested clinically; it can be seen that this is in reality a stereo threshold.

Several common stereoscopic tests are available on the market where circles, lines, or pictures are presented to each eye separately, using polarizing glasses and targets that are correspondingly polarized (e.g., Titmus, Bausch & Lomb, TNO plates, AO Vectographic slides distance and near). To understand how these work, a little knowledge of polarization is required.

Recall that in Fig. 1-1 light was said to have electric and magnetic planes that were perpendicular to each other. If the source is random, the direction of the electric fields are randomly arranged with respect to each other. Some materials have their molecular structure so arranged that as light passes through them, only those electric fields with their orientation in the same direction are transmitted. These fields may emerge all in the same plane, e.g., horizontal or vertical, and are said to be *plane polarized* when they emerge. Similarly, they may be *circularly polarized* due to transmission of only helical or circular fields. Mirrors, glass, even water and the atmosphere have polarizing properties that can be eliminated by polarizing filters, such as Polaroid, which allow only the light opposite to the plane polarized reflected glare to penetrate. Crystals such as calcite are very effective polarizers, as are pigments such as xanthophyll (a macular pigment), which polarizes light to present to central photoreceptors. This is the basis of the propeller in the Haidinger brush entoptic test determined clinically by rotating a polarizing filter in a uniform blue field to determine macular position and function.

If one places a horizontal polarizing filter over one eye and a vertical polarizing filter over the other eye, one can selectively project polarized objects to one eye or the other with both eyes open. If a horizontal or axial disparity is induced between these objects, one can also measure the angle of stereoacuity. As shall be seen later, this is very useful not only for stereo testing but also for binocular balancing, fixation preference, penalization, and malingering.

In stereoacuity the thresholds measured vary with the test procedure. The Titmus "stereo-fly" subtends 1000″ at 13 inches while the circles range from 800 to 40″ ("Nine out of nine" or "9/9"). AO stereoslides range from 240 to 30″ at 20 feet. Other tests are as specified by the manufacturer's instruction manual supplied with the test. It should also be pointed out that any process which would decrease monocular acuity will have an even greater effect on stereoacuity (since the latter is an inverse exponential function of the testing distance and not linear, as in Snellen acuity).

Under some circumstances the visual acuity is reduced, but a surgical procedure such as cataract extraction or corneal transplant is proffered to improve it. The potential postoperative acuity in these cases can be predicted to some extent by clinical tests such as the amount of media opacity, predisease visual acuity, pupillary responses, color vision, perception of the line with the Maddox rod, electroretinography, ultrasonography, and the Haidinger brush phenomenon. In recent years the blue field entoptoscope, laser interference fringes, and the Potential Acuity Meter (Mentor) have been used with varying success.

The blue field entoptoscope is a commercially available resurrection of Sheerer's "flying corpuscles." In a brightly lit blue field, white spots are seen to stand out on the blue background. In the perifoveal area (remember the capillary-free zone) the red blood cell column is queued in single file interrupted only by the presence of white blood cells. The red cells absorb the blue so that the photoreceptor elements are relatively dark adapted beneath in the blood column in this region. As the white blood cells move along, they present as white flying corpuscles in a uniformly blue field. This is presumed evidence of an intact capillary network, which is usually indicative of healthy macular function. Similar tests involve illuminating the sclera with a bright light and perceiving a grainy pattern corresponding to an intact foveal avascular zone. Not all patients appreciate these phenomena, but a positive response in a reliable patient yields useful information about their potential acuity.

INTERFERENCE AND COHERENCE

To understand laser interferometry a digression into physical optics and the nature of the coherence and interference of light is necessary. If two waves of light interact when the maxima of one is equal temporally to the minima of the other, the electromagnetic fields will cancel, if they are of equal amplitude. This is depicted in Fig. 9-4, *a*, with waves (*1*) and (*2*).

If the waves are as described, they are separated by half their wavelength. If

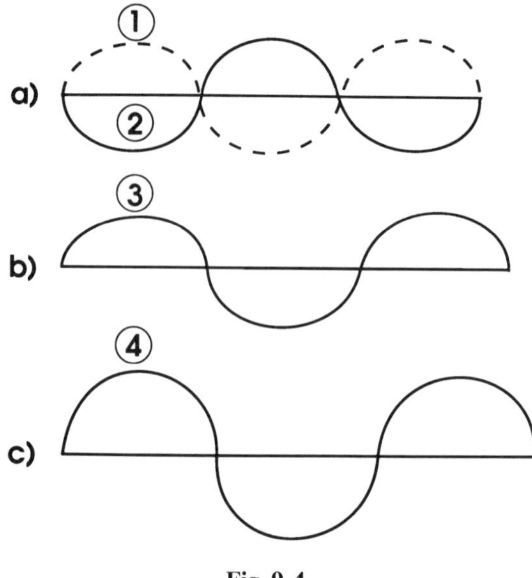

Fig. 9-4

they are in phase or one full wavelength apart, the maxima of one corresponds with the maxima of the other, and a condition of *constructive interference* occurs (*4*). The former entity is then known as *destructive interference.* If a single light source of monochromatic light (same λ) is influenced by a double slit, a parallel plate of glass, a biprism, or some other doubling source, two wavefronts will be formed that will interact with each other. Where constructive interference occurs, a bright band is seen, and where destructive interference occurs, a dark band occurs. This gives rise to *interference fringes. Coherence* is simply a measure of how well two light beams will interfere. The laser, as shall be seen later, is highly coherent. These interference fringes can be projected through cataracts and corneal opacities relatively unaffected by the dioptrics of the eye. The ability to discriminate various fringe widths and contrasts can be roughly correlated with visual acuity. In this way a ballpark figure of potential acuity can be obtained.

The *Potential Acuity Meter (PAM)* is a newer device that projects a visual acuity chart through an aerial aperture of 0.1 mm and focuses the chart with an optometer to neutralize the refractive error. This is mounted to a standard slit lamp and can be focused through minute windows in a corneal or lens opacity. A Snellen fraction visual acuity can be determined.

BEST CORRECTED VISUAL ACUITY

Thus far a point has been reached where one is now capable (and culpable) of determining the "best corrected" visual acuity with our refraction process. This concept intimates the natural converse, i.e., uncorrected visual acuity. The concept of uncorrected acuity is important for ministries of transportation, aviation, law enforcement, fire fighting, and other occupations with the propensity for dislodgement of correction. Under some circumstances certain occupations demand a level of vision that is necessary to preserve public safety and the safety of the individual. This is often the reason this entry is required on many of the forms we must fill out.

On the other hand, best corrected visual acuity is central to our professional existence and if reduced it demands a careful search as to the etiology. In one's vigilance to determine this, don't forget that in children visual maturity is not reached until somewhere between 6 and 10 years of age. A 3-year-old child with only 20/30 visual acuity is normal for this stage of visual development. Newer objective preferential looking and electrical cortical response data are now refining our knowledge of this maturation process.

Please see Part II: Problems and Part III: Solutions for typical examination questions pertaining to the material in this chapter.

CHAPTER 10: ACCOMMODATION AND CONVERGENCE

PROCESS OF ACCOMMODATION

Despite knowledge of the deficiencies of near vision testing, one is continually presented with problems that are primarily manifest at near. To approach these problems, the process of *accommodation* must be examined.

Accommodation is a response. The stimuli that elicit this response are blurred retinal imagery, possibly contributed to by the reversal of the color blur circles secondary to chromatic aberration, bitemporal retinal disparity as an object of regard approaches, and the sensation of near. This has led to its label as a psychooptic phenomenon. Just as bitemporal retinal disparity may affect the orientation and effectivity of the photoreceptors, it is also a potent stimulus for convergence. Accommodation, convergence, and miosis form the synkinetic triad of the *near response.* Each one of the components can occur without the other under dissociating circumstances, such as the addition of prisms or plus lenses. The act of accommodation and miosis cause movement of intraocular structures, i.e., the iris, ciliary body, lens, and possibly even the retina. No other aspect of seeing does this.

Consider now the structural changes that occur in accommodation. As the ciliary muscle contracts and shifts anteriorly, the tension on the zonules of the lens is relaxed. The lessened stress on the equatorial capsule causes an increase in the anteroposterior diameter of the lens and a decrease in the transequatorial diameter. With this increase in the lens diameter, the radii of curvature of the anterior and posterior refracting surfaces are reduced, the former more than the latter. This increases the convexity of both surfaces and results in more plus power being added to the lens. In addition, relaxation of the zonules and decreased transequatorial diameter allows an anterior shift in the lens position, which increases its effectivity. (In a susceptible individual this may provoke an angle closure glaucoma attack and is part of the prone-reading–dark room provocative tests that were more popular in the past.) The accompanying miosis decreases spherical aberration and other peripheral lens aberrations and increases depth of field but adversely affects retinal illumination.

The ability to accommodate decreases from the day we are born. Fortunately, in early life one has much more ability than required. From Table 10-1 and other data on accommodative amplitudes, the rate of accommodative loss can be estimated. The etiology of this is multifactorial. With aging the ciliary muscle is seen to sclerose histopathologically. Histochemically and biochemically the lens proteins are altered and become less deformable with a given change of ciliary muscle tonus. With the ongoing addition of lens fibers, the anteroposterior and transequatorial girth of the lens increases so that zonular tension is decreased, leading to a shift toward myopia. The index of refraction of the nucleus of the lens further shifts the lens in the myopic direction. It is as if these are physiologic compensa-

Table 10-1

Age (Years)	Accommodative Amplitude Change Every 4 Years (Diopters)
8 to 40	−1.00 D
40	6.00 D (±2.00 D reference age)
40 to 48	−1.50 D
48 to 68	−0.50 D

tory mechanisms for the declining accommodative ability. Unfortunately, these compensations occur too late in life to aid the 40-year-old experiencing problems with diminishing powers of accommodation—presbyopia.

MEASUREMENT OF ACCOMMODATION

The measurement of accommodation primarily involves the *amplitude and range of accommodation* (or interval of clear vision). The amplitude of accommodation is commonly measured monocularly but can be performed binocularly. Keep in mind that the latter is more physiologic, is more affected by convergence, and is usually greater in value. It is a measure of the total accommodative power of the lens expressed in diopters. With the distance correction in place, the far point of the eye being tested is at infinity. An accommodative target such as small print, two fine lines or two small dots are brought as close to the eye as possible until the target blurs. This determines the near point, which in emmetropia can be automatically converted to diopters of accommodative amplitude. If the eye is overcorrected or uncorrected, the refractive error will affect both the near point and far point but the difference will remain dioptrically equivalent to the amplitude. This can also be performed with the Prince rule, which measures on a ruler the near point and the far point with +3.00 D lenses. The lenses bring both points closer together, but again the dioptric difference between them remains equal to the amplitude. Alternatively, accommodation can be stimulated with minus lenses until surpassed and then relaxed with plus lenses until blurred. The difference between the two break or blur points is the amplitude of accommodation.

The range of accommodation is the distance between the near point and the far point, and therefore in any given problem the near point, far point, or the amplitude can easily be determined. The implication of the amplitude of accommodation is comfort. For any task it is a good general rule that, if half the amplitude is left in reserve, the patient should remain asymptomatic. If less than half remains in reserve fatigue, asthenopia and recession of the near point will occur. Consider the following examples.

1. A 44-year-old patient is +3.00 D hyperopic. His accommodative amplitude measures 5.00 D. His current glasses are +1.50 D. What would one prescribe to make him comfortable for work at 40 cm?

Accommodative amplitude = +5.00 D

For comfort store +2.50 D

+2.50 D of amplitude remaining (but +3.00 D hyperopia)

Additional distance requirement +0.50 D

For near at 40 cm require +2.50 D/+3.00 D needed for comfort

R_x: single vision glasses +3.00 D

2. A −4.00 D myopic patient has an accommodative amplitude of +6.00 D. What is the interval of clear vision without correction?

$$\text{Far point} = \frac{100}{4} = 25 \text{ cm}$$

$$\text{Near point} = \text{Myopia} + \text{Amplitude} = +6 + 4 = +10.00 \text{ D}$$
$$= \frac{100}{10} = 10 \text{ cm}$$

Interval of clear vision is between 10 and 25 cm.

CONTROL OF ACCOMMODATION

As seen in the refraction sequence, a battle with accommodation control is always being fought by various fogging techniques. Accommodation can be pharmacologically inhibited by a process called *cycloplegia,* and the agents that perform this task are called cycloplegics. Pupillary dilatation is called *mydriasis*, and preparations responsible for this are called mydriatics.

Cycloplegia is an important aspect of refraction and is of diagnostic importance in the differentiation and diagnosis of latent hyperopia, refractive esotropia, pseudomyopia, and refractive errors in the young and infirm. Since accommodation is irrevocably lost for the remainder of the patient's visit, tests that require intact accommodation should be performed before their instillation, i.e., near vision testing, amplitude and range of accommodation, accommodative-convergence relationships, pupillary responses, and gonioscopic determinations. Cycloplegia is compatible with both objective and subjective refinement techniques but is not without its hazards.

As with any pharmacologic preparation, cycloplegics are associated with side effects in susceptible individuals. The basis of their action is their parasympatholytic action involving blockade of the postganglionic response associated with acetylcholine. The nasolacrimal drainage of topically applied agents introduces them to the highly vascular and absorptive surfaces of the nasal mucosa. This absorption results in systemic side effects of the anticholinergic variety similar to those of systemic atropine. Like all medications, the distribution and dosage depend on body weight or surface area, hence the increased susceptibility of children to their effects. Absorption may be partially curbed by occlusion of the common canaliculus with digital pressure. Compression of the lacrimal pump mechanism may result in more negative sac pressure, which on release yields a rebound influx with

Table 10-2

	Maximum Cycloplegia	Duration of Action	Residual Accommodation
Cyclopentolate 1%	15 to 45 minutes	6 to 8 hours	occasionally 1 to 2.00 D
Atropine 1%	2 hours to 2 weeks	2 weeks	<1.00 D
Tropicamide 1%	20 to 25 minutes	2 to 6 hours	1 to 2.00 D

subsequent increased absorption. This is not an easy task to perform in a child after the instillation of an eye drop!

The major cycloplegics used in North America are atropine 1% or ½%, cyclopentolate 1% or 2%, homatropine 2% or 5%, and tropicamide 1%. These differ in their onset and duration of action, peak effect, and induced mydriasis. Their side effects, however, are all about the same: nausea, dry mouth, flushing, fever, tachycardia, psychic stimulation or depression, hallucinations, and possibly circulatory collapse in a serious overdose (such as a child's accidental ingestion of an entire bottle). Topical side effects include immediate or delayed hypersensitivity and punctuate keratitis from their preservatives. The mydriatic effects are all amplified by concomitant administration of topical sympathomimetics, such as phenylephrine or neosynephrine 2.5% and 10%. The pretreatment use of topical anaesthetics such as proparacaine enhances the absorption of all preparations because of its corneal epithelial toxicity so that often only a single drop of any preparation is required. Clinically, atropine 1%, cyclopentolate 1%, and tropicamide 1% are used most commonly. Table 10-2 compares their properties.

Notice that the time for maximum cycloplegia in the shorter acting agents is crucial if the residual accommodation is to be effectively reduced.

Some practitioners find that in older or presbyopic individuals, 2.5% neosynephrine administered before seeing the patient exerts insignificant effects on cycloplegia. This theoretically provides adequate mydriasis for fundoscopy yet preserves sufficient cycloplegia for near vision testing. The major objection to this practice is the alteration of the depth of focus provided by the larger pupil size.

ACCOMMODATIVE-CONVERGENCE/ACCOMMODATION RATIO

The synkinetic near response and the close relationship that exists between accommodation and convergence have already been noted. Logically this must be so, since orientation of the visual axes must be altered in changing fixation from a distant to a near target. This relationship can be measured and compared from time to time in the same individual, from individual to individual, and from one distance state to another. In clinical practice this measurement is the *accommodative-convergence/accommodation ratio* (AC/A ratio) and is a routine segment of the orthoptic work-up.

Although usually found within the domain of strabismologists, several optical principles are involved in the various measurement techniques. The two standard methods of evaluation of the AC/A ratio are the heterophoria and lens gradient methods. Marshall Parks (*Ocular motility and strabismus,* Harper & Row, Hagerstown, MD, 1975) has popularized a distance-near phoria testing that is proposed as the "clinical method" of AC/A determination.

For example:

$$\text{Distance} = 10 \text{ P.D. esophoria}$$

$$\text{Near } 1/3 \text{ m} = 25 \text{ P.D. esophoria/tropia}$$

$$\text{Accommodative convergence} = 25 \text{ P.D.} - 10 \text{ P.D.} = 15 \text{ P.D.}$$

$$\text{Accommodation} = 100/3 = 3.00 \text{ D} \qquad \text{AC/A} = 15/3 = 5/1$$

As shall be discussed later, this clinical method will reveal an increased AC/A ratio. Naturally, if the distance phoria is equal to the near phoria, the AC/A will be zero. This is thus equivalent to a normal ratio.

The lens gradient method simply alters the accommodation requirements with plus or minus lenses and measures the phoria difference. For example:

At 6 m distance = 10 P.D. esophoria	At 0.33 m = 25 P.D. esotropia
−1.00 D sphere = 15 P.D. esophoria	+3.00 D = 10 P.D. esophoria
Accommodative convergence = 5 P.D.	AC = 25 − 10 = 15
Accommodation = 1.00 D	A = 3
AC/A = 5/1	AC/A = 15/3 = 5/1

The method that has most people confused is the formula involving the pupillary distance (PD) that deals with *meter angles,* i.e., the heterophoria method. This concept evolved from Nagel, who initiated it in the nineteenth century. As the eyes converge to fixate a near target, the two visual axes subtend an angle at the target. The unit chosen to represent this angle was the reciprocal of the distance, i.e., the same as the diopter; numerically it is equal to the accommodation required at the same distance. A near target at 0.33 m transcribes 3 meter angles between the visual axes and also requires +3.00 D of accommodation. The problem is that not everybody has the same PD, so the unit is not an accurate measurement of the angle to be measured. Fig. 10-1 depicts this problem. Angles α and β are both at 0.33 m and therefore are 3 meter angles, but clearly angle $\alpha \neq \beta$. Fortunately a relationship exists whereby:

$$\text{Prism diopters of total convergence required} = \text{Meter angle} \times \text{PD}$$

For object O in Fig. 10-1: P.D. = $3 \times 5 = 15$ P.D. for α; P.D. = $3 \times 6 = 18$ P.D. for β. This therefore includes tonic (and fusional) as well as accommodative convergence. Look again at the first example if the PD was 60 mm. Distance (tonic) deviation = 10 P.D. esophoria; near (tonic + accommodative) = 25 P.D. esotropia; near = 0.33 m forms 3 meter angles and requires +3.00 D accommodation.

To keep the eyes straight, a total convergence of 3 meter angles × 6.0 cm =

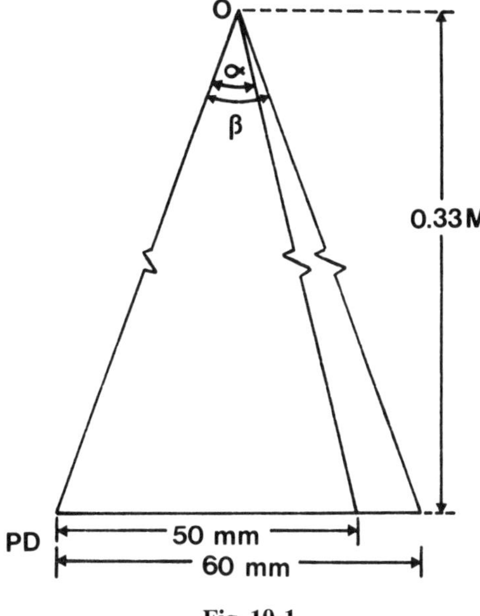

Fig. 10-1

18 P.D. would normally be required. To find the accommodative component to the deviation at near, the tonic or distance deviation must be subtracted: accommodative convergence = 25 P.D. − 10 P.D. = 15 P.D. In other words, the eyes required 18 P.D. convergence to stay straight at 0.33 m but continued to converge an extra 15 P.D., i.e., they overshot their mark. The total accommodative convergence is thus the total of the normal plus the overshoot, or in this instance 18 P.D. + 15 P.D. = 33 P.D. The AC/A ratio for +3.00 accommodation is thus 33/3 or 11/1.

This method gives higher values than the lens gradient method (3 to 5:1) because the latter does not undergo the added influence of proximal vergence unless tested at near with the 3.00 D method. If the patient is more exodeviated at near, the exodeviation represents an undershoot and must therefore be subtracted and not added to the normal convergence. If the tonic deviation was zero (orthophoria for distance), the accommodative convergence would be 18 P.D. and the AC/A = 18/3 or 6:1.

A general formula can thus be derived:

$$\frac{AC}{A} = \frac{(PD \times \text{meter angles}) + (P.D._N - P.D._D)}{D(\text{ACCOMMODATION})} = \frac{PD \times MA}{D} + \frac{P.D._N - P.D._D}{D}$$

Since meter angles = D accommodation numerically:

$$\frac{AC}{A} = PD + \frac{P.D._N - P.D._D}{D}$$

where: PD = pupillary distance (cm)
$P.D._N$ = near deviation
$P.D._D$ = distance deviation
D = accommodation in diopters
Esodeviation +
Exodeviation −

The first or clinical method has simply ignored the value of the PD and considered only the second, more significant, portion. As can be seen, this is not the numerical equivalent of the true AC/A ratio but will clinically show exactly the same abnormalities that the expanded form will demonstrate.

The AC/A is very plastic and is altered under certain conditions so that eye deviations do not occur. The uncorrected myopic eye requires no accommodation for near but still must converge, and conversely the hyperopic eye may accommodate for distance but does not need to converge. If the AC/A is unable to change, a deviation occurs.

Please see Part II: Problems and Part III: Solutions for typical examination questions pertaining to the material in this chapter.

CHAPTER 11: PRESCRIBING

Before undertaking the spectacle correction of the ametropias and the factors that influence the final prescription, it is an opportune time to consider the *acquired ametropias*. In practice, these entities should be reviewed and a mental checklist satisfied before the patient leaves the office.

Acquired hyperopia may result from a retroorbital tumor indenting the globe from behind. This results in an effective reduction of the axial length and a secondary hyperopia, which is progressive from one visit to the next with tumor growth. Central serious chorioretinopathy with neurosensory detachment of the retina elevates the photoreceptors and again decreases the effective axial length. In posterior lens dislocation the vertex distance of the lens has changed and so has its lens effectivity. Contact lenses can temporarily flatten the cornea and result in a hyperopic shift. This is the basis of orthokeratology.

Myopia can be acquired in a multitude of disease entities. Systemic diseases such as diabetes, galactosemia, and uremia have an osmotic effect on the lens, resulting in the imbibition of more fluid. This increases its plus power and hence creates an induced myopia. The reduced index from the imbibed fluid may conversely cause a hyperopic shift. Sulphonamides and their derivatives, such as acetazolamide (Diamox), have also been noted to be associated with myopia. Nuclear sclerotic cataracts increase the index of refraction of the lens and make it more myopic. Miotics such as pilocarpine and the anticholinesterases such as phospholine iodide induce a spasm of accommodation when first instilled, which causes an induced myopia. Anterior lens dislocation alters the effective power of the lens toward the myopic side. Axial length changes in retinal detachment surgery and keratoconus make the eye longer and more myopic. Keratoconus and anterior lenticonus alter the radii of curvature of the refracting surfaces, increasing their plus power. Steep contact lenses can also mold the anterior corneal surface to induce more myopia by a similar mechanism. Retinopathy of prematurity, the vitreoretinal degenerations, and prematurity itself are associated with myopia, as is their treatment with cryotherapy.

Astigmatism can be acquired from lid hemangiomas, ptosis, even chalazia and other lid tumors. Pterygia, limbal dermoids, marginal corneal degenerations, keratoconus, cataract surgery, keratoplasty, and radial keratotomy, can cause astigmatism.

"Premature" presbyopia or accommodative insufficiency can result from a severe debilitating illness, diphtheria, botulism, and even mercury poisoning. Head injuries, third nerve palsies, Adie's syndrome can all be associated with loss of accommodation. Another major cause are tranquilizers, presumably on the basis of their anticholinergic side effects.

This is by no means a complete list, but it does reinforce the multiplicity of the acquired ametropias and our responsibility in their identification and treatment.

The actual *prescribing for ametropia* is not difficult now that objective and subjective techniques are familiar, accommodation is understood, and the principles of far point, magnification, and vertex distance are mastered. What follows is a short discourse on each ametropia and the factors that influence the final decision as to the spectacle correction.

HYPEROPIA

Hyperopia, whether axial or refractive, has its correction placed such that the secondary focal point of the lens is coincident with the far point plane. The fact that hyperopia can, in many cases, be compensated for by accommodation clearly links symptoms to the ever fine balance between the amount of hyperopia and the accommodative amplitude. This is the basis of the classification of hyperopia into manifest and latent. The manifest hyperopia is that amount of hyperopia which can be accepted by the patient without cycloplegia to maintain or obtain 20/20 (6/6) visual acuity. The absolute portion of this is the part that cannot be compensated for by the available accommodative amplitude. The facultative, on the other hand, is the remainder that is compensated for by accommodation. Under cycloplegia the latent component is made manifest. The total hyperopia is the sum of the manifest and the latent.

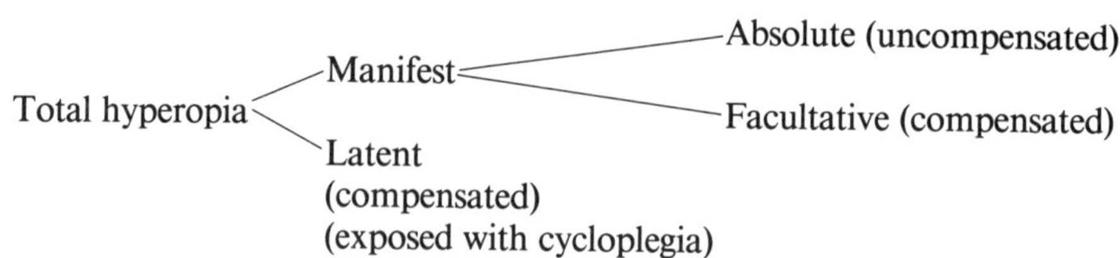

Consider the following example. A patient during refraction reveals the following: vision without correction 20/40; with +2.00 D he obtains 20/20. He accepts up to +4.00 D and still maintains 20/20. Under cycloplegia with cyclopentolate 1% his refractive error is +7.00 D with 20/20 vision.

Summary: 0 to 20/40
+2.00 – 20/20—Absolute (+2.00 D)
+4.00 – 20/20—Facultative (+2.00 D)
+7.00 – 20/20—Latent (+3.00 D)
Manifest = Absolute + Facultative = +4.00 D
Total = Latent + Manifest = +7.00 D

(It is from this classification that the term manifest refraction became synonymous with a noncycloplegic subjectively refined refraction.)

In deciding the amount of correction to be given, consideration must be given to the severity of symptoms, visual needs, occupation, ocular motility status, and of course age and amplitude of accommodation. As general guidelines the following are sufficient:

1. If the patient is young, asymptomatic, and orthophoric with a good amplitude, no correction is necessary.
2. If the patient is young with a large esophoria or intermittent esotropia, the amount of correction is that which controls the deviation while maintaining best visual acuity. In frank esotropia, this may be the full correction of the total hyperopia.
3. If the patient is young with an exophoria or exotropia, the least amount (i.e., only the absolute hyperopia) is corrected. There is some evidence that if there is a large exotropia a trial of full correction is in order (Kushner).
4. If the patient is presbyopic or has accommodative insufficiency (low amplitudes) for any reason and is orthophoric or esophoric, the amount

of correction is such that half of the amplitude is held in reserve to maintain comfort.

5. If the above patient is exophoric, a comfortable balance between accommodative reserve and motility control is attempted.
6. If the patient is prepresbyopic, the total hyperopia is corrected before bifocals are prescribed.
7. If the patient is prepresbyopic and contemplating contact lenses, the entry into bifocals may be delayed with the contacts.
8. If the patient is young with anisometropia, the difference between the two eyes is prescribed to balance the accommodative demand. Once the patient is older, follow the other guidelines.
9. If the patient is young and symptomatic with little hyperopia and adequate amplitudes, correction is probably equivalent to a placebo.
10. Hyperopic patients are used to very clear distance vision and are intolerant of any overcorrection. If refraction is undertaken at 4 m, +0.25 D accommodation is required and compensation for this is necessary to bring the far point to infinity. Even if the refraction is performed at 6 m, undercorrecting the hyperopia slightly is more desirable than overcorrecting.
11. Don't forget the acquired hyperopias.
12. Fresnel Press-on lenses are sometimes useful when you are not sure about the acceptability of a change in lens or bifocals.
13. Remember the prismatic effects of plus lenses on heterophorias and on the measurement of eye deviations.

MYOPIA

Myopia is a progressive disease (in most cases) that is easily corrected optically by employing the same principle of imaging the secondary focal point of the correcting lens to the far point. The reduced accommodative demand leads to a frequent association with exodeviations, in which case full correction or even overcorrection may be indicated. These are probably the only aspects of myopic treatment that are not controversial.

Some modalities of treatment can be easily dismissed as probably of no value. These include exercises such as blur recognition, vitamin and megavitamin therapy, dietary regimentation, and hormonal therapy. Other modalities involve the control of ciliary muscle tonus and accommodation under the philosophy that this is either the etiology or a contributing factor to the progression of the myopia. Many adherents undercorrect the myopia; stronger adherents prescribe bifocals and cycloplegia. Oakley and Young (Bifocal control of myopia, *Am J Optometry* 52:758–764, 1975) found that over 2.7 to 4.0 years bifocal wearers had virtually no documented progression of their myopia, whereas controls had approximately 0.50 D more myopia. This is certainly a harmless approach and at least has some basis with a controlled study.

Night myopia is an anomalous myopia similar to instrument and empty field (space) myopia. It has been recognized for over 200 years but has only been speculative until the advent of laser speckle optometer style refractors capable of measuring it. Laser speckle phenomena (Rigdon and Gordon) result from laser light reflecting from a granular surface. Speckles are formed from interfering wavefronts at the photoreceptor. They are always in focus and thus do not stimulate accommodation. Their movement is one way in myopia (with) and opposite (against) in hyperopia. Wide ranges from 0.40 D of hyperopia to −4.00 D of myopia with a mean of 1.71 D (S.D. 0.72 D) (Leibowitz and Owens) have been reported. In the absence of a laser speckle optometer, dark retinoscopy has been recommended in absolute darkness at 25 to 100 cm. All of these methods and theories now seem to converge on the concept of a *dark focus,* which is the true resting state between distance and near. Under scotopic conditions, one tends to overaccommodate for distance and underaccommodate for near. Previous theories of spherical aberration, pupil size, accommodation, absent Stiles-Crawford effects, and chromatic aberration shifts have now been supplanted by the dark focus. The correction is difficult. With the laser speckle optometer the dark focus can be measured and correction of half to full dioptric value given. With dark retinoscopy the dark focus $= \dfrac{\text{dark retinoscopy} - 0.25\text{ D}}{0.64}$ and similar amounts are prescribed. There is still the factor of intrapatient variability, so a few determinations before prescription may be prudent. Minus lenses in the form of clip-ons or separate driving glasses at night are prescribed if this is a clinically significant entity.

Orthokeratology is a technique of flattening the radius of curvature of the anterior surface of the cornea by a flat contact lens (or series of flat lenses). It is expensive, potentially dangerous, and requires a long-term retainer lens to maintain the newly acquired curvature. The goal is often to achieve an uncorrected acuity standard for entry to a profession or vocation.

The remaining approaches are surgical. It must be remembered that any operation performed is done so for a nonthreatening disease entity. The majority are 20/20 eyes, and all operations have a potential of extending intraocularly with all the attendant implications and complications. The earliest procedure performed was a lensectomy under which circumstances it was soon discovered that the cure was worse than the disease. The Japanese (Sato) were the first to approach radial keratotomy but did so from the endothelial side with radial partial thickness incisions designed to flatten the cornea. The modified radial keratotomy, as popularized by Fyodorov, involves a variable number of 90% thickness radial incisions from the epithelial side of the cornea. The prospective evaluation of radial keratotomy (PERK) studies have shown that radial keratotomy is a satisfying, predictable, and relatively safe procedure for a certain subset of myopic patients. It is now the standard against which other refractive surgical procedures are measured.

Excimer laser photokeratectomy (193 nm) flattens the central cornea by sculpting with ultraviolet light. As in radial keratotomy, the central flattening reduces the refractive power of the cornea and hence reduces the myopia. Solid state technology with harmonic progression into the same wavelength range will undoubtedly replace excimer technology in time.

Keratomileusis, as performed by Barraquer, involves the removal and controlled lathing of a lamellar "autolenticule," which is flattened and returned to its original bed. This flattens the cornea but is not without risk and also must be classified as a purely experimental procedure.

With experience, all of these procedures will have their algorithms refined, predictability enhanced, and safety improved. Patience, not patients, seems to be more of a problem in slowing down the introduction of new technology.

Don't forget the acquired ametropias. It is also useful to consider the minification, prismatic effects on the heterophorias, and the measurement of eye deviations before the final script is given. The practitioner should also be cognizant of the association of myopia with other eye disorders, such as peripheral retinal degenerations, vitreoretinopathies, retinopathy of prematurity, cryopexy with retinopathy of prematurity, prematurity itself, and choroidal neovascularization through myopic lacquer cracks with its attendant and potentially treatable threat to central vision. These facts dictate meticulous direct and indirect ophthalmoscopy to include the retinal periphery in every case of myopia. The association with chronic simple and pigmentary glaucoma requires diligent examination to facilitate early detection and initiation of treatment before irreversible visual loss ensues.

ASTIGMATISM

Astigmatism has been the focus of much discussion to this point. Consideration has been given to its imagery, classification, method of optical correction, problems with distortion and meridional magnification, objective and subjective techniques of refinement, and its acquired causes. In light of these findings, what is its final correction? The following guidelines may prove helpful. (These guidelines have been modified from Guyton DL: Prescribing cylinders: the problem of distortion, *Surv Ophthalmol* 22 (3):177-188, 1977.)

1. In children requiring correction, the *full* astigmatic correction is given. If the child is amblyopic from unilateral astigmatism, a trial of lenses is indicated before occlusion therapy. It is becoming apparent with more young children being examined that many infants and especially premature infants have against the rule astigmatism. This has been postulated to enhance myopia, and many are now advocating its correction even in the very young. Cortical readaption is accomplished so readily in children that distortion is not a significant problem.
2. In adults who are asymptomatic, be wary of changing the axis of their correcting cylinder even if apparently incorrect. They have achieved adaption to distortion and blur and will often be unhappy with a change.
3. If an adult was previously fully corrected and the amount of astigmatism has changed, he will probably tolerate full correction, especially if at 90° or 180°.
4. If an adult was previously undercorrected, i.e., not corrected for the full amount of astigmatism, distortion may present a real problem. The only way to predict this is with the full correction in place in the trial frame under binocular conditions. (Remember that monocularly distortion arises only from meridional magnification, but binocularly the distortion increases markedly in an exponential and not a linear fashion.) If the full correction is well tolerated, it may be prescribed. If it is not well tolerated, occlude one eye to establish distortion as the etiology of the problem. If distortion is the problem, it can be reduced by several manoeuvres:
   a. Reduce the power of the cylinder. This automatically reinstates astigmatic imagery and creates an interval of Sturm. The best vision usually occurs when the circle of least confusion is on the retina, so the spherical equivalent must be maintained with rechecking and refining the sphere. Since the spherical equivalent remains the same, one has in fact removed a cross cylinder and not just reduced the correcting cylinder. Under bin-

ocular balancing conditions the correct balance between blurred vision from astigmatic imagery and distortion from the correcting lens can be achieved.

b. Rotate the cylinder axis toward 180° or 90° or the old axis. (Remember that the distortion is a function of the correcting lens and not the eye error.) Vertical and horizontal distortion is more tolerable, but a new axis is formed between the obliquely crossed cylinders (corrective and eye error cylinders). The power at the new axis can be optimized using cross cylinder testing even though it is the "incorrect" axis.

c. Minus cylinder spectacles, minimal vertex distance, and contact lenses all reduce distortion.

5. Forewarning a patient about distortion and adaption problems reassures the patient when this occurs and reinforces his confidence in the practitioner prescribing the lenses. The anticipation allays anxiety and affords adequate time for cortical readaption to occur.

If the patient is intolerant of the cylinder correction, contact lenses will reduce the distortion associated with the correction of the astigmatism. If the astigmatism is all corneal, one can use hard bitoric, gas permeable, or soft toric contacts. If the astigmatism is both lenticular and corneal, soft torics are preferred. If the patient is incapable or intolerant of contacts but equally intolerant of the distortion, consideration of refractive surgery should be given. Various T, L, and curvilinear keratotomy procedures can be used to reduce or eliminate the corneal astigmatism. Elliptical excimer photokeratectomy may reduce myopic astigmatism.

Some patients have never had their astigmatism corrected as children and have bilateral amblyopia as a result. They are often disappointed when attempts to pass driver's tests are repeatedly met with failure. This subset of patients should be identified *before* all of the above measures are performed. Unfortunately, this diagnosis is often made retrospectively to the chagrin of physician and patient alike.

Another group of patients beginning to reap the benefits of refractive surgery and the surgical manipulation of corneal astigmatism are cataract patients. Procedures combining refractive keratotomy with implant surgery and also principles of altering the site and closure of the wound are becoming more popular. The question that has not been answered is whether the patient is happier with their "old" astigmatism or no astigmatism at all.

PRESBYOPIA

Presbyopia is another problem that reinforces many of the principles that have already been discussed. Especially pertinent are the concepts of image jump and displacement, induced prismatic effects in bifocal lenses, and the waning of the accommodative amplitude with age. As David Michaels, M.D., says: "The onset of presbyopia marks the old age of youth, the interlude between time marching on and time running out." (Visual optics and refraction, ed, 2, St. Louis, 1980, Mosby.)

When prescribing, consideration should be given to the following factors:

1. Single vision reading glasses may be preferred when bifocals have failed, cervical disc disease precludes changing head positions, anisometropia induces large prismatic effects and when tightrope walking is required.

2. Bifocals are preferred at all other times, especially if any distance correction is worn.
3. Undercorrection is much better than overcorrection. With higher adds (> +2.00 D) the interval of clear vision is condensed to clear zones, one far and one near. The intermediate zone is lost and may be of occupational importance. Under these circumstances trifocals with half the near add expands this interval. Progressive add bifocals with a continuum of increasing plus power from distance to near also perform this function. These are much easier to adapt to if started as a first bifocal and not introduced when high add requirements are well established. Newer progressive lens designs have significantly reduced the number of failures with them.
4. Flat top or executive style bifocals minimize image jump and displacement for myopic patients.
5. Round top minimizes displacement (executive) and flat top or executive minimizes jump (waiter) for hyperopic patients. (See section on prisms.)
6. The induced prismatic effect in anisometropia can best be handled with slab off prism or single vision readers. Mixing segments (round top one eye, flat top the other), although theoretically correct, looks like someone made a mistake.
7. Bifocals in children with accommodative estropia should be of the executive style and set high so that the segment bisects the pupil. If this is not done, the segment will not be used. In trifocals the intermediate segment should be at the lower border of the pupil.
8. Keep old bifocals to use for shopping, playing music, or whenever a stronger add is not functional.
9. Occupational bifocal varieties can be tried first with Fresnel Press-On lenses to assess their acceptability before a definitive pair is ground.
10. Aphakic patients with normal visual acuity seldom require adds greater than +2.50 D.
11. When you are measuring bifocals in high plus or minus lenses, the glasses must be reversed from their normal position in the lens meter, a new front vertex distance measurement done, and the power in the segment read.
12. It takes 1 to 6 weeks to adjust to bifocals, and fewer than 5% of patients will be unable to tolerate them. Like new shoes, they take a while to break in.
13. Bifocal contacts are difficult to fit and often have variable vision, but designs are improving. Overplusing one lens (usually the nondominant eye) may be tolerated by some individuals willing to sacrifice their binocularity for cosmetic reasons. This is called a monofit.
14. An add of less than +1.00 D is difficult to find and is of questionable value. Just because it's their first time, don't be too gentle! Myopic patients tolerate more correction in the segment than do hyperopic patients. This reduces with time.
15. When nuclear sclerosis produces myopia, the reading distance becomes closer and the patient adjusts to the proximity and magnification it affords. If the myopia is corrected for distance, a boost of the add to this nearer position is better tolerated.
16. The power of the bifocal add can be given empirically by age if no special occupational or visual consideration is necessary. Table 11-1 is better as a

guideline to start your near examination than to definitively prescribe from.

Table 11-1

Age	Power
45 years	+1.00 − +1.25 D
50 years	+1.50 − +1.75 D
55 years	+2.00 − +2.25 D
60 years	+2.50 − +2.75 D

The amplitude of accommodation can also be used (as illustrated previously) to maintain half the amplitude in reserve. The "method of limits" places a reading card with the fine print at the desired reading distance. Midway between the blur induced by excessive plus and minus spheres is the power of the add that leaves approximately half the amplitude in reserve.

17. Remember the acquired causes of accommodative insufficiency.

18. If the power of the add is different from eye to eye, recheck the distance correction and rethink number 17, above. Asymmetric adds can be an alternative to trifocals for some patients.

CONVERGENCE INSUFFICIENCY

One cannot separate the problems of accommodative insufficiency and presbyopia from *convergence insufficiency* problems, which share many of the same asthenopic symptoms at near.

Convergence is a disconjuge (nonparallel) monocular or binocular eye movement to maintain the object of regard on corresponding retinal points. According to newer servomechanism models (e.g., Schor, Kotulak) both accommodation and accommodative convergence have fast (50° to 70°/second) and slow components sensitive to retinal disparity, looming (size), and blur. Fast components have peripheral drives and slow components have foveal drives. The initiation of accommodation and accommodative convergence is in areas 18 and 19 of the occipital cortex, where synchronization also originates. A "near" nuclear center coordinating the near response is somewhere around the third nerve nucleus to stimulate the medial recti for convergence, the Edinger-Westphal nucleus for miosis, and the ciliary muscle for accommodation. Negative feedback loops, including input from the hypothalamus, influence the central nuclear pathways and the α and β receptors influencing accommodation. Insufficient accommodation or insufficient convergence can result from a breakdown anywhere in the system. Headaches, diplopia, blurring, eyestrain, loss of concentration, and sleepiness accompany recession of the near point of convergence and a low AC/A ratio. Less than double the phoria is measurable as the horizontal fusional amplitude (Sheard's criteria). Most afflicted individuals are young adults or early presbyopic patients altering their AC/A ratio with readers or bifocals. This latter group have their accommodation replaced with plus lenses and reduce their accommodative convergence in response. Both groups end up with insufficient convergence and an exodeviation at near.

Treatments have involved everything from jump and step vergence exercises to push-ups with pencils. It would appear that short, more frequent training works best. Variety seems to maintain interest. Computer self-paced models are becoming available to individualize therapy. Surgery is reserved for the extreme nonresponders.

It is often forgotten that monocular patients have no need for convergence, since reading material can be brought along the optical axis of the remaining good eye. These individuals will often tolerate an extra +0.25 to +0.50 D add because of their reduced convergence demands. Similarly, high adds bring binocular patients to a closer near point and increase convergence demands. These individuals may have an insufficiency relative to their add and require prism in addition to plus power. In myopic patients the reading segment can be set at the pupillary distance to get some base-in prism effect for relief.

This is a very plastic relationship that alters with and without correction in myopia and hyperopia. A myopic patient without correction must converge at near but not accommodate. With correction, both accommodation and convergence are required. Some myopic persons are more capable of altering their AC/A and CA/C ratios than others. The myopic person who insists on reading with glasses may not be crazy, just incapable of altering these ratios. The situation with hyperopic persons is the reverse.

Just as things can be insufficient, they can also be overactive. Spasm of the near reflex, accommodative spasm, or convergence spasm all exist and are very difficult in some cases to manage. Often treatment fosters the psychologic crutch on which the patient leans. As anxiety can lead to peptic ulcers, so too can it manifest symptomatically in the visual system by any of these entities. One must first rule out the central causes, which are especially common after trauma but can be present from more sinister pathologies. Treatment ranges from explanation and reassurance to cycloplegia and bifocals. Often a cycle will be entered with accommodative spasm where minus lenses are prescribed, overaccommodation occurs, and the patient returns again requiring another −1.50 D. Probably the best treatment is clip-on minus lenses for driving only. The least amount of minus that meets the driver's license requirement is advised.

ANISOMETROPIA

Anisometropia is another common refractive error that has been dealt with in some depth already. The induced anisophorias (different eye deviation according to what position of the lens one is looking through) have all been covered in detail, as well as the aniseikonia that results from this entity. Some prescribing guidelines follow:

1. Amblyopia is very common in young anisometropic patients. It is more common in hypermetropic anisometropia than in myopic anisometropia possibly because of the use of the more myopic eye for near vision. The lack of binocularity promotes strabismus and is presumed the etiology of the common association between the two. Treatment consists of patching the less hypermetropic, nonamblyopic eye followed by correction of the differ-

ence between the two eyes with spectacles. For example +7.00 D hyperopia OD with +3.00 D hyperopia OS would require +4.00 D OD once vision was equalized by occlusion. Concomitant esodeviations would influence the amount of partial or full correction of the remaining hyperopia. In myopic anisometropia, occlusion of the good eye with immediate correction of the myopic eye is indicated. The parents must always be warned that with any form of occlusion the risk exists for a strabismus to become manifest. Although the prognosis for binocular vision with fusion and stereopsis is very good, many will fall into a monofixational pattern. The general rule is that if young anisometropic patients require correction, they should have their full anisometropia corrected.

2. The amount of aniseikonia produced is approximately 2% for every 1.00 D of anisometropia. (This, of course, depends on whether the refractive error is axial or refractive. Since in the majority this is not known, this estimate is quite sufficient.)
3. The amount of aniseikonia that a patient can tolerate is an individual phenomenon. Most people seem to be able to tolerate the 6% or so aniseikonia associated with the contact lens correction of aphakia, whereas others complain about small amounts. In a 10-year study of binocular fusion with spectacles in monocular aphakia, Lubkin and Linksz (*Am J Ophthalmol* 84:700-707, 1977) reported on phakic and aphakic simultaneous correction and found that previously thought impossible amounts of aniseikonia can be tolerated by some individuals (26%).
4. The amount of anisometropia correction to maintain fusion is the desired amount of correction in adults. The balance between the comfort of binocularity has to be weighed against the tolerance for aniseikonia. This again must be individualized. A monofixator may not require bilateral correction. Sensory testing is useful to determine if this is so.
5. Nonpresbyopic adults can avert any induced anisophoria by using the optical centers of their distance correction.
6. Presbyopic adults are forced to look through an eccentric position of their lenses when using bifocals. This, as already seen, can induce anisophorias, which obey Prentice's rule and can be calculated with ease. They can, of course, be measured by prism and alternate cover testing in the reading position or with the Maddox rod (although this is not an accommodative target). Segment decentration, temporary Fresnel Press-On prisms, bicentric grinding (slab-off), or single vision lenses can all be prescribed according to these findings. If a patient is found to look eccentrically (i.e., away from the optical center) with his distance correction with no discomfort, then he has adapted his fusional status, via his amplitudes, to the induced anisophoria. This patient will probably require nothing in the way of prism with bifocals.
7. Give prisms only to symptomatic patients.
8. Always divide the prism equally between the two eyes unless a restrictive or paretic strabismus problem exists.
9. Iseikonic spectacles can be made by altering back and front curves (see section on telescopes) but are expensive and seldom indicated (and even less often prescribed).

PRISMS

Prisms may also be prescribed for entities other than anisophorias induced by anisometropia with bifocals. The following principles and uses of prism therapy are rendered for consideration:

1. Give prisms only to symptomatic patients.
2. Always give a temporary prism in the form of clip-ons or Fresnel Press-On prisms before facing spectacle incorporation. Often a deviation will change or the patient will derive no benefit from therapy and the prism will either have to be changed or discontinued. Spectacle prism is heavy, cosmetically unattractive, and expensive and causes spectral dispersion and acuity reduction.
3. Always give only the amount of prism necessary to control symptoms.
4. Decentration is efficacious in high myopia and hyperopia.
5. Prisms may be used to shift the null point in nystagmus patients when an unacceptable head turn is present. This may be of predictive value as to the surgical benefit of procedures such as the Kestenbaum procedure. Base out prisms can induce convergence, which may also dampen the nystagmus.
6. In convergence insufficiency patients, horizontal fusional amplitudes can often be augmented with orthoptic exercises utilizing base out prisms. (Remember that to neutralize base out requires base in with apex out so that the induced deviation is an exophoria.) The induced exophoria requires convergence, and by training this can be progressively increased.
7. In comitant horizontal deviations such as congenital esotropia, some strabismologists use a prism adaptation test to try to establish binocularity preoperatively. By eliminating the deviation with prisms, the sensorial adaptions (suppression and anomalous retinal correspondence) are theoretically prevented. Unfortunately, several changes are often necessary because of the instability of the angle of deviation. A clinical trial on a multicenter collaborative basis has been undertaken by the National Eye Institute to assess this modality of treatment.
8. Surgical overcorrections, especially of acquired exodeviations, can be salvaged with prisms to eliminate the diplopia of the secondary esotropia.
9. Incomitant strabismus may require different amounts of correction in different positions of the gaze. In this event only primary position and downgaze are corrected.
10. Purely vertical deviations are more bothersome because of reduced vertical fusional amplitudes but the principles of management are the same. Cyclovertical disorders cannot be corrected with prisms. A double maddox rod test is useful to demonstrate a torsional, cyclovertical component to the deviation.
11. Combined horizontal and vertical prisms add vectorially. Combined horizontal and vertical deviations can be alleviated with a single vector prism specified by base and axis, remembering that each meridian has two dimensions when specifying the base.
12. Patients "eat-up" prism as their fusional amplitudes are relaxed with prism therapy. The power often has to be increased to adjust for this at a subsequent time. Prescribing too much prism weakens the fusional ampli-

tude too much. If surgery is contemplated, it is very useful to have the best fusional amplitude possible to tolerate any potential overcorrection or undercorrection.

13. Bedridden patients may benefit from 15 P.D.-25 P.D. base down prisms for reading or watching television. This displaces the image up (towards the apex) alleviating some of the neck and eye strain of sustained downgaze.
14. Monocular occlusion may be the only respite in prism failures with bothersome diplopia.
15. Remember plus lenses decrease the deviation and minus lenses increase the measured deviation (see section on optics of prisms). Recall also that glass prism's are held in the Prentice position and plastic are best held in the frontal plane position.
16. Diplopia is a symptom that demands a diagnosis. To simply treat it is inadequate.

APHAKIA

Aphakia is a condition whose spectacle correction is riddled with aberrations and perceptive phenomena that require major visual adaptions before complete rehabilitation can be achieved. Analysis of some of these will aid the practitioner in understanding the problems encountered by such a patient and hopefully engender a little more empathy and sympathy for his plight.

The aphakic condition is comparable to a large minus eye error with a less powerful correcting lens at a set vertex distance. This, as has been explained in the past, is a Galilean telescope whose magnification is 15% to 25% as derived by $\frac{D_E}{D_O}$. In most instances under monocular correcting conditions this leads to insurmountable aniseikonia, which lies outside the limits of tolerable retinal disparity. Intractable diplopia ensues. If binocular aphakia is corrected, the smaller portion of the visual field of each eye now covers a larger retinal area and everything appears closer and taller. This leads to two interesting phenomena—the ring scotoma and the jack-in-the-box. If this were not bad enough, square objects such as doors and tables undergo pincushion distortion so that they not only appear closer and taller, but all four edges appear bowed inward.

Consider Fig. 11-1, *a,* which reveals an area corresponding to the ring scotoma. If ray O is considered as the theoretical ray that is just next to the most peripheral ray that can be refracted by the lens, then it undergoes the maximal prismatic effect of that lens. (Peripheral pencils are also of course subject to all the other aberrations such as astigmatism of oblique incidence, coma, and spherical aberration that all peripheral and oblique pencils are subject to.) The image point for O is displaced toward the apex by the prismatic effect to point I. Point P_1 is the most central ray that is unaffected by the lens yet still is refracted by the eye and corresponds to the most central portion of the uncorrected visual field. As ray I travels that infinitely small distance to become the most peripheral refracted ray, its image I approaches point P_1. It is therefore quite evident that all object points between point O and P_1 gain no access to either the central or peripheral field. If plotted on a tangent screen or Goldmann perimeter, this area corresponds to an absolute scotoma with a ring shape (Fig. 11-1, *b*). If the images on the retina are

(a)

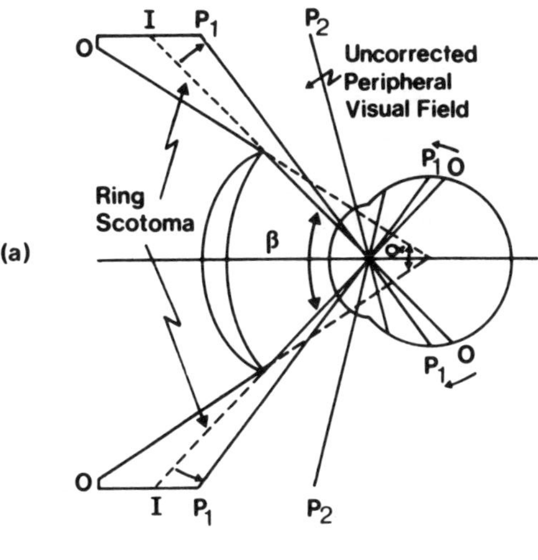

(b)

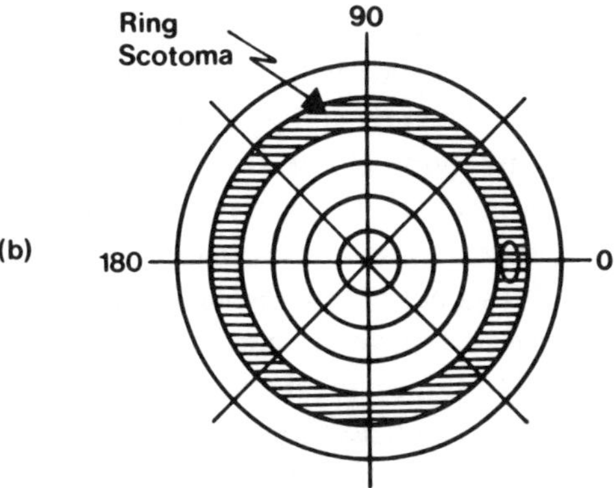

Fig. 11-1

considered, as O reaches that position as the most peripheral ray refracted, it becomes immediately juxtaposed to the position on the retina corresponding to P_1. In other words, object points between O and P_1 have no retinal representation and therefore are not perceived. This is because the central field (0-0) is magnified on the retina (P_1-P_1) and crowds out the peripheral field. (The refracted rays subtend a greater angle β than they would if not influenced by the lens, i.e., angle α).

This is a difficult concept but so striking clinically that it is worth understanding. Consider a situation in which the scotoma is about 10° (this depends on the power of the lens, vertex distance, and size). This 10° at a distance of 30 feet represents a large object space. With the eyes looking in the straight-ahead position, a pedestrian may be seen in the peripheral unrefracted field. Suddenly he disappears as he enters the scotoma, only to reappear some time later just as suddenly, like a jack-in-the-box. To the uninitiated, when a peripheral object is seen, the eye changes position to take up fixation. Now the eye is looking through a different part of the lens and the ring scotoma is now in a different spot—a roving scotoma. This contributes even further to the jack-in-the-box effect. The patient soon learns that the head is better moved than the eyes; only one scotoma has to be dealt with. This is also more comfortable, since the roving scotoma, as well as other image displacements, gives the illusion of movement to the environment or a swimming effect. These phenomena affect both the patient's confidence and safety in the

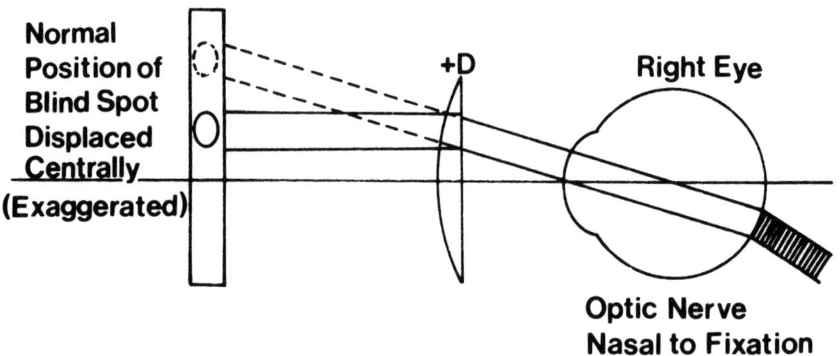

Fig. 11-2

operation of a motor vehicle. Once the patient is adapted to the aberrations, confidence and safety are restored.

The scotoma found during visual field testing has been alluded to, but other artifacts can also be elicited during perimetry. Fig. 11-2 depicts a vertical view of the tangent screen with the normal position of the blind spot corresponding to the optic nerve. Through a high plus lens it can be seen that this corresponding scotoma is now found closer to fixation. In a similar manner, all the tested isopters will be found closer to fixation. All tested isopters are found to be condensed, so the field appears smaller. (Converse reasoning will show that a highly myopic field is larger with a peripheral displacement of the blind spot.) This should not be considered pathologic or be confused with a progression in a glaucoma field, for instance. This is purely an optical phenomenon and should be recognized as such when found. The field should be tested with the aphake wearing contacts if at all possible. This eliminates the above problems.

Another testing artefact is found in visual acuity testing. The visual angle is altered by the magnification of the lens so that the minimum separable angle is expanded from 1.0′ to 1.15 to 1.25′, making it more easily distinguished. In other words, 20/25 visual acuity becomes 20/20. Naturally, with a contact or introcular lens implant this is not seen, so the visual acuity will still be 20/25 or appear less than with spectacles.

When a bilaterally spectacle-corrected aphakic person attempts reading, the base out effects of the lenses require extra convergence to overcome. This can be improved immensely by segment decentration and design. When the person is looking eccentrically, the vertex distance effectively increases. This blurs all but central fixation. This again can be improved by altering the lens design. Some of these design characteristics are worthwhile reviewing.

The primary developments have centered around the principle of *asphericity.* An aspheric lens has different radii of curvature as the periphery of a lens is approached. This helps correct several of the aberrations present in spherical high plus lenses. The amount of asphericity depends on what the desired effect may be. If it is desired that when the eye fixes eccentrically in the lens the power is correct for central vision, a lenticular design emerges (foveal rationale). If, on the other hand, one desires that while the eye is looking through the optical center the peripheral rays are well focused, a full field aspheric lens design emerges (peripheral rationale). The Welsh 4 Drop and Hyper Aspheric are examples of this type of lens. Another new design is the Ful-Vue lens, which claims to retain both of these characteristics. Further consideration of aspherics will be found later in the materials section.

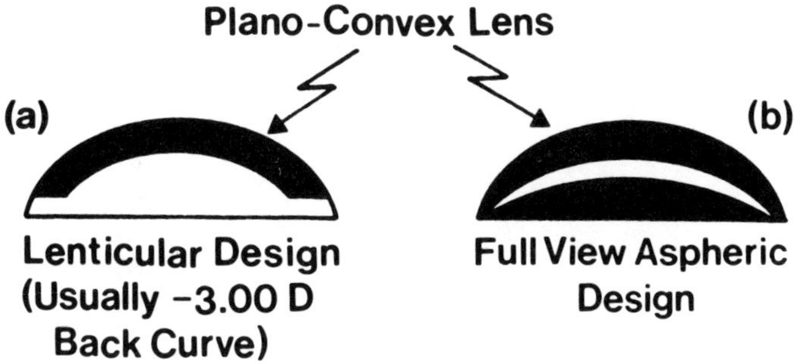

Fig. 11-3

One advantage of all of these types is the great weight-reducing combination of plastic and asphericity. Cosmetically, the full field aspheric lenses are superior and afford larger lens diameters, which can be set in more modern style frames while also increasing the visual field and decreasing the ring scotoma. They do not have the bubblelike appearance of the lenticular lens, but even they can't get away from the magnified appearance of the patient's eye. This is inherent in any plus lens of this strength (Fig. 11-3).

Possibly one of the greatest advantages of dealing with these lens types is the availability of kits with temporary lens blanks of known spherical power. By overrefraction at the correct vertex distance with a properly fitting frame, the final perscription is much more precise. This is performed with the use of clips (Halberg, Janelli), which are placed on the frames to hold the overrefracting lenses. The final combination can be determined on the lensmeter. Overrefraction can also be performed behind a phoroptor or with some of the automated refractors.

Of course, if all of the problems encountered were cured with these lenses, there would be no demand for contact or intraocular lenses. The popularity of these latter entities yields some comment as to the imperfections that still remain with spectacle lens correction.

PSEUDOPHAKIA

Pseudophakia, or aphakia corrected with an in situ intraocular lens (IOL) implant, has revolutionized cataract surgery. This technique exquisitely displays how the science of optics has affected the art of ophthalmology.

After extraction of the cataractous lens, an implant of prechosen power is inserted into either the anterior chamber, iris plane, or posterior chamber of the eye Fig. 11-4. The position chosen is dictated by the surgeon's preference. The unique aspect of implant surgery is that the power of the lens must be derived preoperatively. From what is already known, it becomes evident that the power required will depend on:

1. The refracting power of the cornea
2. The position of the retina
3. The position of the implant relative to the cornea

The power of the cornea as a refracting surface is easily determined with the keratometer. The position of the retina can be determined by A-scan ultrasonography or laser Doppler interferometry. This is the axial length of the eye.

The end position of the implant will vary from one implant type to another and from one eye configuration to the next. An average value can be substituted

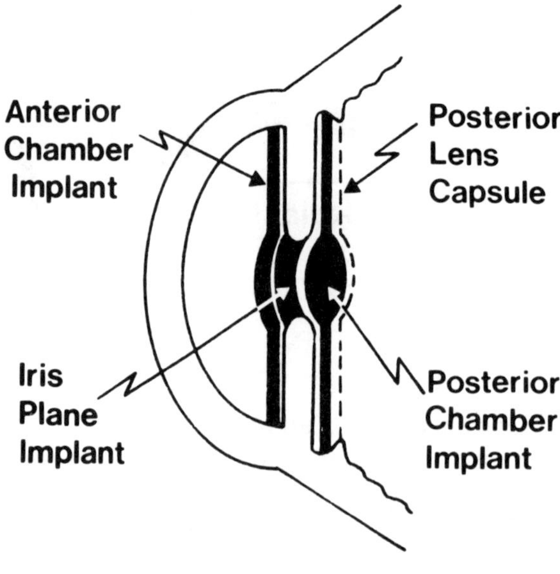

Fig. 11-4

from A-scan ultrasonography from postoperative patients for each type of implant. With knowledge of these three variables, the power of a second thick lens in a two lens combination whose focal point coincides with the retina can then be determined. Various reduced formulae, nomograms, and computer programs are used rather than calculation for each independent case. With this technique the final spectacle correction can be determined to within ± 3.00 D in virtually every case.

Several factors can vary from surgeon to surgeon and lens design to lens design. The final implant position is critical. Each 1 mm of anterior displacement results in a 1.00 D change in IOL power. Similarly, each 1 mm error in the axial length can result in 2.50 D of refractive error. Intuitively the factors of importance are the surgeon, the IOL type and position, the axial length, and the *K* readings. Sanders, Retzlaff, and Kraft (SRK) have established a simplified formula with standardized constants for all manufacturers.

$$P = A + (-2.5 \times \text{Axial length}) + (-0.9 \times \text{Average } K)$$

where: P = IOL power for emmetropia
A = IOL surgeon specific, manufacturer specific, variable from anterior to posterior chamber and lens shape (convex-plano, biconvex, meniscus)

Modifications to this basic formula have been made to improve predictability. An anterior chamber depth factor (ACD) estimating the distance from the iris to the principal plane of the IOL (Holloday), variable A constants for varying axial lengths (SRKII), and exponential factors in regression analysis of long eyes (Thompson) have all been modifications to the simplified formula. They become particularly useful for short eyes where calculated values tend to be too strong and long eyes where they tend to be too weak. As yet, the correction of astigmatism or accommodation cannot be achieved with intraocular lenses, although toric foldable implants and new bifocal implant designs are addressing these problems.

It may not always be desirable to have no postoperative refractive error (emmetropia). In this case, the power of the IOL (D_{IOL}) can be altered from emmetropia (P) by a correcting factor according to the desired postoperative refractive error (R).

$$D_{IOL} = P - \frac{R}{1.5}$$

where: D_{IOL} = new IOL power
P = power for emmetropia
R = desired postoperative refractive error

For example, to achieve a refractive error of −3.00 D postoperatively, what strength of IOL is required if the SRK formula predicts +20.00 D for emmetropia?

$$\begin{aligned} D_{IOL} &= +20.00 - \left(\frac{-3.00}{1.5}\right) \\ &= +20.00 + 2 \\ &= +22.00 \text{ D} \end{aligned}$$

Occasionally during a procedure, conversion from a posterior chamber IOL to an anterior chamber IOL is necessary. Since the axial length and K readings are fixed, the only important change is in the A constant. The anterior chamber lens power is simply the posterior chamber lens power minus the A constant difference.

For example, a +19.50 D IOL is planned for a posterior chamber implant with an A constant of 118.0. The posterior capsule ruptures and inadequate fixation for a posterior chamber lens is present. An anterior chamber lens with an A constant of 115.0 is selected. What power for emmetropia should be used?

$$\begin{aligned} D &= +19.50 - (118.0 - 115.0) \\ &= +19.50 - 3.0 \\ &= +16.50 \text{ D} \end{aligned}$$

(Remember CAP = closer add plus, so the posterior chamber IOL always has the higher dioptric value when compared to the anterior chamber IOL.)

The shape factor of the implant also contributes greatly to the IOL power and specifically to the A constant. Theoretical models favour biconvex implants for minimizing spherical aberrations and suffering less image degradation if decentered. They also appear to reduce posterior capsular opacification rates. The A constant requires about +2.00 D of change to compensate relative to a meniscus style IOL. Check each manufacturer's A constant carefully before final selection.

Although accommodation cannot be achieved, attempts have been made to produce bifocal optics by diffractive and refractive means with implants as well as contact lenses. The principle involved is to have both distance and near focused simultaneously on the retina. The brain will select whether to focus on the near or the distant object of regard and ignore the other image. A trial of a similar design contact lens on the better eye to simulate this style of viewing seems prudent. Some patients will be unhappy, and this may select them before surgery. Pupil size, centration, postoperative astigmatic and refractive predictability, and design become very important to maximize acuity. Contrast sensitivity reduction seems to be the price for simultaneous perception. Time will tell whether the products are worth that price.

An interesting phenomenon may emerge with the intraoperative manipulation of corneal astigmatism. Consider preoperative corneal astigmatism that is spectacle corrected. Cortical adaption has occurred to compensate for the distortion. An IOL is inserted and the corneal astigmatism is eliminated by suture manipulation such that a spherical cornea results. Postoperatively a period of cortical readaption is required because of the absence of astigmatism. If this is not appreciated, the patient is labelled a complainer, when the symptoms are quite real. Reassurance and a tincture of time are all that is required.

PINHOLE AND DIFFRACTION

While discussing the spectacle correction of aphakia mention was made of overrefraction technique. The simplest method of overrefraction is the *pinhole*. Consider first its basic principles and then its uses.

Fig. 11-5 illustrates what the effect of a pinhole is on both myopia and hyperopia. By limiting the system to only paraxial rays, the blur circle on the retina is considerably reduced to almost stigmatic imagery. When the aperture is small, as it is with the pinhole, the circle of least confusion is also small and the vision is improved. In essence, the pinhole is capable of reducing any refractive error, and in so doing improving the visual acuity. It is, as Melvin Rubin, M.D., likes to call it "the universal corrective lens constant" (*Optics for clinicians,* ed 2, 1977, Triad). But as do all good things, it has its limit. The limit is created by a process called *diffraction.*

Diffraction literally means to break apart. To understand this concept, another departure from geometric into physical optics must be made. When light waves encounter an aperture or any opaque edge, they are bent. The original wavefront continues through the central portion of the aperture undisturbed. Those on the edges are bent to take on a new configuration different from the original waves (Fig. 11-6). These newly formed waves interfere with the originals and form a diffraction pattern. If the aperture is round, dark rings are formed that correspond to the areas of destructive interference. Where constructive interference occurs, bright rings are formed. The diffraction pattern thus formed is called an Airy disc, after the astronomer who first described it. The smaller the aperture, the broader the central portion of the disc.

As the central portion increases, it spreads its intensity over a wider area and

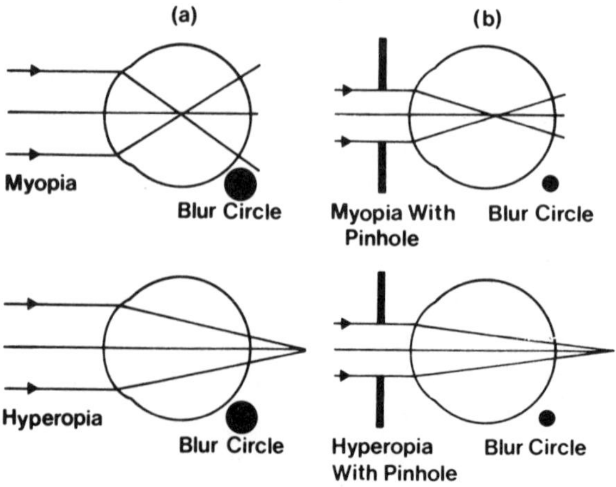

Fig. 11-5

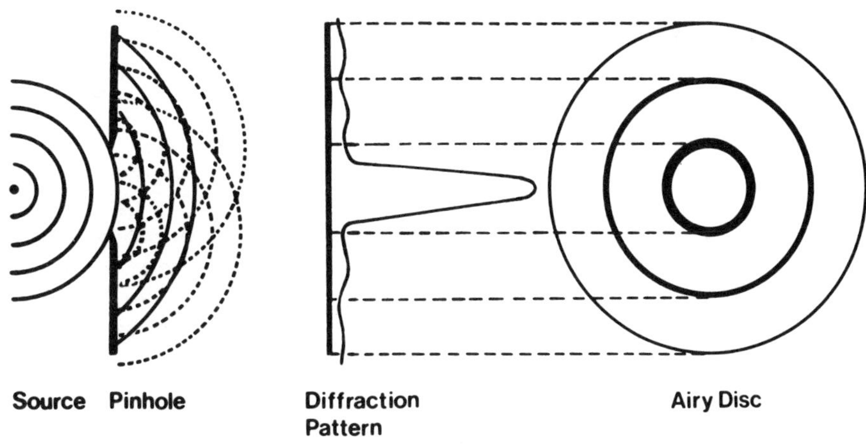

Fig. 11-6

becomes a less effective stimulus, i.e., its ability to be resolved is diminished. If this were applied to the eye, the blur circle would be larger as a critical size of pinhole is reached. At this point the system is said to be diffraction limited. Pupil size that has the highest resolving power by theoretical considerations is 2.5 mm. Clinical data, however, suggest that 1.2 mm is ideal for general neutralizing of refractive errors.

It was mentioned that the pinhole is effective in overrefraction. If the patient is wearing his best correction and the pinhole is placed over it (preferably one with many holes, making localization easier), the vision may improve. If it does, the correction may be inadequate, irregular astigmatism may be present, media opacities of a focal nature may exist, or the pupil may be dilated leading to spherical aberrations. If it diminishes the visual acuity, retinal or diffuse medial opacities may exist and the reduced illumination negates the better focus.

More commonly the pinhole is used as a screening procedure to determine quickly (as in the emergency room) if the reduced acuity is on a refractive basis. The diffraction effects will, however, reduce an emmetropic person's acuity to 20/25. Similarly, very high hyperopia and myopia will experience only minimal improvement. This can be greatly augmented when ± 5.00 and ± 10.00 D lenses are used in conjunction with the pinhole. To decide whether the patient is myopic or hyperopic, move the pinhole while the patient fixes an accommodative target. If the target moves in the same direction, the patient is myopic and the minus lens with the pinhole is used.

The pinhole can also be used as a presbyopic correction for a patient who has forgotten his glasses. Similarly, an accidental cycloplegia in medical personnel or family members can be conveniently corrected in this fashion. As shall be seen later, a double pinhole is an effective refraction method employed in automated refraction—the Scheiner principle.

Of course, the natural pinhole is achieved by squinting, as is so readily seen in uncorrected myopia. This actually forms a slit but has the same effect. The stenopeic slit can be a useful adjunct in refraction. Isolating the two best meridians with the slit and then neutralizing them with the appropriate sphere for the best visual acuity yield a power cross that can easily be converted to a spherocylinder. Retinoscopy is so vastly superior that this technique is seldom employed.

Please see Part II: Problems and Part III: Solutions for typical examination questions pertaining to the material in this chapter.

CHAPTER 12: MATERIALS

During the discussion of aphakia the subject of *spectacle lens design* was touched upon to deal with various ways of improving aberrations. Patient inquiries frequently revolve around lens tints and coatings, and the practitioner is often faced with problems and errors in dispensing to which she must be attuned.

Spectacles can be made out of various substances with differing weights, impact resistance, reflection properties, and scratch resistance. The patient wishes to fill his prescription with glasses that comply to the specifications of the prescription and fit his face properly. This process is a great enigma to many ophthalmologists, let alone patients. The following is an explanation of the materials and process involved in the manufacturing and dispensing side of the industry.

LENSES

Lenses are made of many materials, including crown glass, high index glass, plastic, and high index plastics. Each has unique properties, advantages, and disadvantages that make it the material of choice for some patients.

Glass

Glass is an amorphous, inorganic substance with atoms that are strongly bound by covalent bonds yet randomly arranged. This random assortment does not form molecules, crystals, or grains. The raw materials are often combinations of various oxides of silica, aluminum, barium, etc. Unlike metals, salts, and crystals, no definite melting point is present. Instead, one speaks of softening and annealing points as important temperature barriers. Industrial quality glass uses natural raw materials, but for optical grade lenses synthetic materials are needed. It can be colourless ("white") or added to for tints or photochromaticity (photochromism).

One optical grade is referred to as *crown glass.* It has an index of refraction of 1.523. Crown enjoys a natural scratch resistance. Welders, however, will note that it does pit with splatter (plastic does not). Glass was cheaper, but recently costs have risen dramatically. Part of this cost is the damage done to diamond bits used by the generator for grinding the back surface. Surfacing tools for glass might last only 1 month, whereas similar plastic bits might last up to 2 years. Crown weighs 50% more than plastic and warps less but does require impact resistance treatment.

High index glass has greater vergence for less curvature. This allows the lens to be thinner. Materials such as lanthanium, lead, and titanium can be used to bring the index up to 1.800 or more. Although thinner, they are more refractive, have greater color dispersion, are more brittle, and are more difficult to work with in the lab. Fused segments in bifocals and thinner edged high minus lenses are possible uses. They can be thermally or chemically tempered for impact resistance.

Photochromic glass changes colour on absorption of visible ultraviolet (UV) light. Elemental silver dissociates from AgCl on absorption of a photon of light, i.e., $AgCl \rightleftarrows Ag^+ + Cl^-$. The speed of darkening varies directly with the absorption of UV and inversely with the temperature, i.e., the hotter the temperature, the slower the change. For calibration purposes a 2 mm block at 20° is used to measure the transmittance. Fully faded after a night's rest, it may transmit 65%, which is reduced to 20% when fully darkened. This is said to be a "swing of 65/20." High plus lenses might reach 4 mm center thickness, which reduces this to 65/10. Some other examples are PhotoGrey 85/50, PhotoSun 65/20, and PhotoGrey Extra 87/22 (Corning).

In addition to the AgCl one can integrate a tint if desired. A UV coat on the back can block the remaining UV but on the front would prevent the process. Treating a fully darkened lens traps the darkened state permanently. They are compatible with antireflection coatings. The process for chemical hardening is slightly different from that for crown (with a lithium bath and slightly different temperature). When first dispensed they may have a yellowish tint until a few cycles have passed. This early yellow cycle can be simulated with a UV lamp.

Corning has introduced high index 1.600 PhotoGrey 16 and PhotoBrown 16. These block 98% of the UVA and 100% of the UVB and are antireflection coating compatible. For retinal degenerations and dystrophies, filtration into the visible blue (511, 527, 550 nm) with CPF lenses is possible. CPF 550 21/5 is red when darkened, amber when lightened.

New borosilicate and aluminophosphate glass, e.g., Reactolite, PhotoGrey Extra, and Colormatic, claim to fade twice as fast; 50% in 2 to 5 minutes; 90% in 15 to 20 minutes.

Newer patents weave photochromatic glass fibers into a 0.01 to 0.02 inch thin laminate and bond it to CR-39 (allyl diglycol carbonate). The old laminates crazed into a honeycomb pattern as stress built up internally from plastic expanding 10 times faster than the photochromic glass. The woven pattern dissipates the internal stress. Colormatic Hard Resin and Transitions are new photochromatic plastic lenses. Hopefully they will prove more durable than previous types. Apparently, problems with antireflection coating and leaching of the photochemicals may be new problems yet to be completely surmounted.

Another new response to the variable coefficients of expansion of laminates is the use and provision of composite technology. This binds a central plastic polymer to an outer glass lens without the use of bonding agents. It is hoped that polymeric bonding between materials will achieve the stability laminates failed to achieve. The advantages are that they are light as plastic, thin as glass, and available as a photochromic lens (CS Composite).

Another new photochromic lens (Transitions 80/28) is a polymer made from a monomer different from CR-39 ($n = 1.50$). The photochromatic material is integrated into the front surface rather than laminating/bonding. About 94% of UV to 380 nm and 63% to 400 nm is filtered relative to photochromic glass, which filters only 72% to 380 nm. The use of antireflection coatings does reduce the performance of most photochromic plastics. The projected lifespan is 2 to 5 years with less (potentially) darkening with time than photochromic glass. These lenses may not darken as much in a car with windshield UV absorption and may darken indoors with UV from fluorescent lighting. At 2 mm center thickness, no impact resistance treatment is required.

Plastic

Plastics are macromolecular (up to 300,000 atoms/molecule), organic (milk, coal, or cotton) polymers that can be shaped when heated. Thermoplastics can be shaped and reshaped, but duroplastics are destroyed when reheated (bond breakage).

CR-39 was patented by Pittsburgh Plate Glass, and now plastic constitutes 80% of the lenses dispensed. The index of refraction is 1.498 with a relatively low colour dispersion (Abbe number 56 is a measure of dispersion). At about ±6.00 D the weight differential between crown and plastic is less a factor because of the increased thickness of the plastic lenses. It is easier to work with in the lab and now cheaper to work with as well. There is inherent impact resistance with slightly (2%) more transmission. Welder spatter does not easily pit plastic, but the lenses warp more than do crown lenses.

Attempts to reduce thickness for cosmetic and weight purposes have led to the development of *high index plastic* (HIP) lenses. Thus far the expense makes it a consideration for high myopia $> \pm 6.00$ D only, although others may consider it. As the index is increased, the curve is flatter and the lens is thinner. Current HIP lenses have an index of refraction of about 1.600. Composites used in tennis racquets, car parts, and medical prostheses are glass on the outside with plastic on the inside. The polymer core is covalently bound to the glass shell by carbon = oxygen bonding. The glass can be photochromic 91/55 if desired. The lens is lighter than glass, as impact resistant as plastic, and as scratch resistant as crown.

To date most HIPs are manufactured as semifinished blanks in Japan (Hoya, Pentax, Asahi, Nikon, Seiko) and cut/edged/mounted at the local lab. As the Abbe constant decreases, the chromatic dispersion increases, which is a problem with HIP relative to CR-39. Table 12-1 gives some insight into the density of each HIP relative to CR-39 (the lower the density, the lower the weight).

All HIPs filter all UV <380 nm. The surface is softer than CR-39 so scratch coating is necessary. As will be seen later there is considerably more reflection, necessitating antireflection coating and wash coating. Absorption of water by the surface and differential expansion with heat can lead to coatings crazing into honeycomb patterns in the sauna. Newer generations claim to have solved this problem.

Polycarbonate of old had many problems (n = 1.586). It was very soft, too thin, and would flex and warp when mounted in a tight frame. This necessitated the center thickness being 1.8 mm just for stability. The colour dispersion was high. The surface was hard to work. Edging had to be done manually. Significant warpage would occur with injection moulding, and the lenses maintained a slightly bluish tint.

The "new" polycarbonates such as Sola (n = 1.589) can be cast in glass moulds

Table 12-1

	n	V	Density (g/cm^2)
CR-39	1.498	56	1.32
Polycarbonate	1.586	30	1.20
HOYA HI LUX II	1.560	40	1.27
SEIKO 16	1.600	33	1.38

and are less flexible, allowing the center thickness to reduce to 1.3 mm. Regular surfacing generators can be used, but special edging and scratch coating are still required. Other surface coats are all similar in use to CR-39. This is becoming very popular.

Where edge thickness is a problem for the myopic person, the center thickness is a problem for the hyperopic person. Aspheric lenses reduce the curvature from the center to the periphery of the lens. By reducing the curvature, the lens thickness is reduced and the field is improved. Aspheric plastics (e.g., Hyperal, Cosmolit) are available, but the market is awaiting HIP aspherics expectantly. Newer aspheric lenses not only flatten a lens and reduce oblique astigmatism, they also are now available in larger sizes (e.g., 75 mm Hyperal) for more fashionable frames. High index glass for high minus lenses are now almost approaching a flat front surface. The residual myopic halo rings can be reduced by colouring or polishing the edges with a light pink or Cruxite tint or selecting darker frames.

Special high index glass (n = 1.800), such as Index 8 (formerly Hidex), is used for x-ray absorption. For x-ray protection, a minimum center thickness must be maintained with or without side shields applied. Dress wear to goggles can be made of this material. Other manufacturers (Zeiss, Essilor) have index 1.800 lenses for regular dress wear.

Impact Resistance

A lens subject to a blow or projectile must display sufficient impact resistance to protect the eye from the threat and from its own shards on breakage. The standards are different if the lenses are for dress wear versus industrial or safety wear. Different countries have different standards for center thickness and impact resistance. The U.S. Food and Drug Administration has established a drop ball test. A steel ball of ⅝ inch diameter weighing 0.56 oz (about 16 g) is dropped from a height of 50 inches (1.27 ms). Dress wear lenses must not break during this test. To be classified impact resistant lenses, the drop ball test is done with a 1 inch steel ball of 2.4 oz (about 68 g) dropped from 50 inches (1.27 m), i.e., approximately four times the weight. In Canada the drop ball test is performed only on industrial and safety lenses, not on dress wear lenses. To pass the test, the lens must not break.

Further consumer protection is conferred by ensuring minimum standards for center and edge thickness. For example, for heat hardened crown the minimum center thickness must be 2.0 mm; chemically hardened lenses can be reduced to 1.8 mm. Industrial safety crown must be 3 mm with an edge thickness of 2.5 mm. The edge thickness standard becomes important for hyperopic plus corrections where technically the edge could be reduced to razor thin. Lenses of dubious origin will not necessarily adhere to any safety standards, and caution must be exercised.

The standards are met differently with each material used. For glass or high index glass, heat or chemical hardening is required. For CR-39 and HIPs, including polycarbonate, no treatment other than the minimum center/edge thickness is necessary.

Heat tempering is a 5-minute process with readily available inexpensive materials. The glass is heated to between its annealing and softening point, which is about 650° to 700° C. This is determined by weighing the polished, ground, and edged lens and heating it for a specified duration according to the finished weight. This is quickly air cooled or quenched, which cools the outside faster than the inside of the lens. The slower inside cooling contracts the harder outside and results in compression of the outside surface into a toughened shell. The inside remains under internal stress, which is a problem when the lens is scratched. A deep scratch can reduce the impact resistance by up to 44%. There have also been cases of spontaneous explosion or breakage of a lens when the external compressive forces are exceeded by the internal expansive stress.

When heat treated lenses do break, they shatter into similar sized, small pieces with smoother edges than ordinary glass (which tends to splinter and shard). They are less likely to inflict injury for this reason.

Since a treated lens cannot be reworked in the lab without chipping or shattering during edging, it is occasionally useful to determine if a lens has or has not been heat treated. The treatment process leaves the lens with different indices of refraction in different regions of the lens. This yields a phenomenon called birefringence, or the ability to rotate polarized light, which can be detected before the lens is worked on.

Frames that require the lens to be drilled, grooved, or slotted create foci of weakness incapable of withstanding the high internal stress. This precludes heat tempering for this type of frame selection.

Photochromic lenses can be treated, but it may darken the lens permanently in the process. This occasionally proves useful in matching a replacement lens to an older counterpart on the other side.

Chemical tempering offers the advantages of lower minimum center thickness requirements and preservation of impact resistance with scratching. This latter property is especially important for children.

The process involves immersion of a preheated lens into a bath of 99.5% potassium nitrate and 0.5% silicone acid at 842° F (460° C). Photochromic lenses require a lithium bath at 752° F (400° C). The principle is to replace the smaller sodium ions on the lens surface with larger potassium or lithium ions. This exchange occurs slowly over 12 to 16 hours. By cramming the larger ions into the smaller slots, the outer surface enters a state of external compression similar to heat tempering. Drilled, grooved, or slotted lenses can be treated this way in addition to the photochromics. The major disadvantages to the lab are the expense, long turnaround time, and the handling of hazardous chemicals. The advantage is that the lenses can be reworked for edging and surfacing considerations.

Safety frames, temples, hinges, sideshields, and bevels are equally important to impact resistance and radiation filtration in industrial design and dispensing. The International Organization for Standardization and the Canadian Standards Association are involved in developing standards for eye protectors.

Tints

The transmission of visible and invisible irradiation by a lens can be altered by a tint. This can be integrated into the material during its manufacture (integrated tint) or deposited on its surface in a vacuum (metallic tint). For plastic the surface can be dyed by immersion in a dye bath (dyed), or for glass a tint can be fused or cemented as a layer to white glass (equitint or graduated tint). An integrated tint will have the depth of colour of the tint vary with the thickness of the lens. In hyperopia the plus lens would be darker centrally; in myopia the periphery would be darker; in anisometropia the two lenses would be different colours. Photochromic lenses with the AgCl integrated will display this same phenomenon. With glass the fusion of an equitint or graduated tint layer to the surface distributes the colour as desired, irrespective of the prescription.

Metals or metallic compounds can be deposited on the surface of glass by a vacuum deposition process. This alters the reflected light rather than the absorption spectrum. Only specially equipped laboratories can do this to plastic lenses. These metallic mirror finishes can be gold, silver, zinc, or chromium and are costed accordingly. They commonly reduce transmission by an additional 30% and can be used in conjunction with other types of absorptive glass.

Plastic lenses in a heated (210° F or 99° C) immersion bath can be surface dyed according to the surface characteristics of the lens and length of time in the bath. A lens that is older may have a surface substantially different from a new lens. Dye lots may vary and lead to different colours on replacement lenses. It is often better to bleach both lenses and start with them both white rather than attempt a colour match. Graduated tints can be achieved by a dipping process. These processes do not significantly alter the ultraviolet or infrared absorptive properties of the lens. Older lenses coated with antireflection coating(s) must first be chemically stripped.

Tinting can be functional, cosmetic, or both (sunglasses versus funglasses). Functional tints filter ultraviolet, infrared, x-ray and a percentage of the visible spectrum. Ultraviolet filtration can be an integrated chromophore that absorbs the UV light or a coating that achieves the same goal. Manufacturers may state that 100% of UV is absorbed but may not include the wavelength of the cut-off. If there is concern, this can be specified on the prescription, e.g., filter $<$400 nm. Many over-the-counter sunglasses now have UVA filters and may go to 380 nm. These can be checked by an optician owning a spectrophotometer.

Infrared tints with ferrous oxide, x-ray, and other industrial absorptive lenses are specified by the industrial user and various standards organizations.

Preference for neutral grey, brown, amber, yellow, or green is often simply a personal preference. Care must be taken on the adverse effects of colour matching, especially with respect to traffic lights and signals. This is very important when dealing with protanomals and deuteranomals, where their colour perception may degrade from colour defective safe to unsafe with certain tints. Neutral grey has certainly proven safe for colour balance for over 50 years.

A new synthetic melanin called Melanite (Gal-Tech) uses a laminate of synthetic melanin with standard CR-39 as a "natural" tint.

The potential harmful effects of sunglasses are theoretical rather than proven. The argument goes that reducing visible transmission reduces those rays controlling pupil constriction. If no UV filter is present, increased UV access to the crystalline lens and retina will be experienced with potentially enhanced phototoxicity. It would seem prudent to ensure UV filtration with any absorptive filter that reduces visible transmission.

Antireflective Coatings

In 1892, Dennis Taylor noticed that tarnished lenses with an oxidized surface reduced reflection and increased transmission. By 1904 a chemical patent was issued and the race began. The advent of high index materials was accompanied by enhanced reflections demanding a solution. The multilayer coating was born.

Fresnel's law of reflection states that the reflection (R) is such that:

$$R = \left(\frac{n-1}{n+1}\right)^2 \quad \text{where: } n = \text{index of refraction of the reflecting interface}$$

For example:

Crown glass $n = 1.523$

$$R = \left(\frac{1.523 - 1}{1.523 + 1}\right)^2 = 0.043$$

or 4.3% of incident light is reflected

This is true of each interface between any two media of differing indices of refraction. If 4.3% is reflected from the first surface, the remaining 95.7% is transmitted and encounters the second surface. If 4.3% of this 95.7% is reflected, 91.5% is transmitted. For crown glass, the total transmission is therefore approximately 92% of the incident light. Table 12-2 illustrates the effect of altering the index of refraction on the reflection.

Clearly, the arrival of higher index materials was accompanied by the troublesome feature of reflection. Curiously, the lower dioptric strengths of myopic correction feature reflected images that are most bothersome. They are nearly in focus and closer to fixation, making them very difficult to ignore.

It became clear that, if the reflected light from the first surface was 180° out of phase with the reflected light from the second surface, destructive interference would cancel them both out. Coatings were found to achieve this phase shift. Unfortunately they are good for only one wavelength of light, hence the necessity for multilayers. By searching for coatings that affect the middle region of the visible spectrum, the most bothersome reflections would be eliminated. The red and blue regions would still reflect and yield a magenta hue to the reflected light.

Table 12-3 illustrates the antireflective efficacy of current multilayer coatings on CR-39.

There are several trademarks and names, such as SC-99, Super T coating, T-star, High Fidelity Transfer, that can be applied to glass, high index glass, CR-39, HIP, and polycarbonate.

The lenses must be impeccable. This requires an ultrasonic cleaner until the lenses are particle free. They are then preheated to improve the coating adherence. Any moisture is removed and an electron beam gun evapourates MgF_2, $MgCl_2$, sodium, or lithium metals as a series of proprietary coatings. The material is held

Table 12-2

	n	Transmission (Total %)
CR-39	1.49	92
CROWN	1.52	91
INDEX 6	1.60	90
INDEX 7	1.70	87
INDEX 8	1.80	84

Table 12-3

CR-39	Transmission
NO COAT	92%
SINGLE	96%
DOUBLE	97%
FIVE	99.5%

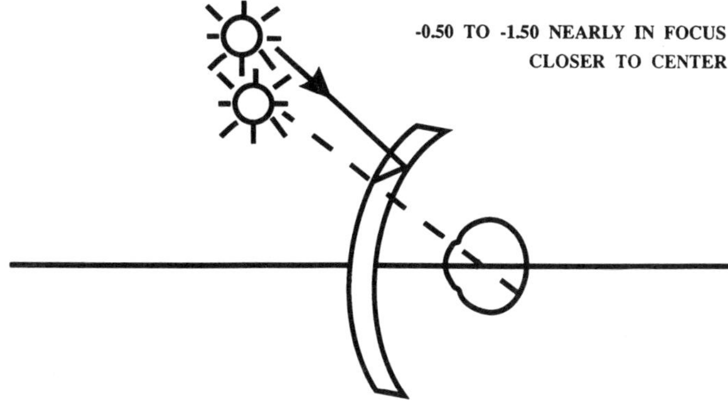

Fig. 12-1

in a copper crucible, water cooled, and vapourized with the electron beam. The vacuum chamber transports the vapour to the lens, which accepts the deposit. A computer controls the timing and the sequence of the multilayers. The lenses are processed in batches with a control lens of quartz whose frequency changes as weight from the layer is deposited. The computer monitors this frequency modulation. The final layer is a quartz or silica coat, which confers some scratch resistance and protection for the underlying coatings. Once complete, the lenses are flipped and the other side is treated.

Since this takes place at high temperatures, laminates, polarized lenses, thermal segments, and thermal lenticulars would be destroyed. This also implies glass and plastic lenses must be separated into different temperature batches.

Most antireflective coatings are stable to acetone and solvents but labile to hydrochloric acid. The coatings can be stripped chemically from CR-39, crown and photochromic glass but cannot be removed predictably from polycarbonate or HIPs (only about 80% success).

Applied Vision has developed a newer, faster, cheaper method of coating using magnetron sputtering. Magnetic confinement of particles displaced by colliding argon ions are deposited on mirrors or lenses.

Other Treatments

Prior to undergoing antireflective coating, an *antiscratch coat* can be applied (Hard cote, PLX, Supershield). This is a cured hard resin that is baked for 7 hours onto the surface of the lens. A new 3M oven uses a chemical/thermal process that achieves similar curing in 7 minutes.

After antireflective coating a *wash coat* or *superphobic* treatment can be applied. With multilayer antireflective coatings one often feels the lenses are dirty all the time and laden with dust particles and fingerprints. These newer applications preserve the antireflective properties of the lens even when dirty, reduce dust, and facilitate cleaning the lens. It is still advisable to recommend avoidance of caustic solutions, hairsprays, and ultrasonic cleaners on antireflective coated lenses even with these newer applications. A gentle dishwashing detergent with warm water and a soft cloth is still best for cleaning.

Fogging is a nuisance when wearing glasses. It occurs when prolonged exposure to cold lowers the lens temperature less than the dew point of the inside air. Condensation of water onto the lens occurs. The antifog sprays and antistatic cleaners reduce the droplet size of the condensate, improving visibility under such circumstances. Some of these have a silicone component that actually works poorly with the multilayer antireflective coating.

Finally, engraving or decal painting can be added to the lens. This is a fashion statement but must be done with care so as not to interfere with any of the previous processes.

FRAMES

Glazing is the process of mounting lenses into frames. Frames can be made of almost anything, including metals, plastics, shell, leather, horn, ivory, ceramic, and graphite. There are advantages and disadvantages to each that contribute to the decision as to which material is appropriate for each individual patient. Before reviewing the materials themselves, the actual glazing process is worthwhile to understand.

The organic materials such as plastics expand when heated. This used to be done in a bath of hard rock salt (salt bath), which was heated to soften and expand the frame to pop the lens in. Today uniformly round glass beads are heated and the frame is actively rotated in this bath. If the beads are in contact with a stationary frame, small pits are impressed into the frame surface. Constant motion reduces this likelihood. A hot air blower can achieve the same result. When shell frames are chosen, a shell heater or blower is used to work the shell.

If a lens is off axis by a few degrees, an attempt to heat the frame and rotate the lens might correct the axis alignment. The type of lens must be considered. Rotation of a bifocal might alter the optical center of the reading segment, replacing one problem with another. The shape of the lens may also be such that rotation creates internal stress on the lens and results in damage or warpage.

Metal frames are worked with screws of various materials to fasten the lens into the frame. Rimless spectacles use a nylon line in a groove around the lens for fixation. Another alternative is to screw the lens directly to the frame. A diamond drill is best. The hole is drilled halfway from the front and then halfway from the back. The risk of breakage is much less this way. The edges are smoothed or chamfered before the screw is set in the hole.

The actual nomenclature that is used to describe the different parameters of the frame and lens varies slightly from country to country, but the basic principles are the same. Fig. 12-2 gives an overview of the important parameters that influence how the frames and lenses conform to the patient.

The effective diameter of the lens (EDL) is the widest part of the lens and hence will influence the size of the lens blank selected to grind the lens. The larger the frame, the larger the blank and the greater the cost.

The distance between lenses (*DBL*) and the patient's pupillary distance (*PD*) will determine how much the lens blank is decentered to fit the frame. For example, consider Fig. 12-3. If horizontal lens diameter is 44 mm, the optical center (*OC*), if not decentered, equals 22 mm. Therefore a decentration *IN* of 3 mm of both *RIGHT* and *LEFT* would be required for the mechanical *PD* to match the patient's *PD*.

These must all be calculated before the lens is ground. Any disparity between the patient's PD and the mechanical PD will induce prism according to Prentice's rule. The amount of decentration is another fact that determines the size of the

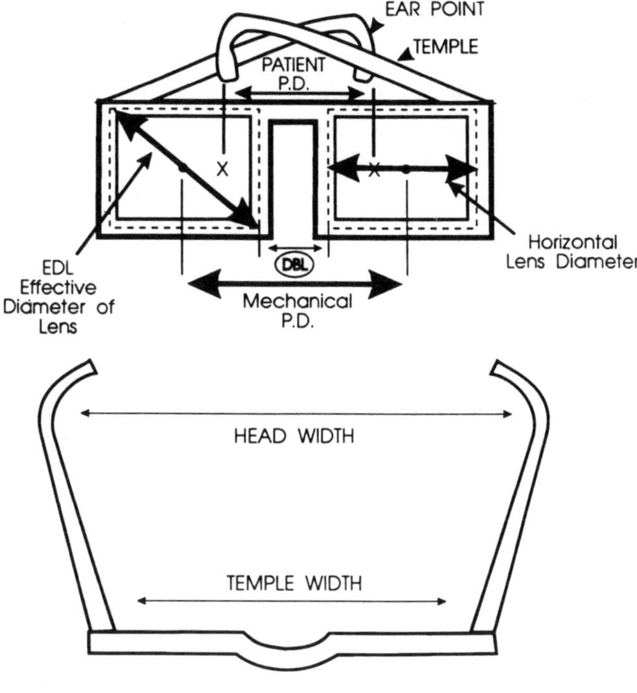

Fig. 12-2

Patient PD = 60 mm
DBL = 22 mm

∴ 38 mm of lens required
19 mm RIGHT and 19 mm LEFT

IF Horizontal lens diameter is 44 mm
the optical centre (OC) if not decentered = 22 mm

∴ a decentration IN of 3 mm of both RIGHT
and LEFT would be required for the
mechanical PD to match the patient s PD°

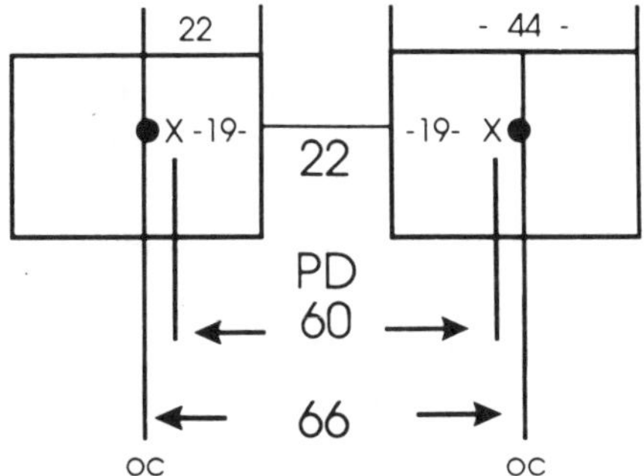

Fig. 12-3

lens blank selected. Matching the PD of the frame to that of the patient minimizes this decentration. This is turn reduces the cost. Conversely, the decentration for intentional prismatic induction has the opposite effects.

The other considerations important in frame selection are features such as the bridge configuration. Whether it projects, indents, or is flat, or whether the frames sit directly on the nose or do so with nose pads are all style selections necessary for the frame to conform to the patient. Newer silicone nosepads are very soft and inert yet resist corrosion, can be adjusted, and are not as slippery when wet as other materials. Adjustable nosepads for high dioptric prescriptions allow vertex distance and segment height adjustments, simplifying the dispenser's job. Children, Asian, blacks, and whites with flat bridges have difficulty with bridge fitting; this can be simplified with nosepads. The downside is that the weight bearing is focused on a small area of nasal skin that in keyhole type configurations would otherwise be distributed over a larger area. This may be poorly tolerated by some patients.

Plastics

Frames can be made of natural or synthetic plastics. *Natural plastics* are materials such as horn, ivory, and tortoiseshell. Species endangerment prohibits their use in most jurisdictions and has led to newer synthetic imitators. The original was not tortoise at all but rather hawksbill turtle. The shell is easily worked and has unique natural properties, including the feature of bonding strongly to itself with the application of heat and pressure. The old sheller's kettle has been replaced with blowers, but the principle is the same. The ease of repair to a damaged frame is a strong feature in its favour. The synthetics attempt to simulate these features.

Synthetic plastic frames are made from a host of plastics. Some common ones are methyl methacrylate (Plexiglas, Lucite), allyl diglycol carbonate (CR-39), cellulose nitrate (Celluloid), cellulose acetate, acrylic resins (Perspex, Optyl), cellulose propionate, nylon, carbon-nylon, and carbon fiber graphite. These can originate as small granules that are heated and then injection moulded or as a molten liquid that is cast in a dye. A solid or laminate can be formed from sheets of the material and shapes cut or pressed to desired configurations.

The first plastic used was *cellulose nitrate* (Celluloid). It is an organic compound utilizing the cellulose from the cell wall of plants. Cotton is the best natural source of cellulose, which must be cleaned and bleached before nitration by the addition of nitric and sulphuric acid. This nitrocellulose is mixed with camphor, which is a natural "plasticizer," giving the substance much of its desirable workability. This dough can then be rolled, pressed or cut as desired. Unfortunately this material is very flammable, limiting its use.

Acetylation of the cellulose with glacial acetic acid and acetic anhydride yields *cellulose acetate.* This necessitates the use of a different plasticizer (phthalate and acetone) but yields a product that is almost as easy to work with as the nitrate but much safer, since it is less flammable. Most plastic frames today are made of cellulose acetate. A pantograph machine cuts the material into the desired eye shape with the appropriate lens groove to hold the lens. The hardware is installed and any refinements necessary are performed. They are then tumbled for 5 days in wooden barrels to achieve a polished sheen. The temples are cut, wires driven, and edges tapered, bevelled, bent, and tumbled for polishing. The temples are mitred to the front and hand assembled, and a final polish is given. Many of the other plastics address one advantage or another but all are compared to cellulose acetate as the standard.

Cellulose propionate is more elastic and shock resistant and weighs 10% less. Acrylic resins are more transparent but more brittle. Copolyamid is more elastic and adjusts more easily to over- and undersized lenses.

Carbon based materials such as carbon fiber graphite and Carbonplus are combinations of carbon, carbon fibers, and nylon. These are the same materials tennis rackets and golf clubs are made of. They are 15% to 25% lighter (depending on the proportions) but more brittle than cellulose acetate. The lenses are mounted similarly to those in metal frames and can be finished with a protective bonded enamel finish. Colour and finish are dramatic, but flexibility and adjustment/ replacement features are more difficult.

Nylon has reentered the market with an improved product that is thinner, stronger, and much easier for lens insertion than the old product. It has an inherent memory lock for any adjustment. It is coloured prior to moulding, and high fashion colours can be achieved (Bolle).

Each year newer and better materials emerge, but nobody is ever quite sure what the dictates of fashion will be. This is true not only of plastics but also of metal frames.

Metals

Metal frames are the most durable product and have many features that make them the first choice of many spectacle wearers.

Gold is corrosion resistant, acid resistant, tarnishes with difficulty, is easily worked, and can be alloyed to change its colour and strength. It is expensive, so attempts to reduce the gold content but maintain its properties have been tried. In view of the great expense, measurement systems to judge the purity and quantity of the precious metal have arisen. One is called the Troy system after the city of Troyes in France. An imperial measure of quantity is the carat, which is 3.16 grains or 205 mg of pure gold. The metric equivalent carat is 200 mg. Fine or pure gold is 24 carat and is used to compare alloyed gold (whose proportion of gold is less than pure) to pure gold (e.g., 12 carat gold is 12/24 or 50% gold and 50% alloy). The same unit to compare both quantity and proportion is, needless to say, quite confusing for the patient and dispenser alike. To make matters worse, gold filled or rolled gold are bronze, nickel, and silver base metals with a thin plate of gold fused by high heat bonding to the surface. These are rolled into wire or strips to work the frame. The gold in these is marked in quantity and quality (e.g., $\frac{1}{10}$ = 18 means one tenth of the weight is 18 carat gold. Other times the measure is parts per thousand: $\frac{75}{1000} = \frac{100}{1000} \times \frac{18}{24} = \frac{1}{10} = 18$ carat. These measures are more to protect the wholesaler/retailer than the patient.

Gold alloys can be with silver, copper, nickel, or zinc, and various proportions alter the strength and colour from white to yellow. Electroplating 0.5 to 4.0 μm of 14 to 24 carat gold is an alternative.

Aluminum is light but loses its strength with bending. It is anodized to alter its surface to the oxide form, which is more resistant. It can be painted or coloured as desired. Since it is a high heat conductor, it gets especially cold in the winter and is best insulated with plastic end covers around the ears.

Titanium is flexible, corrosion resistant, and light with excellent memory retention. It is useful for individuals who sweat and thus corrode their frames quickly. Heat resistance means that it cannot be soldered for working and repairs.

Stainless steel has 74% iron but does not rust. The combination with 18% chromium and 8% nickel made H. Brearley a wealthy man in 1913. It is nonmagnetic, corrosion resistant, and flexible. It can be worked very thin but cannot be soldered because of its heat resistance.

Nickel/silver (formally German silver) has little nickel and no silver! It is 18%

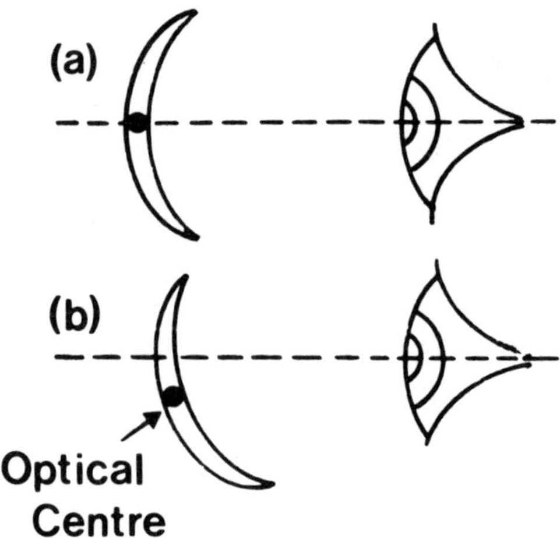

Fig. 12-4

nickel, 64% copper, and 16% zinc. It is useful for eye wires requiring high shock resistance yet little propensity to damage the lens. It can be electroplated with nickel or rhodium for effect.

The selection of which metal is dispensed often is as much an esthetic decision as a functional one.

Occupational and industrial safety frames often specify the tolerances of the type of metal or plastic that are acceptable to that particular industry. Requirements for special temples, sideshields, hinge construction, and bevel configurations may vary according to the needs of the job. The vertical positioning, or the pantoscopic tilt, also is very important when it comes to the position of the optical centers. Fig. 12-4. illustrates the fact that, whenever a lens is tilted down, the visual axis looks through an eccentric position above the optical center. The rule of thumb is that for every 2° of tilt the optical centers must be adjusted 1 mm to compensate for this.

The question arises as to what the most accurate way is to measure the PD. One simple way is measuring with a ruler the distance between the corneal light reflexes fixing a near light; 4 mm is added to the near measurement to give the distance PD. Alternatively the nasal limbus or pupillary border of one eye and the temporal limbus or pupillary border of the other is measured while the patient fixes a distant target.

To measure the vertex distance, a small gauge called the distometer or lenscorometer is used. An adjustment for closed lids is about 1 mm but read the instructions with your instrument. Each refractor has a vertex guide, but over about ±4.00 D an additional measurement independent of this is indicated and should be included on the final prescription notation.

SUMMARY

The sequence of events from the frame selection to the final product is now understandable. In the modern laboratory the frame parameters are received physically or by modem. A computer measures the existing frames or lens for the contour, total circumference, and effective diameter of the lens and selects the correct lens blank to accommodate the prescription. It also measures the lens groove and relays this information not only to the layout section of the lab but also to the edger. In the case of a frame, it can transpose the mirror image of the intact side to create the parameters for the broken side. Similarly, broken or loose lenses can be matched for rimless spectacles and their replacement.

The prescription is then prepared for layout. The program selects the ideal size lens blank (e.g., 71, 76, or 80 mm), and the layout process orients the surface saver tape. At this point a semifinished blank of chosen size has one finished surface and one uncut surface with the layout information imprinted onto the tape. Once the layout is verified, a working block is created by using an alloy with a low melting point that fixes a metal working piece to the finished, protected surface. The alloy must have a melting point less than plastic or glass to prevent any damage to the lens blank. The working block is necessary to fix the lens in position for grinding the uncut back surface and subsequent polishing sequences. It is then forwarded to the generator that works the uncut back surface.

The newer generators work the back curve from plano to −20.00 D. There is now automatic compensation for tangential, sagittal, elliptical, and astigmatic errors for different curves in the higher corrections. The same generators can work both plastic and glass, but the cutting tools require diamond bits of differing grade. As mentioned earlier, the plastic cutters can last 2 years compared to only 1 month for glass cutters. The process generates a crude cut back curve with a blocked, protected, finished front surface.

A mould is then selected to exactly match the back curve. Under water, the surface is ground to finer and finer quality. A velvet surface with a fine polishing compound (for either plastic or glass) is then used to yield the optical quality back surface. The finished blank is then placed in a reclamation tank that heats the blank to 130° F (54° C). The blocking alloy melts at 117° F (47° C), so the alloy is reclaimed in liquid form and recycled to the layout blocking chamber. The surface saver tape is removed and the finished blank is ready for edging.

The computer program that initially selected the blank now selects the final edging parameters. This process, when done manually (e.g., polycarbonate), requires the selection of a "former," which is a template of the selected frame style. From this template the edge is ground with the former as a guide. Features such as a hide-a-bevel edge can be programmed to be performed automatically.

A finished blank with the final shape and correct bevel is now in hand. A hand wheel is used to chamfer any sharp edges that remain. The lens is dyed or tinted if desired. This is followed by heat or chemical tempering. The lens is then cleaned by an exacting ultrasonic process until particle free. The antiscratch coat is applied (if desired), as is a metallic mirror finish. The multilayer antireflection coating is then applied. A wash coat or superphobic treatment is added. The lens is mounted in the frame. If holes in the lens are required, they are drilled before chemical tempering. Any engraving or decorative decals are added.

The finished, mounted lenses and frames are then adjusted to suit the temple width and head width. The nose pads (if present) are adjusted to obtain the correct vertex distance and segment height. The prescription is verified and the lenses inspected for defects or deformities. If the quality is within the limits of tolerance, the finished product is given to the patient.

Buying glasses is like buying a car. You always end up paying more than you expected to, and everything seems to be extra, e.g., tints, coatings, mirror finishing. As a prescriber one must always consider whether a change in prescription warrants these costs. It is always useful to demonstrate the refractive change with loose lenses over the current prescription to determine if the patient feels it is a significant change relative to the anticipated costs. Changes for cosmetic, damage, or insurance reasons do not bear the same degree of scrutiny, but if there is little anticipated benefit the patient should be clearly told this fact.

The quality of the finished product depends on the standards and rejection rates of the dispensing laboratory. Some patients are willing to accept seconds for reduced costs; others are not. When a mistake has been made, a careful examination of the product will usually reveal the responsible professional. It is the financial responsibility of the party at fault to rectify the problem to the patient's satisfaction. For a patient having problems with a recently prescribed pair of lenses, the following guidelines may be of assistance:

1. Neutralize the lenses with the lensmeter. Check if any prism is incorporated. Mark the optical centers. Recheck the original prescription and compare it to the old glasses if they are available. Reverse the glasses to measure the add in high powered lenses.
2. Put the glasses on the patient. Take the visual acuity monocularly and binocularly. Check motility for induced phorias at distance. Check the position of the segment to determine if it is too high or too low, whether centered or decentered correctly, and whether a phoria or tropia is present in the reading position. Check the pantoscopic tilt and vertex distance. Measure the patient's PD and compare to the mechanical PD. Assess the appropriateness of the style. Compare old to new base curves with the lens clock.
3. If the vision is not as expected, retinoscope over the present lenses and subjectively refine this refraction. Measure the final combination in the lensmeter. Recheck the visual acuity. Give a "walking around" trial if a change is to be made.

Please see Part II: Problems and Part III: Solutions for typical examination questions pertaining to the material in this chapter.

CHAPTER 13: CONTACT LENSES

Contact lenses have been mentioned time and again as a method that eliminates many of the optical problems associated with spectacles. Many excellent texts and fitting manuals deal with the actual fitting of contacts, but few deal with the optical considerations that are the basis of this mode of correction. What follows is an attempt to explain the theory and not the actual fitting aspects of contacts, although the former is extremely valuable when it comes to fitting, especially when the first trial lens doesn't fit.

ADVANTAGES AND DISADVANTAGES

Consider the optical advantages of contacts over spectacles. Cosmetically there is no doubt that they are superior and hence their popularity with young and active women and men. They don't fog in changing environments and they don't fall off or break with simple activities like stooping or bending. The fact that they move with ocular excursions means that the optical center of the lens follows the visual axis. For activities such as sports, eye movement can supplant head movement for optimum acuity. This phenomenon also eliminates the induced prismatic and spherical aberrations associated with spectacle eccentric viewing. If fitted with a proper optical zone, the aperture through which clear viewing is obtained is no longer limited by the size of the spectacle lens or frame, so the viewing field is enlarged. The reduction in vertex distance reduces magnification and minification and their subsequent aniseikonic effects on retinal imagery. The correction of astigmatism in this plane virtually eliminates the distortion effects previously noted. Reduced accommodation demands in hyperopia may offer a temporary reprieve, delaying the need for bifocals or near correction. Irregular corneal astigmatism can benefit from the new surface the lens induces, and even regular astigmatism can be eliminated or ameliorated from cylindrical incorporation onto the lens.

Just as in life, there is always the other side of the coin to consider. Lenses move and decenter with lid movement, which may affect the lens curvature and the position of the optical zone. Since the lens is on the corneal surface, the oxygenation and the metabolism of the cornea are affected, which may induce changes in corneal thickness and epithelial regularity. The cornea may mold to the curvature of the lens and in so doing temporarily alter its power. When the lens is removed and glasses worn, the vision is not perfectly corrected until the old corneal curvature, for which the spectacle was prescribed, is regained. This leads to spectacle blur for a variable amount of time. If the lens itself is not of perfect quality, it may warp and induce astigmatism that did not exist before. If the astigmatism is corrected on the cornea, the rotation and movement of the lens vary the axis of correction and may not provide stable vision. If the refractive error is very high, as with monocular aphakia, the aniseikonia might not all be corrected and the condition improved but not eliminated. Being applied to the body surface, it is an antigenic substance which can interact with the immune mechanism to cause problems. It can also act as a focus of infective organisms and the site of deposition for proteins, salts, and mucus. In other words, although an excellent mode of correction, it is not the panacea to all refractive woes.

The lenses are classified as to the material and oxygen permeability characteristics of the lens. Primarily this encompasses hard lenses, gas permeable or semipermeable lenses, and soft lenses. Hard lenses are polymethylmethacrylate (PMMA). This plastic polymer has less than 3% water content and is virtually oxygen impermeable. Oxygen transmission to the cornea is thus dependent upon the tear exchange, which occurs beneath the lens. Silicone derivatives and cellulose acetate butyrate (CAB) lenses are more oxygen permeable but have fewer desirable optical characteristics than hard lenses, especially in the case of silicone. Newer derivatives have markedly improved wetability, gas permeability, and optical quality. Less adaption time is required, but since the lenses are small, contact with the lids is about the same as with hard lenses. This factor, and not the water content, is the major determinant of patient comfort (or lack thereof). Soft lenses are made of hydroxymethacrylate (HEMA) and related polymers and have a water content that can vary from 25% to 80%, depending on the type of lens and the manufacturer. High water content and ultrathin varieties are suitable for extended wear; ultrathins may also be disposable.

FITTING AND DESIGN

Before dealing with different types of lenses available, it is useful to review a few essential principles about contact lens fitting and design. The ultimate aim of these lenses is to adapt to the contour of the anterior corneal surface in such a way as to neutralize the eye error in the ametropic state. To achieve this end, the original contours must be known. From our clinical armamentarium one knows that the keratometer will provide these data, but in dioptric form. Recall that the relationship from which keratometry is derived is the refracting power of a smooth refracting surface:

$$D_s = \frac{n' - n}{r}$$

where: $n' = 1.3375$ for the cornea

$n = 1.00$ for air

The refracting power is the K reading

$$K = \frac{1.3375 - 1}{r} = \frac{0.3375}{r}$$

(Note: $n' = 1.3375$ is the index used for calibration in keratometry.)

This illustrates the crucial relationship that exists between the K reading and the radius of curvature. Consider the information in the following box:

K	**Radius of curvature (mm)**	
40.00 D	8.434	Flatter
42.00 D	8.036	
45.00 D	7.500	
48.00 D	7.031	Steeper

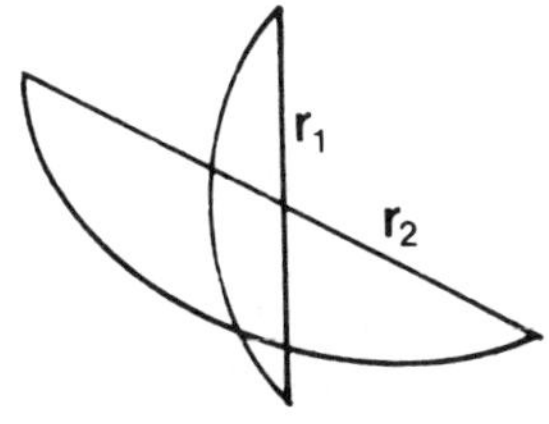

Fig. 13-1

Depicted diagrammatically in Fig. 13-1, a toroidal surface is transcribed with the meridian of steepest curvature being the most convex and hence having the greatest refractive power. In this way one has a contour map by radii of curvature of the front surface of the cornea.

These readings are in meridional power. Recall:

K 40 @ 90 = 40 × 180	Eye error
48 @ 180 = 48 × 90	= +8.00 × 90

This corresponds to the eye error in plus cylinder form. If a contact lens smoothed out this surface, some of the astigmatism would be eliminated. This would be equivalent to adding minus cylinder at that axis. The convention for contact lenses is to express all spherocylinders in minus cylinder form. This is also one reason why cylinder is ground on the back surface of the contact lens. In this way complementary contouring adds to the stability of the lens about the correcting axis.

Unfortunately, this contour applies only to the central few millimeters of the cornea or about one third of the corneal surface. As the less apical portions of the cornea are approached, the radii of curvature begin to lengthen as if to physiologically correct for spherical aberration. This change must be taken into account when fitting a less flexible lens such as a hard or a gas permeable lens. This gives rise to the different zones that are spoken of in reference to hard lenses (Fig. 13-2).

The posterior optical zone is constructed to conform to the central corneal contour as outlined above. The peripheral curves adjust for the radii of curvature in the periphery. The junctions of the three different curves are called blends. These can be adjusted to blend to the natural changing radii.

It is therefore evident that if the posterior surface is responsible for fitting and minus cylinder application, the front surface curvature is the major power variable. To this surface plus cylinder can also be ground, making the correction of

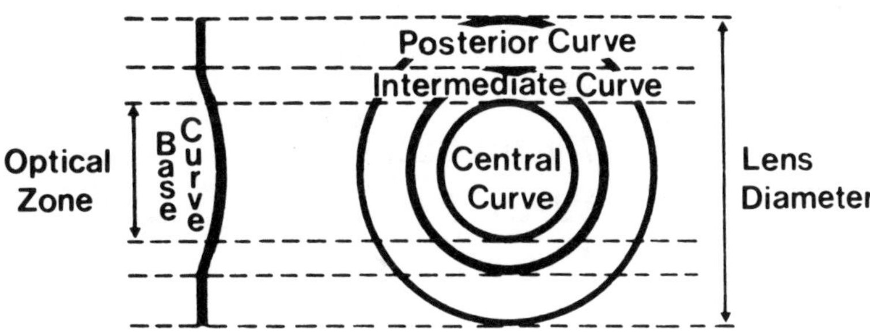

Fig. 13-2

even more astigmatism possible (at 90° to the minus cylinder, of course). The size of the optical zone is such that it will not limit the natural aperture—the pupil. The curvature of the posterior optical zone must be such that it forms a meniscus lens (of a certain thickness and index of refraction [1.49]) with the chosen anterior central curve to obtain the power of the lens desired.

This method of fitting hard or rigid gas permeable contacts is called *fitting on K*, where the flattest *K* (lowest *D*, longest radius) is used and the lens fitted parallel to it. If one looks back again at Fig. 13-1, it becomes evident that if a rigid sphere of radius r_2 (i.e., the longest or flattest radius) were placed over this surface, the tears would fill in the difference so that the combined surface would approach a sphere of radius r_2. A minus cylinder effect occurs. The problem with this technique is that the lens touches the epithelial surface for its entire radius. This doesn't allow adequate tear exchange and causes edema, moulding, and secondary spectacle blur from inadequate oxygenation. Clinical experience shows that, if the lens is fitted 0.50 to 1.00 D steeper than the flattest *K*, the corneal apex is just cleared and a much better physiologic exchange occurs. When this is done, tears fill this space and create an additional refracting meniscus, which will alter the power. If the lens is steeper than the cornea (Fig. 13-3, *a*), a plus tear meniscus is formed that will require less plus or more minus power in the contact lens. The mnemonic for this is SAM (steeper add minus). With a flat lens a minus tear meniscus is formed, requiring more plus or less minus power (Fig. 13-3, *b*). The mnemonic here is FAP (flatter add plus).

The rule of thumb is that for every 0.05 mm change in radius, an adjustment of 0.25 D in the appropriate direction must be made. If one is fitting 1.00 D steeper than the flattest *K*, the posterior curve must be $0.05 \times 4 = 0.2$ mm steeper and the lens prescribed must be changed by 1.00 D.

The beauty of a hard lens is that it can be reground and altered to custom fit a given patient. The peripheral curves can be blended, the optical zones widened, and the lens steepened or flattened (within limits) as required. The lens can also be fenestrated (by lasering or drilling small holes) to augment tear and oxygen exchange.

If both meridians are the same radius, the lens is *spherical*. If cylinder is ground on the back surface, it is a *back toric* lens. In addition to this, if cylinder is added to the front surface, the lens is *bitoric*. If lenticular astigmatism is present with a spherical cornea, cylinder can be added to the front surface and a *front toric* LENS is obtained. The axis of the cylinder is unstable with a free spin on the cornea, since there is no "lock and key" effect of matching different radii of curvature

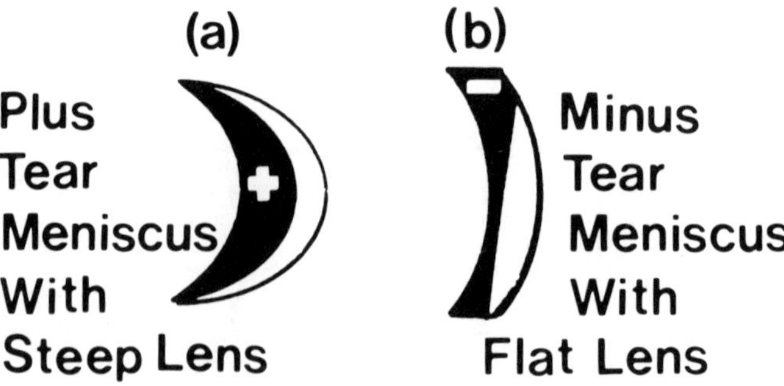

Fig. 13-3

between the lens and the cornea. About 1.5 to 2 P.D. base down can be added to *prism ballast* the lens so that the prism weight will orient the lens by gravity. The image displacement, if equal in both eyes, is no problem. The lens can also be *truncated* so that the portion of the lens which follows the axis of the lower lid angle is removed. This stabilizes the lens in the desired axis. These methods are illustrated in Fig. 13-4.

It is also appreciated that this can be done for any lens which is rotating excessively. Some bifocal contact designs use these principles for stabilizing the position of the segment.

The spherical power of the lens can also be altered a small amount by regrinding. Once the curves are established, a little less plus or more minus can be ground, but the addition of plus sphere is very limited. A lens might have to be reground to achieve the same fitting characteristics.

Often the power of the sphere causes weight and edge changes that can be anticipated. A plus lens of high power will be center heavy and ride low on the cornea. Conversely, a high minus lens will have thick edges that can be trapped by the upper lid and pulled up, causing it to ride high. In a plus lens a minus carrier will add edge thickness, which will elevate the lens (Fig. 13-5, *a*). This is referred to as *myoflange*. The edges of a high minus lens can be thinned to form a *lenticular bevel* (Fig. 13-5, *b*).

Problems with movement and centration are often the result of a poor relationship between the diameter of the lens and the radii of curvature. This concept is integral to fitting both hard and soft lenses. In Fig. 13-6, *a*, the radius of curvature remains constant, but the chord diameter is increased and the apical vault of the lens increases (i.e., it becomes a steeper lens). Conversely, if the diameter remains the same, the lens is made steeper by decreasing the radius of curvature, which increases the apical vault (Fig. 13-6, *b*). To steepen a lens, the diameter is

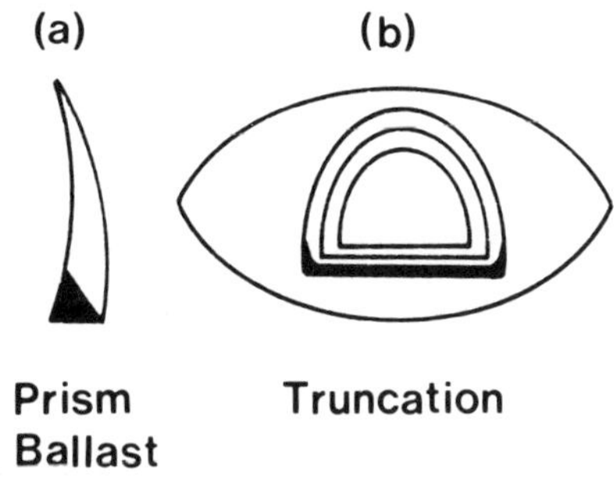

Fig. 13-4

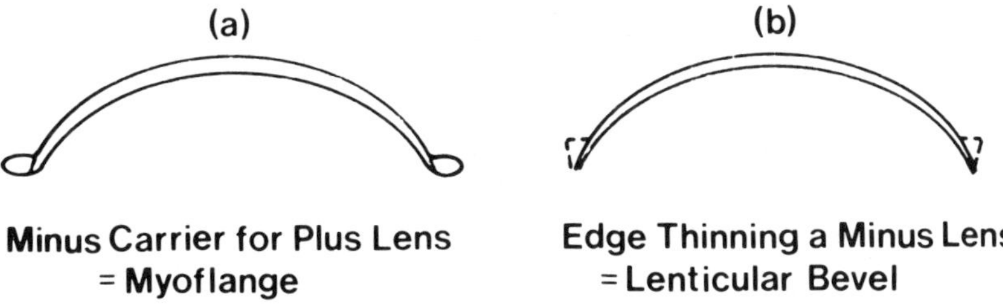

Fig. 13-5

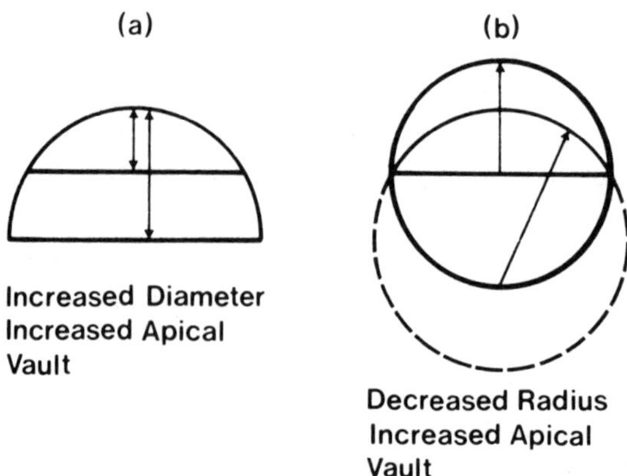

Fig. 13-6

increased, the radius of curvature is decreased, or both. To flatten a lens, the diameter is decreased, the radius of curvature is increased, or both.

The fluorescein pattern under hard lenses and the clinical biomicroscopic appearance of hard and soft lenses will determine in which direction a lens must be changed to optimize the fit. In the assessment of old contact lenses one must be wary of fitting and power changes. With age, the polymers become more rigid and altered from their initial fitting criteria. Corneal changes may be induced, and refractive errors may be temporarily or permanently altered in any direction. Prescribing new lenses or spectacles is not recommended until adequate time has elapsed for stabilization. The power of a minus lens may be changed from the pressure of the lids on a thin central optical zone over a long period of time. This flattening effect may alter centration, vision, and metabolic requirements causing problems for the patient. Often a new lens of the old prescription dimensions is all that is required.

CONSIDERATIONS IN CHOICE OF LENSES

Soft lenses are not only more comfortable for the patient but considerably easier to fit. The only two variables involved are the diameter and radius of curvature of the lens. The diameter is so large to compensate for the high apical vault, the radius of curvature must be increased. This means that the lens must fit flatter than *K* to optimize the fit to the corneal contour. This usually is 2.00 to 3.00 D flatter than the flattest *K* but varies from one manufacturer to the next. Basically the flattest lens capable of good centration and vision is the most desirable end-point. As the water content increases and the thickness decreases, the lens becomes so malleable that it adapts to almost any corneal contour and even the radius of curvature of the lens approaches a "one size fits all." This requires little fitting skill, and virtually anyone can fit this type of lens.

One price to be paid is the virtual absence of astigmatic correction. Since the lens adapts to the corneal contour, whatever regular corneal astigmatism was there beforehand remains with the lens in place. One fortunate aspect, however, is the conversion of surface-induced irregular astigmatism to regular astigmatism. This is quite useful in many conditions such as keratoconus and can even be combined piggyback with an overlying hard lens to correct the residual regular astigmatism. Some of the lower water content (25% to 40%) lenses are firm enough that minor amounts (0.50 to 0.75 D) of astigmatism might be corrected.

The bottom line is that regular soft lenses are not effective in the treatment of anything but spherical ametropia. Under certain circumstances (which are exceptional) patients are willing to accept residual astigmatism and 20/50 vision to have the comfort and low price of standard soft lenses. Generally, a good philosophy is that comfort is the patient's responsibility and vision is the fitter's. One also must keep the driving standard in mind if this is a consideration.

Newer developments in soft toric lenses have considerably eased this burden. One now has the comfort of a soft lens with the power to correct corneal and lenticular astigmatism. Prism ballast and truncation help orient the lens along its axis. The lid angle becomes an important measurement that can easily be accomplished with the cylinder axis on a refractor or trial frame. These lenses are fitted a little steeper than a regular soft lens, so they appear marginally tight. This further decreases lens rotation and helps stabilize the axis. As lens designs improve, these are certainly becoming more popular with both the public and fitters alike.

Generally, the least amount of plastic that maximizes both vision and comfort seems to be ideal. With the increased prevalence of lens- and preservative-induced sensitivity reactions, this consideration also minimizes these problems.

The principles of extended wear lenses are identical to those of high water content and ultrathin lenses. The onus of responsibility for maintenance, however, falls more on the fitter instead of the patient. Since the optical stability of these lenses is so closely allied to their water content, the vision tends to be more variable.

With all types of lenses the final power should be obtained by overrefraction techniques with a similar power trial lens. If this is not available, compensation for the vertex distance is required. As already noted, the prescription is always converted to minus cylinder form. Some practitioners use the sphere to select the lens power in hard lenses and the spherical equivalent for soft lenses. Alterations in steepness and flatness must be considered according to the 0.05 mm = 0.25 D relationship. To illustrate these points consider the following example.

An aphakic patient desires a contact lens. Her spectacle correction is $+11.00 + 2.00 \times 90$ at vertex distance 10 mm. *K* readings are 42.0×45.0 horizontally and vertically. What power of contact lens is required and at what base curve if a hard lens is chosen that is 1.00 D steeper than *K*?

$$+11.00 + 2.00 \times 90 + = 13.00 - 2.00 \times 180 \text{ vertex} \times 10 \text{ mm}$$

(Ignore the cylinder and use only the sphere.)

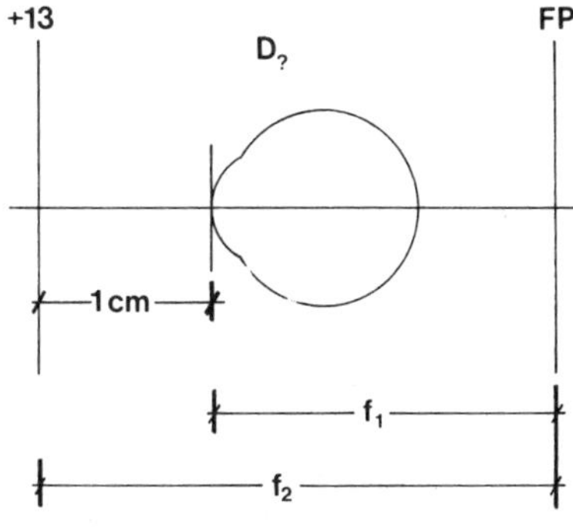

Fig. 13-7

At vertex 10 mm = 1 cm $\quad f_2 = 100/13 = 7.69$ cm

At the corneal plane vertex = 0 $\quad f_1 = \dfrac{100}{7.69 - 1} = \dfrac{100}{6.69} = +14.95$ D

At 1.00 D steeper add −1.00 (SAM): +14.95 − 1.00 = +13.95 D

$$D = \frac{1.3375 - 1}{r} \quad r = \frac{1.3375 - 1}{D} = \frac{0.3375}{D}$$

(Flattest K = 42.00 D,
1.00 steeper = 43.00 D)

$$r = \frac{0.3375}{43} = 7.84 \text{ mm}$$

(Remember the corneal index used to standardize the keratometer is 0.3375 and *not* 0.376, which is usually taken as the n for the cornea.)

Alternatively, using K = 42.00 D $\quad r = \dfrac{0.3375}{42} = 8.04$ mm

Since 0.25 D = 0.05 mm change in radius

For 1.00 D steeper = 0.25 × 4

0.05 mm × 4 = 0.20 mm change in the radius

8.04 − 0.20 = 7.84 mm (A 7.84 mm/+13.95 D lens is required.)

In addition to changes in specifications of the power, diameter, and base curve, one will often switch a patient from rigid PMMA to gas permeable or soft toric contact lenses. The cornea requires oxygen and glucose for its demands of oxidative metabolism to "run the pumps" for corneal clarity. There are many new materials of higher oxygen permeability than PMMA. These gas permeable substances are often silicone based and permeable not only to oxygen but also to carbon dioxide products of aerobic respiration. The relative gas permeability depends on the diffusion (D) and solubility (K) of oxygen. This gives the *DK value* that is often quoted in comparing contacts of varying materials.

DK = Diffusion coefficient × Solubility of oxygen in the material

Quite naturally a thicker plus lens would have a lesser DK than a thinner minus lens. The thickness factor (L) gives an index of *oxygen transmissibility* $\left(\dfrac{DK}{L}\right)$. The partial pressure of oxygen across the lens will also influence the oxygen flux at the corneal level. This becomes important in air transport, where partial pressures of oxygen are reduced relative to ground level. This gives the "red eye special" if the flight duration overwhelms the corneal compensatory mechanisms.

The *oxygen flux* $= \dfrac{DK}{L} \times \Delta P$.

ΔP is the partial pressure of oxygen on each side of the lens. Very little glucose diffuses through the lens, so the corneal integrity depends on the aqueous delivery of glucose. The tear contribution to oxygen and glucose cannot be forgotten.

Other newer extended wear materials have high *DK* values. If they are ultrathin, the *DK* need only be very close to daily wear lenses. If they are thicker but of a material with a higher *DK* value, they often are high water content lenses. Evaporation tends to alter water content between blinks, which may degrade the visual acuity. Their use for extended wear is somewhat controversial. Many extended wear or disposable lenses are "one size fits all" ultrathin, large diameter lenses. They are worn for 5 to 7 days and then disposed of. Exposure to no preservatives makes this lens popular in the sensitive subset of contact lens wearers. One must always be selective in the type of individual fitted with these lenses. The natural bias is for people who wish to neglect contact lens care, and soon 5-day wear translates to 15-day wear. Newer rigid gas permeable lenses are approaching *DK* values suitable for extended wear as well.

Custom lenses manufactured from corneal topography data will undoubtedly meet the needs of the special lenses for irregularly shaped corneas (e.g., Eye Sys). Patients with cosmetic corneal disfigurement can even have a painted prosthesis, cosmetic contact lens, or scleral shell matched to the opposite eye by computer mirror imaging.

The other realm of extended wear is *bandage* contact lens wear. These lenses are traditionally extended wear ultrathin lenses or new collagen lenses. They can be drug soaked. The collagen lenses literally melt away after a predetermined time, e.g., 12 hours. They can replace a patch or be used for other therapeutic means, depending on the circumstances.

One error patients often commit is to think that distilled water is sterile. This was especially prominent when homemade saline with salt tablets was in common usage. Newer ultrasonic, ultraviolet, and microwavable contacts will often further alternatives to the contact lens wearer sensitive to preservatives. One has to reflect on what therapeutic drugs in the future will be precluded by such preservative sensitivities. Many vaccines for hepatitis, influenza, tetanus, and meningitis are preserved with thimerosal and cannot be used without desensitization. Many topical antibiotics, antivirals, and ocular hypotensive drugs are similarly preserved and may pose serious problems for these patients in the future.

Please see Part II: Problems and Part III: Solutions for typical examination questions pertaining to the material in this chapter.

CHAPTER 14: LOW VISION, PENALIZATION, MALINGERING

LOW VISION AIDS

The principles of spectacle and contact lens correction are applicable not only to those patients who can achieve normal visual acuity but also to those with subnormal vision. *Low vision aids* employ these principles to maximize the discriminatory ability of these patients such that normal or near normal functioning is obtained in everyday circumstances. Optical manipulation of the visual angle, accommodation, magnification, and visual demands are all principles that can be employed when dealing with this population.

The central vision may be disrupted by many disorders that reduce the sensitivity or increase the threshold for visual resolution. This is manifest by an increased visual angle required to discriminate visual stimuli and, as usual, is expressed as the Snellen fraction. Another useful device for this very central visual area is the Amsler grid, which tests the central horizontal and vertical 10° of visual field for evidence of central disruption. A study on peripheral visual acuity (eccentricity from the fovea) was performed by Randal, Brown, and Sloan (Peripheral visual acuity, *Arch Ophthalmol* 75:500-504, 1966). Fig. 14-1 depicts their results as they would correlate with an Amsler grid projected onto the posterior pole of an eye. As the distance from the foveola increases, the visual acuity naturally decreases, but not nearly as rapidly as one would expect. Thus a patient with a very focal central lesion may still maintain very good visual acuity. The fixation reflex cannot be changed binocularly. Under monocular conditions, eccentric viewing can achieve these enhanced parafoveal acuities. This often requires some degree of vision training to achieve.

Peripheral vision field defects may result from neurologic, retinal, or glaucomatous optic nerve problems. If the defect approaches fixation, magnification may adversely affect vision by projecting the image into scotomatous regions of the field. Under these circumstances a fine balance between the required and practical magnification is encountered. Retinal degenerations such as retinitis pigmentosa may affect night (scotopic) more than day (photopic) vision secondary to the site of affliction, i.e., rods greater than cones. This can be helped with special night vision aids. Often these patients have restricted fields from rod deficits and central visual loss from cystoid macular edema. This presents an intricate balance with magnification devices similar to that noted above.

When considering the visual aids available, the major concern is with methods that increase the angular magnification as subtended at the nodal point of the eye. The visual angle can be increased either physically or optically. The act of bringing an object closer or making it larger increases the visual angle in a linear fash-

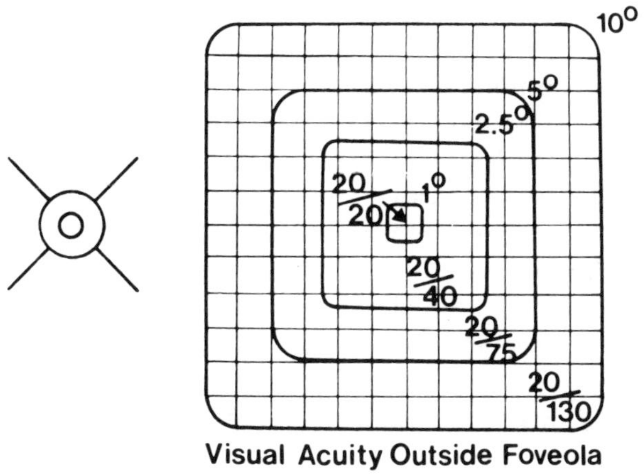

Fig. 14-1

ion. If the standard Snellen letter is brought from 20 feet to 4 feet, it subtends an angle five times as large. Similarly, if it were increased to five times its size at 20 feet, it would also subtend an angle five times as large. These effects are readily appreciable to the low vision patient who is helped greatly by bringing material closer to the eye and using large print materials. Optically, the visual angle can be increased by either simple magnifiers or loupes and telescopes, depending on the visual requirements.

The selection of the type and power of the visual aid depends on the motivation of the patient, visual ability and acuity of each eye, and the visual demands for near and distance. The actual examination and available materials are well summarized by Eleanor Faye (In Safir A, ed.: *Refraction and clinical optics,* New York, 1980, Harper & Row). The optical principles will be reviewed for some selected approaches and visual aids.

For near visual improvement consideration must be given to the age and accommodative amplitude of the patient. Children often have more than 10.00 to 12.00 D of accommodation. They can comfortably accommodate to very near objects such as fine print up to and beyond 20 cm. This functions as a simple magnifier by adding not only more plus power but by increasing the angular subtense. Once a person reaches the teens, however, the amplitude recedes to about 10.00 D, and fatigue and asthenopia must be relieved with bifocal adds to maintain half the accommodative amplitude in reserve.

Reading adds of course depend on the visual demands of the patient, but several general guidelines are applicable. If the visual acuity is reduced greater than two lines in one eye compared to the other, consideration must be given to monocular correction. The disparity of retinal imagery would otherwise present bothersome visual confusion. Similarly, there are limits to convergence that must be considered when prescribing strong reading adds. Recall that at 10 cm not only 10.00 D of accommodation are required but also 10 meter angles of convergence. If the PD is 60 mm, the convergence required is 10 meter angles $\times$ 6 cm = 60 P.D. of convergence. This can be augmented by base in prism (e.g., 12 P.D. base in with +10.00 D Aolite half glasses), but 48 P.D. of convergence is still required. This is about the limit for binocular correction. Naturally, once monocular correction is decided on, the material can be brought straight up along the visual axis requiring no convergence, i.e., effectively dissociating accommodation from convergence.

The amount of initial add to be prescribed can be estimated by Kestenbaum's rule. This states that the reversed Snellen fraction in diopters will correct near vision to J_6 or 20/50 visual acuity if given as an add. (Recall the reversed Snellen fraction is the visual angle.) This is the amount required to read average newsprint. If finer or coarser visual requirements are needed, the power of the add is adjusted accordingly. For example, a 20/400 patient would require 400/20 = + 20.00 D of near add to comfortably read newsprint. This is a 20/4 = 5× simple magnifier. Spectacle correction in this form has the disadvantage of having a very close reading distance, but it also provides a large field with two free hands. Any add greater than +6.00 D is a special order, which makes it more expensive commercially. A trial with a Fresnel Press-On segment will decide if it is worth the price to make this a permanent form of correction.

Many older people find reading at very close distances aesthetically and functionally unacceptable. They much prefer a hand-held or stand magnifier (if arthritis or Parkinsonism precludes steady fixation). Although a reduced field results and one hand is lost to function, it affords adequate magnification for essential and leisure tasks. A +20.00 D aspheric lens makes an excellent 5× magnifier and when held close to the eye, can double as a makeshift monocular reading glass.

Spectacle-mounted telescopes with adds over the objective lens are the equivalent to a surgical loupe. This can have a variable focal length adjustment. The major advantage is the more distant reading distance but at a major cosmetic price. The enhanced distance vision is ideal for students requiring both hands free for note taking. Most prefer the small and inconspicuous pocket telescopes that can be rapidly extracted when required.

An interesting Galilean telescope can be created by an uncorrected aphakic patient with a +4.00 D or +5.00 D lens held at 17 or 12 cm. The eye error is equivalent to an eyepiece lens. This is a nice and easily portable telescope for such a patient. A similar situation could be introduced with a high minus contact lens (e.g., −40.00 D) and a +25.00 D spectacle lens at vertex distance of 15 mm with a bifocal segment. This would be equivalent to spectacle-mounted telescopes with built-in near correction. The same disadvantages of reduced field and depth of focus would exist and mobility would be reduced.

Mention should also be made of the many nonoptical devices such as enlarged telephone dials, increased ambient light levels, and felt tip pens that make life so much easier for the partially sighted.

Night vision infrared range-finder scopes can aid any patient with some remaining rod and cone function in scotopic ambulation. Vertically divided horizontal prisms can help hemianopic patients fix objects in their blind field by displacing them into their seeing field with only a slight ocular excursion.

As in the other areas of ophthalmology, technology has advanced for low vision aids. Computerized reading devices that work by optical character recognition are capable of reading the written page for those unable to benefit from any other low vision aid. Based on Kurzweil technology, these readers have markedly expanded the world of the previously Braille-dependent reader.

Closed circuit television offers a choice of magnification and polarity (white on black versus black on white). This will often make an otherwise impossible reading task possible. It is most useful for use at work to maintain one's ability to function in a normal work environment. Many new telescopic systems have been introduced using newer principles of field enhancement and cosmetics. One is the Amorphic Lens System (Feinbloom). This is a spectacle-mounted telescopic system that minifies the 180° meridian but maintains the vertical perspective. This increases the horizontal field, facilitating awareness of peripheral objects.

The partially sighted often miss driving a car most. The dependence that ensues is a major psychologic factor in visual impairment. Bioptic telescopic spectacles have a bioptic telescope used for driving mounted in the superior portion of a carrier plastic distance spectacle lens. The telescope is used for spotting purposes only and is available in 2.2×, 3×, and 4× magnification. The field of view varies from 6° to 16°. Many states will grant a restricted license to those individuals with 20/40 to 20/70 vision in the better eye with an intact 140° or more of horizontal field of vision. Needless to say, this is a very controversial aspect of low vision therapy.

Other new spectacle-mounted systems include the Bilevel Telescopic Apparatus (BITA—Edwards Optical), Behind the Lens Telescope (Coatings Technology), Micro Spiral Galilean Telescope (Designs for Vision), Vision Enhancing System, (Ocutech), and others. One potential problem is the safety concern if the telescope is thrust posteriorly into the eye. The reduced transmission of light available for seeing through miniaturized optics is another concern. Patient preference will most likely increase the demand for these despite their current high costs.

A new hand-held, 6× monocular telescope by Nikon offers a 7.5° field of view for distance and 32.8° for near in a 3-inch × 2-inch box.

Highly antireflective, hard coated, and aspheric hand-held magnifiers by Zeiss are maximizing hand-held magnifier technology.

The traditional white cane can now have a sonar-type sensor that audibly relates distances by frequency modulation.

Experimental brain implants, similar in principle to cochlear implants, are offering a form of vision previously unthinkable even a few short years ago. The hope that these developments inspire is one of the greatest gifts we can give our blind and partially sighted patients.

PENALIZATION

A reverse situation exists where distance or near vision is purposefully worsened to treat mild to moderate amblyopia. This technique is called *penalization.*

In a child whose amblyopia is not too profound, the good eye can be cyclopleged with atropine and corrected for distance, while the amblyopic eye remains with intact accommodation. Since the majority of a young child's life revolves around near vision, the amblyopic eye is employed maximally. The continued use of the good eye for distance vision guarantees against the creation of an occlusion amblyopia. Some recent evidence suggests impaired accommodation in amblyopia, and some authors propose the use of a bifocal for the amblyopic eye. Don't forget the ultraviolet filter in the glasses if cycloplegia and mydriasis are present.

Similarly, in an older child the good eye can be fogged with plus lenses until distance fixation is maintained with the amblyopic eye.

A very sensitive indication and titration method is one employed by David Guyton. With polarizing lenses on, the AO Vectographic Chart is presented to the patient. Only the letters with the fixing eye are seen. When adequate fogging is achieved, a very abrupt change in fixation is manifest by the other set of letters suddenly appearing. Often only ±0.25 D will interchange this endpoint. Once this is determined, confidence that fixation will continue with the amblyopic eye is heightened. A small piece of tape behind the fogged lens may aid the patient in switching fixation.

The obvious cosmetic advantages of penalization are welcomed by parent and child alike. Some occlusion failures are salvaged by this technique, and maintenance therapy is often facilitated. These advantages, as well as the benefit in latent nystagmus patients, are well summarized by Cibis (Penalization treatment of ARC and amblyopia *Am Orthopt J* 25:79-84, 1975).

HYSTERIA AND MALINGERING

Another unique situation exists when low visual acuities seem inexplicable and uncorrectable by all forms of regular and low vision aids. This occurs in *hysteria* and *malingering.* The unifying concept in both entities is that of secondary gain. Hysteria is a psychoneurosis in which internal psychologic conflict cannot be adequately dealt with by employing ordinary defense mechanisms. A hysterical conversion reaction occurs, which focuses these anxieties in a fashion such that a secondary gain in the form of care and sympathy from family or state is derived. Paralysis and blindness are common manifestations and are characterized by *la belle indifference,* whereby the patient is seemingly unconcerned about an otherwise devastating physical predicament. This is amenable to psychotherapy.

Malingerers, on the other hand, are often sociopathic or have inadequate personality disorders often obvious from the first encounter. They seek some kind of financial gain from state, insurance, or litigational circumstances and are often very astute at any attempt to discredit their claims. These individuals are not often rehabilitatable let alone treatable. Since sound documentation is often their nemesis, a solid understanding of a few testing procedures is necessary.

Probably the most reliable method of diagnosis is not a single test but a composite of behavioral, objective, and subjective testing, which is inconsistent with the claimed amount of visual loss.

Functional or hysterical patients, aside from their indifference, are inordinately cavalier in manipulating their physical environment. Despite their apparent blindness, they seldom bump into things or sustain falls or accidents as a truly blind individual might in a strange environment. Conversely, a malingerer makes it a point to hit everything in his path with an attitude approaching reckless abandon. A truly blind individual approaches new surroundings cautiously and frequently waits for assistance in unfamiliar grounds.

Spatial perception and bodily appreciation such as finger to finger touching and finger to nose testing are intact in truly blind individuals.

With a normal ophthalmologic exam, including pupillary responses, menacing reflexes, optokinetic nystagmus, and visual fields, the diagnosis of blindness is tenuous. A classic hysterical tubular field that is the same size at 1 and 2 m defies normal angular magnification principles. Similarly, acuity that fails to improve with larger or closer targets is highly suspect.

If uniocular disease is feigned, AO Vectographic testing may reveal discrepancies unless the patient is clever enough to quickly alternate occlusion. Similarly, near stereotesting may show a disproportionate amount of stereopsis. Fogging the good eye with plus sphere should be accompanied by decreased distance but not very near acuity. A plus and minus 6.00 D cylinder in front of the bad eye will cause no effect if oriented in the same axis. If off axis, blurring will occur. The patient is asked to turn the dial until vision is clearest. If consistent neutralization occurs, both eyes are being used. With red-green glasses a Worth 4 Dot test should reveal a side preference.

H.S. Thompson uses the red-green glasses with a pink highlighter pen. Letters or pictures of any size can be drawn and appear black on white paper. The letters are only visible with the green side.

Another test is with plus and minus 2.00 D cylindrical lenses over the good eye oriented at the same axes. The vision will be excellent. The examiner stands between the acuity chart and the patient, moves the cylinders 90° apart, blurring the good eye to 20/200, fiddles with a plano lens over the bad eye, steps out of the way, and asks the patient to read the letters again. Anything better than 20/200 is from the bad eye.

Prism introduced in front of a seeing eye is accompanied by a fusional ductional response to maintain binocularity. This is a difficult response to suppress if an accommodative distance target is used. After the bad eye is covered, a light and a biprism are introduced to the good eye. Monocular diplopia results. At the same time as the bad eye is uncovered, the biprism is brought down a few millimeters so that only a single vertical prism is presented. If diplopia remains, binocular vision with diplopia is being experienced.

If all of these tests are noncontributory or equivocal, fluorescein angiography, electroretinography, visual evoked responses, and even computerized tomography of the brain may be necessary to present in a litigational dispute. Electrical testing with pattern visual-evoked potentials can be impaired by a voluntary near response by the patient. It has even been suggested that skin galvanometry (lie detector testing) and sodium amytal ("truth serum") should be administered as presumptive evidence in court.

No matter how proud one may feel about exposing hysteria or malingering, don't expect a flood of gratitude (or even payment) from the patient.

Please see Part III: Problems and Part III: Solutions for typical examination questions pertaining to the material in this chapter.

CHAPTER 15: INSTRUMENTS

LENS MEASUREMENT

All of the techniques of refraction depend on the power of the lenses placed in front of the patient to image objects at the eye's far point. The power of the lenses must therefore be critically calibrated, and a ready method of determining the power of the spectacles must be at hand. To measure the power, just as one measured the eye power, the process of neutralization is used. The principles involved have led to the development of instruments that are an integral part of all aspects of ophthalmic practice, including lens design and dispensing.

Initially, when only biconvex or biconcave lenses were used, by measuring the radius of curvature of each surface, the surface power could be obtained by the $\frac{n' - n}{r} = Ds_1 + Ds_2$ relationship. This could be incorporated into a gauged system, but calibration of course is only for one index of refraction, usually crown glass. This is the basis of a *lens measure* (e.g., Geneva lens measure or spherometer) (Fig. 15-1).

The principle of the basic lens measure is quite elegant and worthwhile to review. It reveals how chord diameters can translate into radii of curvature and hence refractive power.

In Fig. 15-2 where S is the sagittal height of the chord BD, r = radius = OD = OA. The goal is to determine the radius of curvature (r) of the chord BD.

$$\text{Triangle } OCD\text{: } r^2 = y^2 + (r - s)^2$$

$$r^2 = y^2 + r^2 - 2rs + s^2$$

$$2rs = y^2 + s^2$$

$$r = \frac{y^2 + s^2}{2s}$$

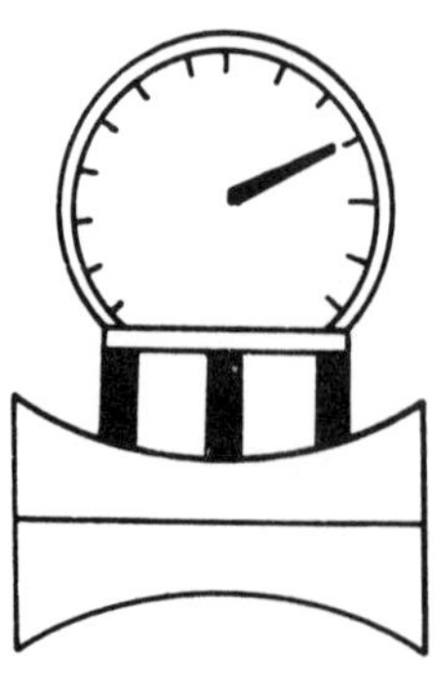

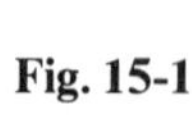

Fig. 15-1

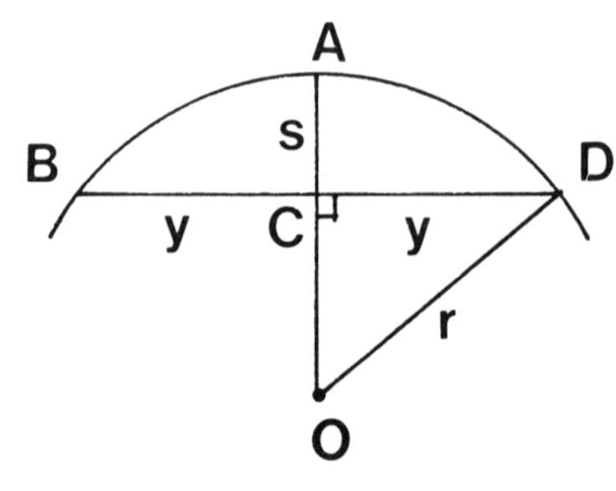

Fig. 15-2

$$r = \frac{y^2}{2s} + \frac{s}{2}$$

$$\text{when } s \text{ is } < y, \frac{s}{2} \text{ is small} \quad r \approx \frac{y^2}{2s}$$

$$D = \frac{n' - n}{r}$$

$$\text{in air} \quad D = \frac{n' - 1}{y^2 / 2s}$$

$$D = \frac{2s(n' - 1)}{y^2}$$

$$\text{if } n' = 1.50, D = \frac{s}{y^2}$$

By fixing the position of the outside pins on the lens measure, the chord diameter $BD = 2y$ is fixed so that y and y^2 are known. By measuring s with the center pin, the refractive power D of the surface can then be read on the dial (Fig. 15-3).

This is calibrated for a single index of refraction but can be calculated with the knowledge of any other material's index of refraction. It is very useful for determining if a patient's new glasses have different base curves relative to their old glasses. It will also detect lens warpage.

When dealing with hard or gas permeable contact lenses, it is necessary to verify the posterior central curve (PCC) on the concave surface of the contact. This is done by the use of a *radiuscope*. The posterior optical zone (POZ) is determined from the chord diameter and radius of curvature. The refracting power of the contact can be calculated. The index of the material, center thickness, and front curvature must be known to determine the total dioptric strength.

When meniscus and plano-concave/convex lenses emerged, vertex power became an important aspect to consider. For biconcave or biconvex lenses the front and back vertex powers are identical, so this was not a consideration.

By placing lenses of known calibration in front of an unknown lens, the move-

Lens Measure

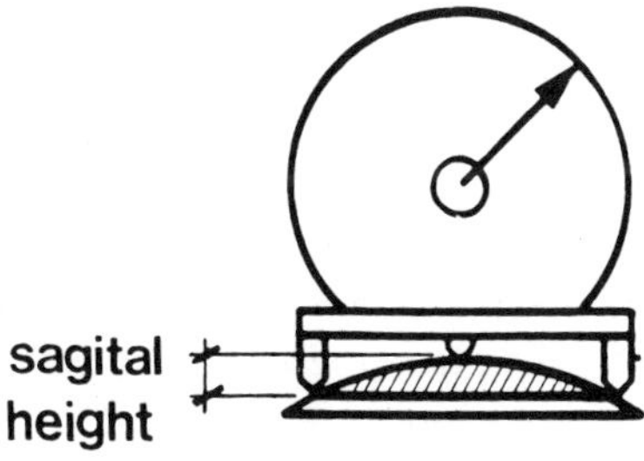

Fig. 15-3

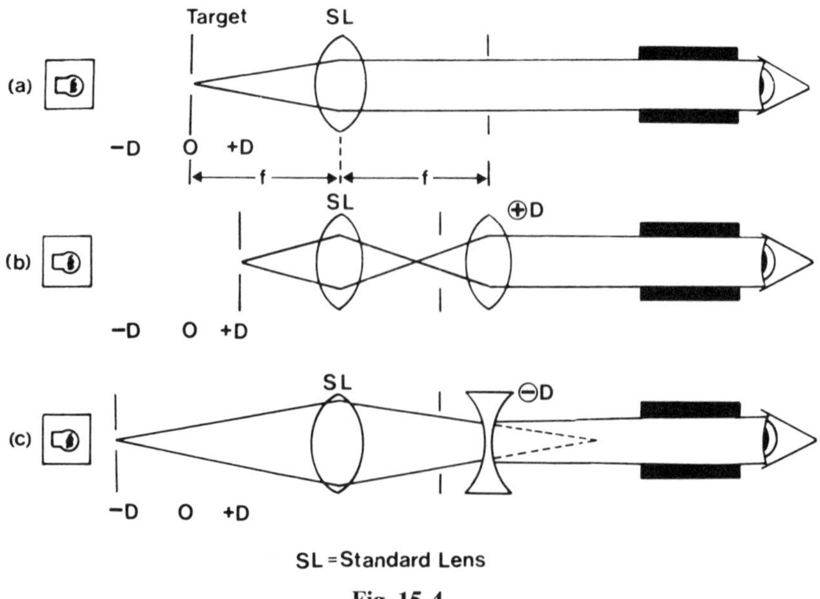

Fig. 15-4

ment with or against can be employed similar to neutralization in retinoscopy—called *hand neutralization.* The problem is that the front vertex power is measured, and with the exception of bifocals all prescribed lenses are measured by their back vertex power. This led to the development of the *lensmeter* (Reichert Lensometer, Bausch & Lomb Vertometer, Zeiss Vertex Refractionometer) as a method to measure the *back* vertex power of a spectacle lens. If a condensing (+) lens or standard lens is placed adjacent to an unknown lens, the combined power of the lenses will focus a target at the new focal point of the system. The problem with this system is that the target image will be at a position on a scale that is crowded at the plus combination end, where very small distances will correspond to wide dioptric variations. Conversely, at the minus end, large distances will correspond to small dioptric changes, i.e., a nonlinear dioptric scale. The image of the target will also be magnified with plus lenses and minified with minus lenses, which can affect the endpoint discrimination of the observer in determining the exact power.

Badal discovered that, if the standard lens was positioned in such a way that its secondary focal point was at the back vertex of the spectacle lens to be measured, not only did a linear dioptric scale result but also emergent rays were parallel. If a telescope with a reticle was used, the parallel rays could be identified as parallel when they came to focus in the plane of the reticle. The target is then moved along a linear scale until its position produces the correct vergence, which, when neutralized by the spectacle lens, emerges as parallel rays that are imaged by the telescope. Observer bias is eliminated, since the target image is the same size all along the scale.

Fig. 15-4, *a,* illustrates the zero position on the dioptric scale. The observer focuses the telescope reticle so that in this position the target is recognized as imagery at infinity, i.e., the emergent rays are parallel. With the introduction of a plus lens, the combination shifts the focal point of the system such that for the target to be imaged at infinity, it must be moved to this new position. The dioptric value corresponds to the power of the lens at this point on the scale. Similarly, the minus

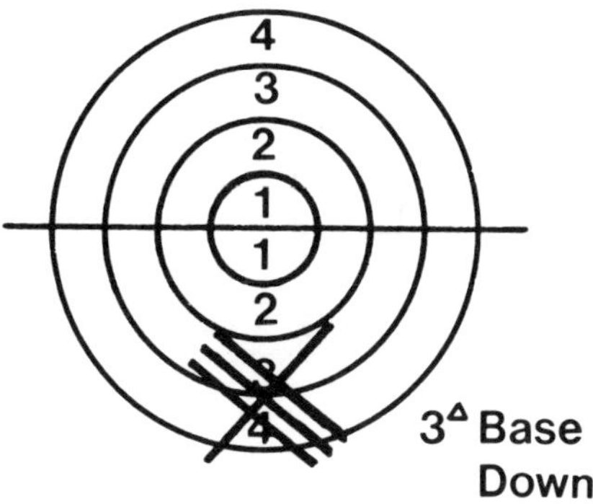

Fig. 15-5

lens power can also be determined. At all positions the image of the target is the same size, so no observer bias can be exerted to influence the endpoint. If the lens is spherocylindrical, by using a target with lines in different meridians a different line will come into focus for each meridian. As seen later, this principle can be used to neutralize the power of the eye, in which case it is called an *optometer.* It is the basic principle used with some automated refractors.

Recent advances in technology have automated the lensmeter so that the above process need not be performed. By analysis of deflection patterns created by different portions of a lens, composite mathematical representations of each portion can be electronically processed to arrive at not only the power of the lens but also prismatic power. Other modifications to the present lensmeter substitute a screen projection device so that telescopic target focusing is not required, and no instrument accommodation is stimulated.

All traditional lensmeters also have the capacity to mark the optical centers with ink and to measure the amount of prism present in a lens. The target mires are centered when no prism is present. Concentric rings or hatch marks on the reticle each represent one prism diopter specified in base direction corresponding to the displacement direction (Fig. 15-5). To expand the scale, known amounts of prism in the appropriate direction can be added over the spectacle.

The problem with bifocal measurement has been addressed previously. Fused bifocals are calibrated as front vertex power, and for actual measurement the spectacle must be turned over and measured. The distance correction should be reread through an equidistant portion above the optical center, and the difference is the power of the add. This is significant when dealing with high plus (e.g., aphakic) lenses. Progressive add styles are very difficult to neutralize in each meridian.

Contact lenses also pose a problem in that their apical vault falls outside the focal plane of the standard lens of the lensmeter. The front vertex power of a contact lens is very close to the back vertex power except for high plus lenses. This means that, if the lens is measured upside down (convex side down), a truer power measurement is obtained. Otherwise, a special lens carrier must be applied to adjust the apical vault to sit in the reference plane of the standard lens.

AUTOMATED REFRACTION

It was mentioned that the Badal system could also be used to neutralize an eye error if the eye were placed where the spectacle lens is placed in the lensmeter (Fig.

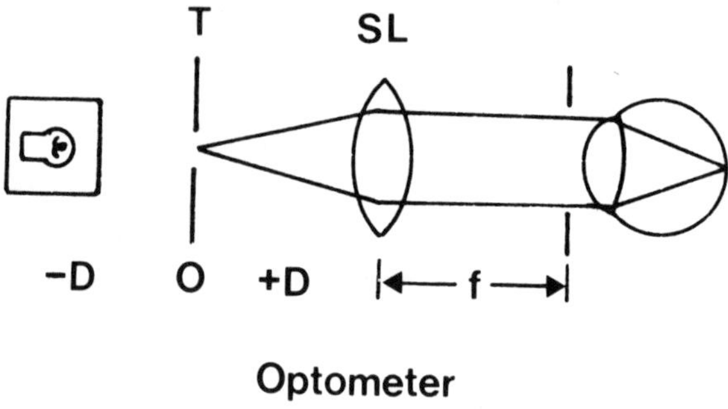

Fig. 15-6

15-6). This optometer principle is the basis of many of the techniques of *automated refraction.* Rather than use a single lens and neutralize the power in two meridians at different times, ingenious methods of continuously variable spherocylindrical lens systems have been developed by Guyton in the Reichert SRIV and by Humphrey in the Vision Analyzer. They allow smooth focusing and simpler mechanics and are the basis of the above cited subjective refractors.

The Scheiner principle is the basis of many refractors and is a very simple double aperture system. When the object of regard is placed conjugate to the retina, a single clear image is formed (Fig. 15-7, *a*). Under any condition of ametropia the image is double (Fig. 15-7, *b*). If the refractor is combined with an optometer, any ametropia can be converted to emmetropia and a single image. This can be done by focusing visible or infrared light on the retina. Different meridians are measured to determine astigmatism. This can be done simultaneously in all meridians with some refractors. The advantage to infrared is that it does not stimulate pupillary constriction. Fixation, pupil size, aperture spacing, and positioning are all important considerations. Infrared light can also be used to

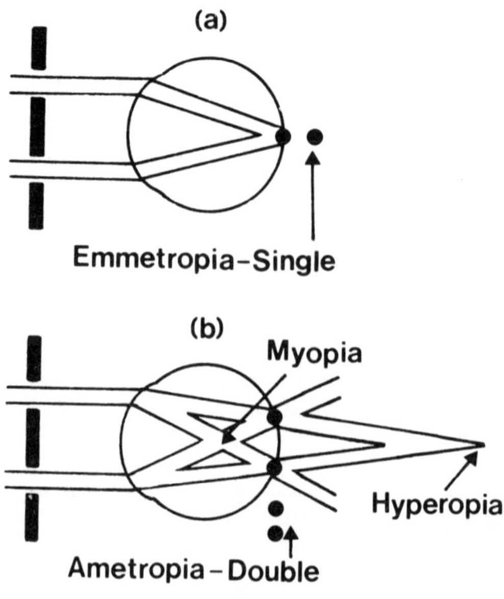

Fig. 15-7

automatically retinoscope a patient and neutralize standard with and against movements (Safir-Ophthalmetron) with an optometer.

Another interesting device similar to retinoscopy is laser speckle pattern refraction using with and against laser speckle pattern movement in ametropia. When an optometer neutralizes the refractive error, movement ceases. (This was discussed under night myopia and the dark focus.)

Photographing the retinoscopic image of a flashed point source of light (Howland) will reveal images of certain shapes and sizes, depending on the refractive error of the eye. Comparing these to standards reveals the nature of the error and has the potential for mass screening and simultaneous group refraction.

Visual evoked potentials test primarily macular function, and when clear imagery is obtained, different potentials are seen (Harter and White). Astigmatic detection is the remaining hurdle.

Other attempts have been made to computerize the refraction sequence (e.g., Marg), automate a standard phoropter (e.g., Möller, Rodenstock), automate an entire refracting lane and equipment (e.g., IVEX System, Bausch & Lomb), automate a normal refracting sequence with special Simulcross cross-cylinder testing (e.g., Reichert SRIV), and refract without any lenses at all in front of the patient (Humphrey). Guyton compares all these systems' advantages and disadvantages in Duane TD, Jaeger EA, eds.: *Clinical ophthalmology,* vols 1–6. Philadelphia, 1992, Harper & Row.

OPHTHALMOSCOPES

Another instrument with a built-in refractive correction is the *direct ophthalmoscope.* A bright light source such as a halogen bulb is reflected by a mirror or reflecting prism, which bisects the pupil. The other half of the aperture is used for visualization purposes (Fig. 15-8). Plus or minus lenses neutralize patient or observer error or both in such a fashion that conjugacy exists between the two retinas. The image formed is upright. The field of view is limited by the small aperture. The magnification is that of a simple magnifier and depends on the eye error. An emmetropic eye of +60.00 D would provide +60/4 = 15× magnification. An aphakic eye of +40.00 D would provide +40/4 = 10× magnification.

In an attempt to obtain an enlarged field of view with stereopsis, the *indirect ophthalmoscope* was conceived. This introduces a condensing (plus) lens between

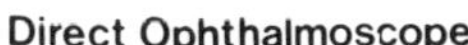

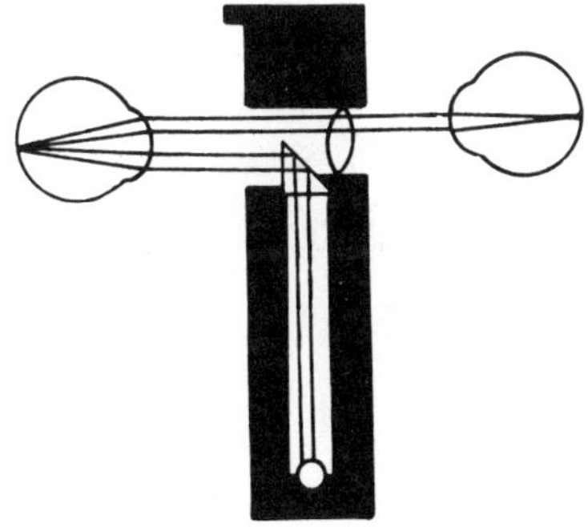

Fig. 15-8

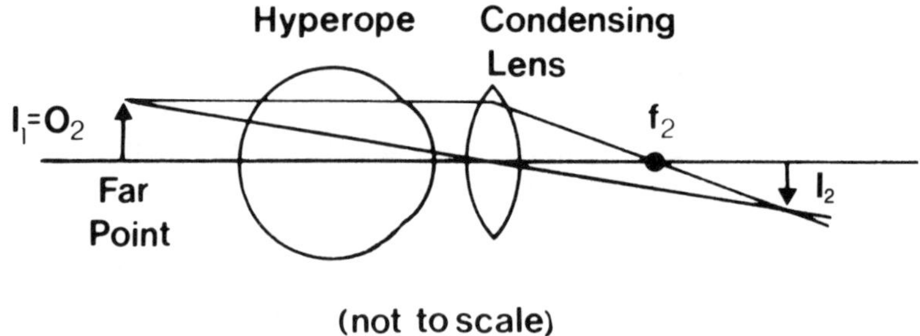

Imagery of the Indirect Ophthalmoscope

Fig. 15-9

the patient and the observer (hence the term *indirect* as opposed to direct, where no such intervention takes place). A bright light source illuminates the fundus. The image then becomes the object of the condensing lens, which in turn forms an aerial image that is larger and inverted (Fig. 15-9). The two plus lenses, the eye, and the condensing lens determine the magnification of the aerial image, which for the emmetropic eye is approximately:

$$M_A = \frac{-D_E}{D_O} = \frac{-60}{D \text{ condensing lens}}$$

The magnification is thus a function of the power of the condensing lens, e.g., $+20.00\text{ D} = \frac{-60}{20} = -3\times$; the image is three times larger and inverted. Fig. 15-9 illustrates the imagery in a hyperopic eye. This is the situation when using a monocular indirect ophthalmoscope. In an attempt to increase the stereoscopic effect, the binocular indirect ophthalmoscope was conceived. Again, the illumination and viewing are both achieved through the condensing lens. The problem exists at the pupil, where the two light pathways must not interfere with each other. This is facilitated by mydriasis to as wide as possible. The next problem is to squeeze a pupillary distance-limited binocular system into this small pupil. This can be achieved by effectively reducing the PD to ¼ (or less in the variable small pupil ophthalmoscopes) or 15 mm by means of reflecting prisms or mirrors. Since the aerial image formed is between the examiner and the patient, accommodation is required that can be compensated for by plus lenses in the eyepieces. Accommodation is accompanied by accommodative convergence, which is equally undesirable; the add eliminates this as a factor as well. These principles are illustrated in Fig. 15-10.

The magnification remains the same, but since a stereoscopic system exists, axial magnification must be considered in the perception of height and depth. For example, with a $+20.00$ D condensing lens $M_A = \frac{-D_E}{D_O} = \frac{-60}{20} = -3\times$, but the axial magnification $= (M_A)^2 = 3^2 = 9\times$. This effect is reduced, however, by the reduction in the PD to $\frac{1}{4}\left(\theta = \frac{\text{PD} \times x}{d^2}\right)$, so the effective axial magnification actually is $9/4 = 2.25\times$.

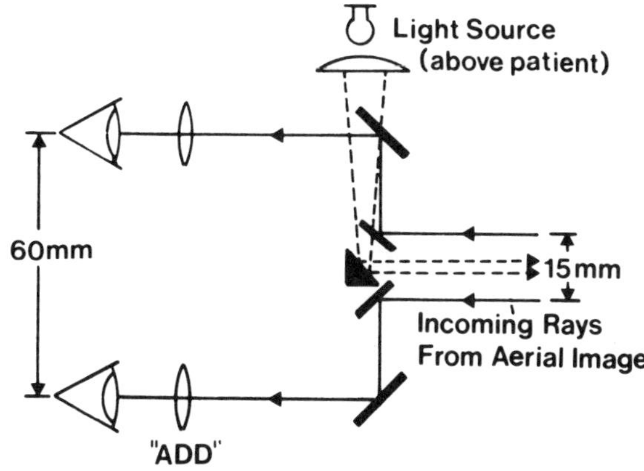

Fig. 15-10

As the power of the condensing lens decreases, the magnification increases and is accompanied by a more marked (exponential) increase in the axial magnification. That is why disk and retinal lesions look deeper or of greater height with lower power condensing lenses.

The aberrations of the condensing lens are markedly reduced by using aspheric lenses, as are now popular. The diameter and power of the lens can also affect the field of view: the higher the power of the lens, the less the magnification and the greater the field of view.

The inverted image of the indirect ophthalmoscope is quite bothersome to the novice observer but is easily adapted to. Attempts have been made to invert the image to upright form, but the inverting prisms used have either been too cumbersome to handle or detrimental to the image quality. Inversion of the remainder of the field of vision is disorienting to the examiner.

MICROSCOPES

The *slit lamp biomicroscope* illuminates and magnifies the eye to allow binocular viewing with preserved stereopsis. Fig. 15-11 traces the light pathway through a Reichert slit lamp to show the complexity of the lenses involved to incorporate variable magnification and upright imagery. The lenses are of the highest optical quality to reduce aberrations and reflections. The magnification is controlled with eye-pieces that can be changed (10×, 16×) or by altering the internal condensing lens combinations by rotating a dial to select variable Galilean telescopes.

The slit lamp biomicroscope can also be used to image the fundus. The image of the eye becomes the object for the microscope and is manipulated with various lenses. Normally the slit lamp is focused on the anterior segment of the eye. To push this focal point back, a minus lens must be introduced. If the most posterior point that can be focused by the slit lamp is about 8 mm posterior to the cornea, it must be pushed back about 15 mm to focus on the retina at 22.6 mm in a normal size eye. About a −55.00 D lens is required. This is the basis of the *Hruby*

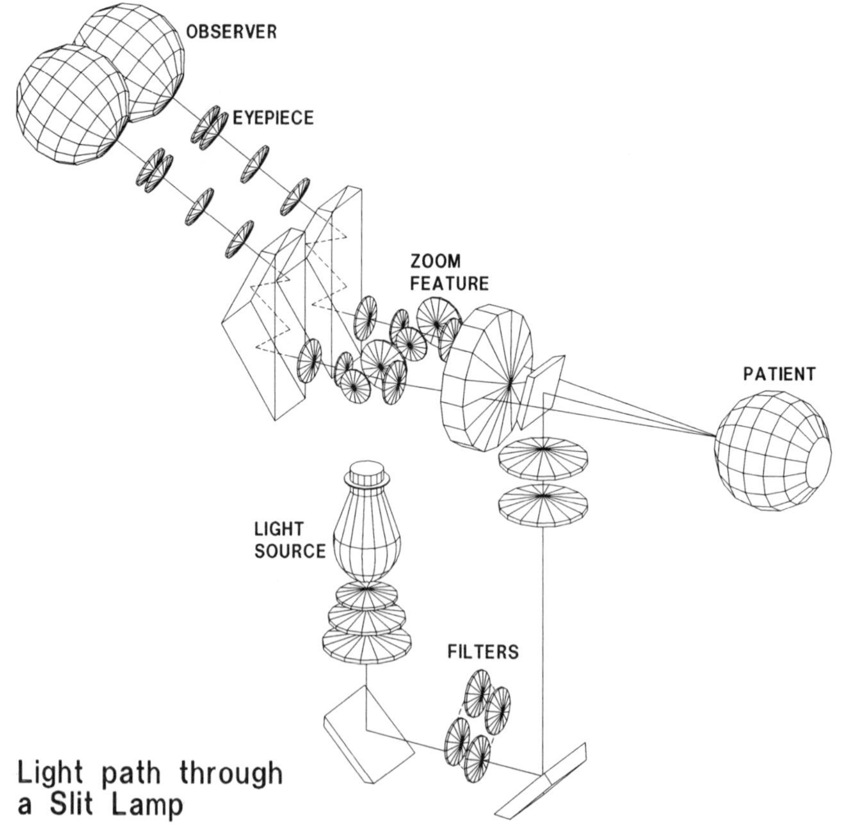

Fig. 15-11 Light pathway through a Reichert slit lamp.

lens (Fig. 15-12). A more valid explanation is to consider the emmetropic eye. The retina will be conjugate to its far point at infinity. A high minus lens (e.g., −55.00 D) will form a virtual image in the anterior focal plane of the lens at 18 mm. This will become the object for the slit lamp, which then presents the image to the observer according to the magnification of the system.

Another method involves corneal contact with a lens and methylcellulose, which effectively neutralizes the refracting power of the cornea. Each interface between media must be considered by the $D = \frac{n' - n}{r}$ formula. If each is considered, the final refracting power approaches zero. This is equivalent to removing a +45.00 D lens or adding a −45.00 D lens at the corneal surface. Optically this presents the same imagery as outlined for the Hruby lens. This is the basis for the *Goldmann lens*, which can also incorporate mirrors for viewing various angles of the retinal periphery and anterior chamber angle.

Similarly, a high plus lens in front of or on the cornea forms a real but inverted image just anterior to the lens. This affords a very wide angle view of the retina useful for examination and laser photocoagulation. Condensing lenses of +60.00, +90.00 D held by hand or mounted to the slit lamp can be used to obtain a stereoscopic fundus view while not disturbing the cornea with gonioscopic gel materials. Contact fundus lenses can give an even larger field of view while preserving stereopsis. This is the basis of the El Bayadi and Rodenstock Panfunduscope lenses. Other high plus, hand-held condensing lenses (+60.00, + 90.00 D) afford a stereoscopic view of the retina with the slit lamp.

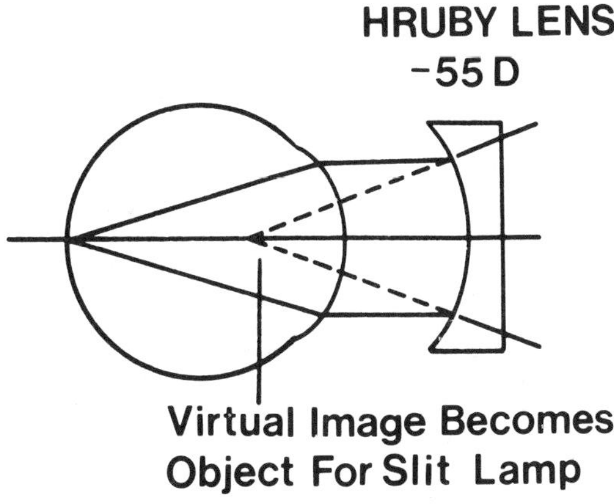

Fig. 15-12

One of the problems that arises with all of these methods of fundus viewing is the variation in depth distortion from one system to the next. The linear or lateral magnification gives the horizontal and vertical parameters, but when the depth perception of normal and abnormal anatomy is compared, one must consider the axial magnification effects. If one examiner uses a direct ophthalmoscope to estimate the cup depth and the next uses a +90.00 D lens, there will be an enhanced depth with the +90.00 D.

To compare the depth enhancement, one compares the axial to the lateral magnification. The relative values (axial magnification/lateral magnification) of some systems with the slit lamp are:

Goldmann	0.93
Hruby	1.02
+90.00 D	0.66
El Bayadi	1.02

These values will vary according to the slit lamp and also the eyepiece used with the lens system.

The *fundus camera* is also capable of imaging the retina and photographing this image. An illumination or flash system is reflected into the patient's eye through a holed mirror similar to the direct ophthalmoscope. The image produced at the far point of the eye is then the object for a condensing lens just as in indirect ophthalmoscopy. Photographs can then be taken of this real image between the holed mirror and the condensing lens. A barrier filter can be interposed to allow only the light of the activated wavelength to be photographed during fluorescein angiography. Wide-angle photographs can be taken using large diameter, high power, aspheric condensing lenses.

The *operating microscope* is similar to the slit lamp in that it is a compound microscope which illuminates, magnifies (but in a zoom fashion), and images the eye (Fig. 15-13).

Each manufacturer has its own strengths and weaknesses. Options from ceiling mounting to voice activation and control are available. The eyepieces have dioptric markings similar to those found on the slit lamp. In both circumstances they

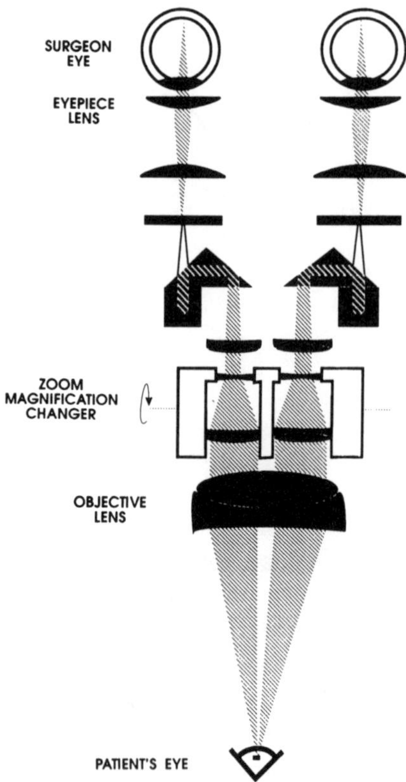

Fig. 15-13

do not correspond directly with the observer's refractive error and should be adjusted according to the manufacturer's instructions. (This is especially critical for laser delivery systems, where the delivery outside the focal point could be related to an adverse outcome, e.g., YAG laser pitting of implants, bleeding, cataract, retinal hole formation.)

When the operating microscope is used for keratoplasties, radial keratotomies, or photokeratectomies, it is critical to establish the line of sight to center the surgery. The most reliable method appears to be to have the patient fix a nonluminous target on the objective lens mount and to sight the center of the pupil with the surgeon using monocular vision (Guyton).

The working distance is controlled by the focal distance of the objective lens (150, 175, 200 mm). This is usually easily changed to suit the individual surgeon's preference. To maintain parfocality (the microscope stays in focus for all zoom settings), the highest setting on the zoom feature is reached. The objective is already in position; the eyepieces are at zero; the object is fine focused; the lowest magnification is set. Each eyepiece is fogged with plus, then minus added until in focus monocularly. Binocular balancing and interpupillary distances are set. The microscope should be in focus throughout the range of the zoom with this strategy.

New *diagnostic confocal microscopes* are now available from several manufacturers (Rodenstock, Heidelberg Instrument, Allergan-Humphrey, Kowa, Topcon, Zeiss). These provide lower light levels by using laser scanning from helium-neon, argon-ion, or diode lasers. An optical section of any material, such as the cornea, can be imaged in real time and projected to a video camera. A 20× applanation cone objective can be used for the cornea to provide a flat field of view. The image obtained is then digitized and recorded for processing. Morphometric analysis, three-dimensional reconstruction, and high-resolution display are all capable with microprocessor image analysis. The natural fluorescence of the lens can be eliminated and focal electroretinogram and VER analysis of retinal function performed. Retinal sensitivity can be quantified using laser scanning ophthalmoscopy. This is like reverse perimetry in that rather than projected scotomata being measured, direct retinal sensitivity can be plotted and followed.

CORNEAL TOPOGRAPHIC ANALYSERS

Similar technology is involved in *corneal topographic analysers* (e.g., Computed Anatomy, Visio, Eye Sys, Par, Nidek-Marco, Kerametrics). Image analysis of 20 to 35 illuminated rings projected from the corneal apex to the limbus is performed by high-speed, high-resolution videosignal processors. The images are digitized and analyzed to give each radius of curvature a value to a resolution of ±0.20 D or greater. A topographic map can be in color or grey scale (e.g., blue = short radius = steep, red = long radius = flat). These instruments are becoming more important with refractive alteration of the corneal topography. Coupling the information to contact lens manufacturing equipment (Eye-Sys) produces customized contact lenses.

Lens opacification and cataractogenesis are also subjects of similar technology. The Opacity Lensmeter (Interzeag) uses a 1.5 mm, 700 nm beam focused on the retina and measures the light scatter from the lens. The value is digitized and age adjusted to yield a numeric reading for following the degree of opacification.

ULTRASONOGRAPHY

When the quality of the ocular media is such that light cannot be effectively used to form an image, the use of sound in the form of *ultrasound* can be employed. Sound can boldly go where no light has gone before.

Sound can be propagated in waveform and be refracted, reflected, scattered, or absorbed. Ultrasound has a frequency greater than 20,000 cps and for ophthalmic use between 8 and 15 million cps or mHz. In 1880 the Curie brothers demonstrated the piezoelectric effect, whereby pressure (*piezo*) or stress of a mechanical nature (or vibrations) could be converted to electrical energy and vice versa. If a quartz or barium titanate crystal, for example, is pulsed with electrical energy from a transmitter, sound waves in the form of ultrasound are transduced. Since the frequency is so high, it is outside the audible range; since the energy pulse is so low, it is incapable of producing tissue damage. If the energy is raised, the vibrations produced from the transducer are capable of fragmentation. If the energy is pulsed at low levels, it can produce ultrasound, which can be used diagnostically. At high levels it can be used therapeutically, e.g., phakoemulsification.

Just as light becomes more divergent from a point source, ultrasound requires a certain distance from the transducer before it is divergent enough and uniform enough to be used diagnostically. Thus in contact ultrasonography the near field extends to the posterior lens capsule, and details anterior to this are lost. This can be circumvented by water bath techniques that place the entire eye, including the cornea and anterior segment, in the diagnostic far field range or with the newer ultrasound biomicroscope technique. When basing clinical decisions (e.g., growth of a melanoma) on the clinical measurements from visit to visit, more objective parameters such as depth on A-scan ultrasonography are more objective. Anterior segment pathology can now be beautifully measured with the ultrasound biomicroscope (C. Pavlin). This uses a modified methylcellulose bath and high-resolution transducer to document regions such as the iris and ciliary body, which were previously poorly accessible.

As the ultrasound encounters different interfaces, it can be displayed visually with a cathode ray oscillograph. The time delay between emission and detection is a function of distance travelled and the density of the substance in which it was travelling: the denser the medium (e.g., the lens), the faster the travel. This is used for axial length measurements, anterior chamber depth, and corneal thickness measurements with corrections incorporated for the varying densities. The size of extraocular muscles and choroidal tumors can also be determined.

Not all sound is completely reflected. Some may be refracted, scattered, or absorbed. The amplitude of the returning wave will then be lessened or attenuated. The amount of attenuation depends on the characteristics of the tissue through which it is travelling. It must, however, be reflected to some extent or nothing is detectable, i.e., it would appear ultrasonolucent. The attenuation characteristics can also be affected by the angle of incidence of the wavefront; the angle of reflection will determine if the echo will reach the detector. At 90° to the interface the detection of reflection is maximal, and only the characteristics of the tissue interfaces will affect attenuation values. Under these circumstances a tissue profile can be created that ideally can distinguish choroidal melanomas from hemangiomas or disciform detachment of the retina on the basis of their attenuation characteristics. This is a time-amplitude study, which is the basis of A-scan ultrasonography and which is maximally useful in both distance and tissue attenuation quantification.

The B-scan is a dynamic study whereby the transducer sweeps across tissue interfaces and profiles them on a grey scale according to their tissue impedance or attenuation. High reflectivity is manifest as white on the oscillograph, whereas lucency is black. The intervening impedance values are given grey values in between. This polarity can be reversed. A two-dimensional picture emerges resembling a cross-section of the eye whereby pathologic anatomy can be pictorially represented. Retinal detachments, vitreous hemorrhages, intraocular foreign bodies, vitreous detachments, choroidal and orbital tumors can all be effectively demonstrated under circumstances that preclude their visualization by other techniques.

The time-motion studies using M-mode ultrasonography are not used in ophthalmology but are vital imaging techniques in obstetrics and cardiology (echocardiology and aneurysm studies).

PACHYMETRY

Mention has been made as to measuring the corneal thickness by means of ultrasonography. A more practical method but less precise is a slit lamp technique

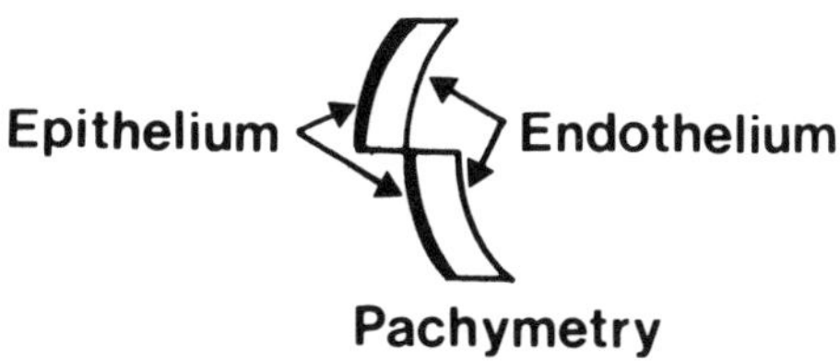

Fig. 15-14

called *pachymetry.* A slit lamp attachment is used so that simultaneous magnification and doubling occur. The corneal cross-sectional image is then adjusted so that the double images are oriented with the epithelial surface of the inferior image juxtaposed to the endothelial surface of the superior image (Fig. 15-14). Distance and therefore thickness can be calibrated and read directly from the dial on the attachment. This can also be performed by specular microscopy instruments, which image and photograph corneal endothelial cells. These cells are considered quantitatively and qualitatively in health and disease states.

APPLANATION TONOMETRY

A similar doubling principle is used during *applanation tonometry.* At an applanation diameter of 3.06 mm it has been determined that the structural resistance to deformation of the cornea is equal to the attractive forces of the surface tension of the tears; these two forces being equal and opposite, they cancel each other out. The intraocular pressure can then be directly measured as the gram force per unit area, which when multiplied by 10 conveniently converts this value to millimeters of mercury (mm Hg) Fig. 15-15. It then becomes crucial to determine when exactly 3.06 mm of applanation has been achieved. As with pachymetry, this distance can accurately be determined by doubling with a split image prism (Fig. 15-15). The cornea may be toric in nature, which can affect the measurement. The prism requires rotation to 43° of the minus cylinder axis or lowest *K,* which is marked by a red line and corresponds to this value. Even if this is not done, an

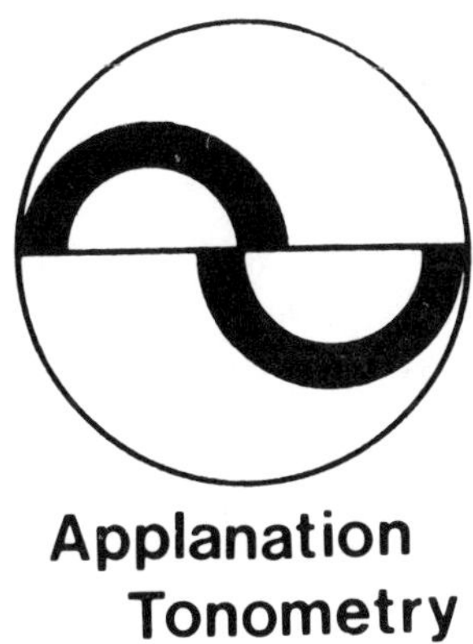

Fig. 15-15

error of only 1 mm Hg occurs for each 4.00 D of cylinder (Holladay). Fluorescein dye and cobalt blue light facilitate visualization and refinement of this endpoint.

KERATOMETRY

This same central 3 mm of cornea is also important in *keratometry,* another measurement technique that employs doubling mechanisms as an integral part of its functioning.

The keratometer or ophthalmometer (Keratometer, Javal-Shiotz Ophthalmometer, CLC Ophthalmometer) is an ingenious device that uses both the reflecting and refracting properties of the cornea to determine the radii of curvature and refracting power of its principal meridians.

As a reflecting surface, the cornea is a convex mirror. It forms an image of an object that is virtual, erect, and minified. This is the first Purkinje-Sanson image. If either the image or object size is kept constant, by measuring the size of the variable in each respective circumstance the amount of magnification can be determined. Once these are known, the power of the mirror $U + D_m = V$ or $U + \frac{2}{r} = V$ can be determined. Once the radii in the two principal meridians are known, the power of the cornea as a refracting surface can then be derived by the $D_s = \frac{n' - n}{r}$ relationship. Since n air $= 1.00$, only the n' must be known. It is known that n' for the cornea is actually 1.336. Since the days of Helmholtz, however, most popular keratometers use $n' = 1.3375$. This actually works out very conveniently because the altered index compensates for the effect of the posterior corneal surface, and this small adjustment gives the total refracting power of the cornea. It also facilitates conversion, since with this value a 7.5 mm radius gives exactly +45.00 D of refracting power. Fig. 15-16 depicts the optics the popular Bausch and Lomb Keratometer. Although at first glance it would appear quite

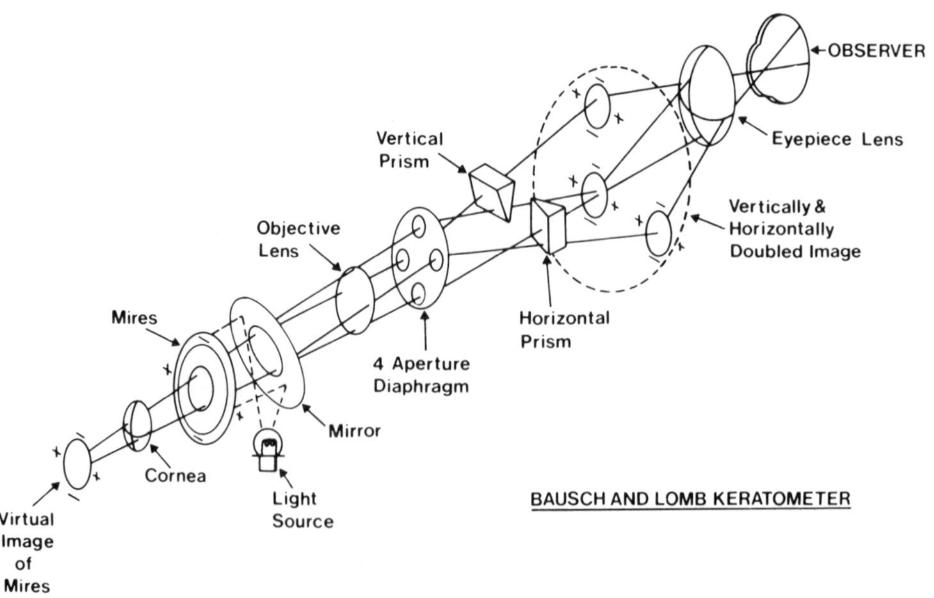

Fig. 15-16

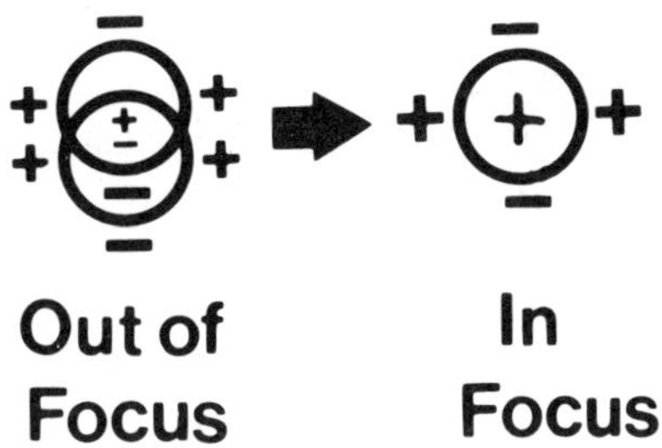

Fig. 15-17

complex, its simple beauty is obvious with a dissection of each functioning segment.

A light source illuminates the mires by reflected light from a mirror. The cornea images these mires behind it as virtual, erect, and minified. Since the object is the mires and its size is fixed, it is the size of the image which is necessary to derive. The virtual image of the mires now becomes the object for the remaining optical components. Object rays pass through an aperture in both the mires and mirror to be projected through a 4 aperture diaphragm. The two central apertures are nothing more than a Scheiner disk. When the image of the central mire is in anything but perfect focus, it doubles the image (Fig. 15-17).

The remaining apertures present the same image displaced by prisms, horizontal and vertical to the central image. In doubling the image two goals are realized: (1) when the eye has unsteady fixation, both images move together, so a measurement still can be taken; (2) the power in two meridians can be resolved simultaneously. To achieve this, the machine must be rotated to find the two principal meridians. This is determined by the positions of the plus (+) and minus (−) components of the double images relative to the central image (Fig. 15-18). Once aligned, the actual measurement of the image size is performed by superimposing the plus and minus portions of the doubled images. The dials are calibrated such that meridional power is directly read from the hatch mark. Using the conversion formula, the radius of curvature $r = \frac{0.3375}{D}$ is found.

The range of the keratometer can be expanded by placing plus sphere over the mire aperture in conditions such as keratoconus, where steeper than normal corneas result. The instrument can be calibrated using a steel sphere of known radius, and the eyepiece must be focused to compensate for the observer's refractive error

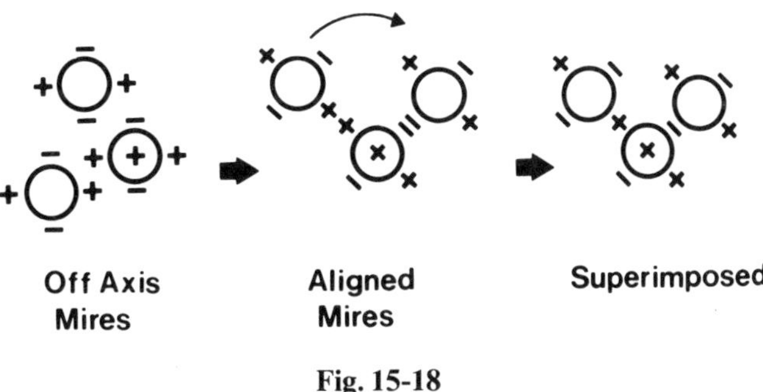

Fig. 15-18

or induced accommodation. The implications and uses of this measurement have been illustrated throughout the text and include contact lens fitting, surgical correction of astigmatism, classifying astigmatism, problems on board examinations, and the determination of the power of an intraocular lens implant. Newer technology couples automated keratometry to topographic analysers, automated refractors, and biometers.

Please see Part II: Problems and Part III: Solutions for typical examination questions pertaining to the material in this chapter.

CHAPTER 16: LASERS

In recent years the *laser* has emerged as an indispensable tool in virtually every medical discipline. Its therapeutic and surgical implications have revolutionized the treatment of retinovascular, neovascular, lenticular, refractive, and glaucomatous disorders of the eye. Newer developments have opened newer horizons for closed laser surgery in various anterior and posterior segment disorders. Since the future holds even greater promise for laser technology, it is incumbent on each practitioner to manifest at least a rudimentary knowledge of laser dynamics.

The word *laser* is an acronym derived from *l*ight *a*mplification by *s*timulated *e*mission of *r*adiation. This process was predicted theoretically by Einstein in 1917, but an operational model was not realized until 43 years later by Maiman's ruby laser.

PHYSICS OF LASERS

The Bohr concept of the atom holds that each atom possesses many energy levels containing orbiting electrons. The more energy the electrons absorb, the further away from the nucleus they orbit. If enough energy is absorbed, the electrons are freed of their orbitals and are stripped from the nucleus. This is ionization and is found in x-irradiation and plasma formation during photodisruption. The amount of energy to move an electron from one orbital level to the next (above or below) is fixed as a quantum of energy. This is like a vending machine that works on correct change only. A photon of ultraviolet light at 193 nm contains 6.4 eV per photon. When an electron absorbs 6.4 eV, it can move to the next highest energy level. When it is excited, it can reduce its orbital and release 6.4 eV as a quantum of energy in light form—a photon. If all of the electrons in the medium go from the same excited to nonexcited state, multiple photons are released at the same time and each has the same wavelength and frequency. The factors to consider and manipulate are the medium that is to be excited, the mechanisms to pump up the energy and excite that medium, and the optical feedback systems to amplify the process to make it medically useful.

Einstein defined three transition processes that occur at the level of the atom under conditions favourable to the absorption of energy. The energy can be *absorbed,* and the atom can go from nonexcited to excited with the absorption of a photon. The energy can be *spontaneously emitted* with the release of a photon, but in a random fashion so that there is no amplification. Or the release of a photon can stimulate a similarly excited atom in a similarly high energy state, to release its energy in phase with the first: *stimulated emission.* Not only is it in phase, but it is also the same wavelength and frequency. If this occurs, the waves will constructively interfere and the resultant wave is thus amplified: the light is *a*mplified by the *s*timulated *e*mission of *r*adiation.

If more than half the atoms are in the excited state (population inversion), amplification exceeds absorption and laser formation is thus favoured. This prerequisite is never achieved with the input of thermal energy, but fortunately it is for light.

If an aluminum oxide crystal has is aluminum replaced by chromium, a ruby crystal (not gem) is formed. If green or blue light is shone onto the crystal, the chromium atoms become excited as they absorb these wavelengths of light energy. If enough atoms are excited, amplification by stimulated emission occurs. If sufficient light activation occurs, the energy will be dissipated as heat or some other energy form. If the activating light continues to pump energy into the system, amplification by stimulated emission is favoured. To further enhance the process, the light already emitted can be reflected back through the excited medium to continue the emission and amplification process. This can be achieved by a resonance chamber with mirrored ends. The resonance chamber must be multiples of ½λ, or the wavelength in length or the reflections coming back will be out of phase and destructively interfere rather than amplify. An aperture or partial silvering at one end allows the escape of the light so amplified. This emergent light is highly directional, monochromatic (since all emitted rays are of the same wavelength), coherent (since all are in phase), and of high intensity (due to the amplification process). This system was the prototype of Maiman's first ruby laser.

Being monochromatic gives laser light the advantage of a single focal point with no chromatic interval. It can be controlled to within ± 0.01 nm, whereas polychromatic white light can be filtered but only to within ± 5 nm of the desired wavelength. Being highly directional implies very little beam divergence as it travels to its target. Most have about 1 milliradian of divergence, so the spot size at the target can be maintained very small. The coherence and linear polarization make its behavior very predictable and allow manipulation and transmission control of the emission. The amplification allows intensities applicable to strategic defense initiatives.

The emission of this light can be continuous wave (CW) or pulsed into short duration, high-intensity releases or bursts. As will be seen, this depends on the type of laser. The parameters or settings one uses on all types of laser control the energy or power, spot size, and duration. To understand some of the nomenclature, it is useful to see the origin of these numbers.

Energy is a form of work and is measured in joules. Power is the rate work is done and is measured in joules per second = watts, 1 W = 1 J/second. To increase the power, one can either increase the work (J) or decrease the time. Mode-locking or Q (quality factor) switching solid state neodymium:yttrium-aluminum-garnet (Nd:YAG) lasers are very effective at this. Mode-locking involves pumping the medium until a passive dye shutter in the resonant cavity absorbs enough light to bleach it. Once bleached, light can travel through the shutter and is reflected, then amplified. The light is locked in phase and released in 7 to 10 pulses over 35 to 50 nsec. Q-switching can be done with rotating mirrors, saturable dyes, acoustooptic modulators, or electrooptic modulators such as pockel cells. These crystals use the linear polarization of the laser light to advantage. When a small voltage is generated across the crystal, a polarity is maintained that prevents transmission of the light in the resonant cavity. A change in the voltage changes the polarity 90° to allow full transmission, reflection, and amplification. The pulse duration is 2 to 30 nsec with a single pulse per burst.

Another variable parameter is the spot size. The same amount of energy (J) over a small spot increases the energy density (J/cm^2) when compared to a large spot, like using a magnifying glass to concentrate sunlight on a dry leaf. It is often confusing using these units, and size perspective can be lost. A 50 μm spot size has a diameter of $\frac{50}{1000}$ cm $= 50 \times 10^{-4}$ cm. Since diameter is twice the radius, $r =$ 25 μm $= 25 \times 10^{-4}$ cm. The area of the spot is $\pi r^2 = (\pi \times 25 \times 10^{-4})^2 = 2 \times 10^{-5}$ cm^2 = 0.00005 cm^2. This is a very small spot!

Not only does each laser have an active medium, but that medium also has a method of pumping that is most effective for it. Gas discharge lasers (argon, krypton, CO_2, excimer) can be excited by the electrons travelling in an electric current between two electrodes. Semiconductor lasers (diode, gallium-aluminum-arsenide) similarly can use conventional electrical power. Liquid (dye) lasers are pumped by argon laser light, whereas some solid state lasers such as Nd:YAG and erbium:yttrium-lanthanum-fluoride (Er:YLF) use incoherent light from xenon arc flashes. The choices are made by which pump is most effective in achieving the necessary population inversion into the excited state to allow the lasing process to begin.

THERAPEUTIC USES

The choice of laser depends on the task to be performed. A clinically useful solid state laser is the *Nd:YAG.* In this laser neodymium ions are incorporated, or doped, into a crystal of yttrium-aluminum-garnet, and radiation outside the visible spectrum—1064 nm, near infrared (IR) is emitted. To be clinically useful, a visible aiming beam (e.g., a nonharmful helium-neon [He:Ne] laser emitting red light at 632.8 nm) is coupled with the emitted light and focused at the same focal length or defocused a controlled amount to protect implants from pitting.

The delivery of the emitted radiation can be pulsed, as in solid state lasers, or be continuous and free running, similar to gas discharge lasers. Pulsing allows very short bursts of power for a very short duration (nanoseconds or picoseconds—billionths of a second). The delivery of multiple pulses per burst theoretically offers some advantage in a suprathreshold burst. As the laser energy density increases, a threshold is overcome where the electrons are stripped from their atoms, and a plasma is formed. This is the electron and baryon cloud that is at the site of the mini-lightning bolt. The intense electromagnetic field disruption is accompanied by complex shock and acoustic phenomena explainable only by complex nonlinear optics. Since there is no coagulation of proteins at the focal point but rather an explosion, this type of laser is a *photodisruptor* rather than a *photocoagulator.* By doubling the frequency, the wavelength is halved ($c = \lambda\nu$). Crystals called frequency doublers can achieve this. The obvious advantage is the conversion of an infrared 1064 nm laser into a visible 532 nm laser with the simple addition of this crystal. (Other harmonics, e.g., 266 nm and 133 nm, have similar potential for utility.) Once into the visible spectrum, absorption characteristics allow photocoagulation similar to other lasers working in this wavelength. With the continuous or free-running mode, thermal effects are also obtained. When defocused about 1 mm from the visible He-Ne beam and targeted 1.0 to 1.5 mm behind the limbus, the ciliary processes can be reached for transscleral photocyclodestruction. Posterior capsulotomy, trabeculopuncture, vitreolysis, iridotomy, trabeculoplasty, anterior capsulotomy, nuclear softening, and with frequency doubling gonioplasty, trabeculoplasty, and traditional photocoagulation of the retina, retinal pigment epithelium (RPE), and choroid are all procedures within the realm of this type of laser (Fankhauser, Aron-Rosa).

Another YAG laser is the *THC:YAG,* doped with thulium, holmium, and chromium. It emits in the near infrared at 2.1 μm and can deliver 80 to 120 mJ through a 90° angulated tip. At 2.1 μm it is better absorbed by water molecules and is potentially useful in creating sclerotomies for full-thickness glaucoma filtering procedures.

Another solid state laser is the YLF (yttrium-lanthanum-fluoride) doped with erbium (1.228 μm) or holmium (1.9 μm). This has similar potential to that of the THC:YAG for full-thickness microfiltration ab externo.

Alexandrite is a solid state *tunable* laser (700 to 820 nm) with a flash pump that promises much greater stability than tunable dye lasers.

Laser phakoemulsification has great marketing potential for laser cataract surgery. Xenon chloride (308 nm excimer), Er:YAG (2.94 μm), and tunable infrared magnesium-calcium-fluoride (MgCaF) are capable of in vivo phakoemulsification. The excimer XeCl uses UV light energy, whereas the others use IR. The UV exposure may have acute endothelial and retinal toxicity and chronic oncogenic/degenerative potential. IR exposure may have thermal toxicity to adjacent tissues. If these turn out not to be harmful, they may indeed provide the laser alternative to ultrasound phakoemulsification.

The more established gas discharge lasers employ media such as xenon, argon, krypton, and CO_2 as the excited substance. The gas is contained in a narrow tube, which is ionized by the application of energy in the form of electrical current. The electrical current excites the medium and initiates the laser propagation. In argon and krypton two or more separate energy levels are capable of laser activation. As the excitation is reduced to the lower energy level, light of two or more wavelengths is produced. Argon produces blue-green light at 488 nm (blue) and 514.5 nm (green), which can be filtered to pure green if so desired. Krypton can produce a number of wavelengths from red to violet, but only red (641 nm) and yellow are currently available. CO_2 emits in the IR portion of the spectrum (10,600 nm). Of the continuous lasers, this is the most efficient and approaches 30% efficiency with high-power outputs. Needless to say, if the most efficient laser is only 30% efficient, the majority of the energy must be dissipated in the form of heat. This necessitates air or water cooling to avert internal disaster. The high efficiency and the fact that virtually all nonmetallic substances absorb the emitted radiation from the CO_2 laser make this a very effective cutting instrument for laser surgery.

The therapeutic efficacy of gas discharge lasers is based on their photocoagulating effects. Each treated tissue is composed of a substance (primarily a pigment molecule) whose absorption spectrum is within the range of the emitted laser radiation. CO_2 is the exception with its absorption by water. The absorption of light energy necessitates energy dissipation in the form of heat. This heat release coagulates the tissue at the anatomic site of absorption.

The intimate association between the pigment absorption spectra and wavelength of the emitted radiation is the current rationale for many therapeutic interventions. Ocular pigments are primarily xanthophyll (lutein), melanin, and hemoglobin. Macular xanthophyll absorbs xenon, argon blue-green, and some krypton yellow. Since this pigment is located intraretinally, thermal damage of this tissue has devastating visual implications. Argon green only, dye, and krypton red are not absorbed by xanthophyll and pass through this pigment unaltered. They are absorbed by the melanin pigment of the choriocapillaris and retinal pigment epithelium. Xenon and argon are absorbed by all three pigments, so in the presence of intraretinal hemoglobin from hemorrhage, thermal retinal damage may also occur. Again, krypton red may prove more efficacious under these circumstances.

Argon laser photocoagulation is used for cutting sutures, iridotomy, gonioplasty, trabeculoplasty, synechiolysis, ciliary ablation with direct viewing, and retinal, RPE, and choroidal photocoagulation for diverse pathologies. Argon green only, krypton, and dye laser photocoagulation are especially useful for juxtafoveal subretinal neovascular membranes and laser photocoagulation of the retina, RPE and choroid in the presence of intravitreal or intraretinal blood. CO_2 lasers are gaining use in orbital and oculoplastic surgery for tumor debulking and bloodless field incisions. The high-energy absorption allows both cutting and coagulation to occur simultaneously.

Excimer lasers are gas discharge lasers whose media are noble gas–halogen combinations (xenon, argon, krypton with chloride, fluoride, bromide). Electrical current is pumped at 90° to the axis of the light transmission. The excited media form *exci*ted di*mers*—diatomic rare gas halides such as argon fluoride (ArF). When a photon is released, it is in the UV range at 193 nm and contains a relatively large amount of energy per photon (6.4 eV/photon). Upon absorption by the target tissue, this amount of energy is beyond the threshold of protein intramolecular bonding. Absorption lyses these bonds, and the tissue is ablated. The cornea can be so treated to alter its refractive power (see later). Working with UV irradiation is technically difficult and requires specially coated lenses and optical systems. The gases are quite toxic, and great care must be exercised when dealing with them. Again, the exposure of surrounding structures such as the lens, corneal endothelium, and retina may show early or late phototoxicity.

Liquid lasers are primarily tunable dye lasers. They use an argon laser to pump liquid organic dyes so that wavelengths 360 to 960 nm can be tuned in like the station on a radio. The advent of combination argon-krypton and frequency doubling lasers has reduced the demand for these higher maintenance machines. A solid state tunable like alexandrite or MgCaF may prove more useful and user friendly.

Semiconductor lasers like the diode or gallium-aluminum-arsenide (GaAlAs) are extensions of light emitting diode (LED) technology on everything from computers to alarm clocks. Their greatest features are their compact size, convection air cooling, standard voltage requirements, and great portability. They are currently in the red part of the spectrum (811 to 900 nm) and can generate over 1 W of power. Judging by the effects of semiconductor technology on the computer industry, this may herald exciting new future potential in ophthalmology.

Phototherapy is already used in perinatal jaundice, and with the aid of hematoporphyrin derivatives (HpD) photoradiation can enhance absorption of light by specific target tissues. Because an intraocular tumor such as hemangioma, retinoblastoma, or melanoma may absorb and retain HpDs, when exposed to the correct wavelength of light, enhanced absorption and tissue phototoxicity can treat it.

Please see Part II: Problems and Part III: Solutions for typical examination questions pertaining to the material in this chapter.

CHAPTER 17: PRINCIPLES OF REFRACTIVE SURGERY

A text on optics and refraction would be remiss without some consideration of the surgical and laser manipulation of the refractive error by alteration of the shape and curvature of the cornea.

Radial keratotomy (Sato, Fyodorov) (RK) involves radial corneal cuts that steepen the peripheral cornea and flatten the central cornea. It is equivalent to moving the pegs out on a round tent—the peak of the dome flattens. This reduces the refractive power by increasing the central radius of curvature $\left(D = \frac{n' - n}{r}\right)$. The end result is a reduction in the amount of myopia. The variables in controlling the amount of correction are several. The deeper the cuts, the more the hyperopic shift. The effect can be enhanced by redeepening the peripheral aspect of the cuts in the event of undercorrection. The number of cuts varies from four to 16. The Prospective Evaluation of Radial Keratotomy (PERK) Study involved eight cuts. Most commonly four cuts are initially performed, and the results are titrated depending on the response. The direction of the cuts can be either from the optical zone to limbus (centrifugal) or vice versa (centripetal). Greater effect is derived with the latter direction. The size of the optical zone is also important. As the number of cuts is reduced so too is the size of the optical zone. The smaller the optical zone, the greater the effect but the greater the incidence of glare. This has become the standard procedure to which other refractive interventions are now compared.

Astigmatic keratotomy involves peripheral or radial cuts that flatten the steeper meridian (Ruiz procedures, intersecting and nonintersecting trapezoids, T cuts, T cuts with RK, RK with elliptical optical zones, phakoemulsification with relaxing keratotomy). As Fig. 17-1 shows, flattening the steeper meridian is accompanied by steepening of the flatter. It is like tightening your belt.

Other surgical interventions involve wound recession to flatten a steep meridian or wedge resection to tighten a flat meridian. These are most likely to be done after penetrating keratoplasty for high astigmatic errors. A tighter, nonabsorbable suture can also be used to tighten a flat meridian.

When combining relaxing keratotomy incisions with cataract surgery, use the surgical keratometer to judge suture tension and keratotomy adequacy. Remember that the steeper meridian has the smallest diameter ($2r$) and hence the shorter radius of curvature (r). It is in this meridian that the relaxing incisions are placed (Fig. 17-2).

The correction of hyperopia by surgical means has been less successful but has proponents. Thermokeratoplasty (Terrien) was simply electrocautery for the astigmatism resulting from Terrien's marginal corneal ulcers. *Radial thermal keratoplasty* (RTK) (Fyodorov) involves intrastromal diathermy with a 34-gauge microprobe inserted to 85% to 95% stromal thickness and heated to 600° C. Six

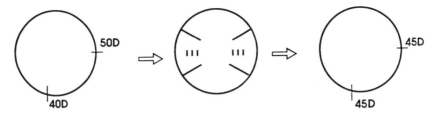

Fig. 17-1 Keratometry readings from the Ruiz procedure. Note the steepening of the flatter meridian.

to 16 radial rays of two to four burns with an optical zone of 5 to 8 mm allegedly corrects up to 5.00 D of hyperopia. If the optical zone is smaller than 5 mm, it will actually flatten rather than steepen the central corneal curvature.

Hexagonal keratotomy (Yamashita, Mendez, Jensen) involves 85% thickness, nonintersecting cuts with a 5 to 6 mm optical zone. T cuts can be added inside the optical zone for astigmatic correction; +1.00 to +5.00 D of hyperopia correction has been achieved. *Hyperopic lamellar keratotomy* (HLK) (Ruiz, Bores) involves the removal of a lamellar disk for 360° around an optical zone. This can be done with a microkeratome and achieves central corneal steepening if 80% depth is achieved.

With RK, long-term fluctuation in the refractive error (Waring) and reduced structural integrity of the globe (Simons, Binder) have continued the quest for other alternatives to keratotomy. The other nonmyopic keratotomy procedures seem even less predictable with greater regression of effect and fluctuation.

One alternative in high myopia is the *phakic anterior chamber intraocular lens* (Strampelli, Barraquer, Choyce). These patients are myopic beyond the range of other refractive surgery. A biconcave, 4.5 mm optic, anterior chamber lens is implanted 2 mm behind the cornea and 1 mm in front of the lens. This is less hazardous (maybe) than lensectomy but preserves accommodation. Endothelial and lenticular damage is the obvious risk.

Intracorneal inlays of Plexiglas and flint (Barraquer) were met with anterior stromal necrosis in rabbits and cats. The advent of newer gas permeable materials has reactivated interest. Intracorneal hydrogels (McCarvey, Binder, McDonald) have the advantage of natural hydrophillic sites, facilitating glucose and oxygen/CO_2 permeability. As with many of these inlays, the interface between the inlay

ASTIGMATIC KERATOTOMY PLACEMENT

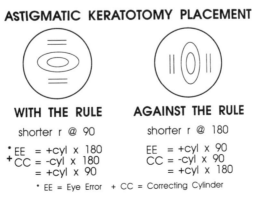

WITH THE RULE	AGAINST THE RULE
shorter r @ 90	shorter r @ 180
*EE = +cyl x 180	EE = +cyl x 90
+CC = -cyl x 180	CC = -cyl x 90
= +cyl x 90	= +cyl x 180

* EE = Eye Error + CC = Correcting Cylinder

Fig. 17-2

and the corneal plane can develop a haze or lipidlike deposits. With polysulphone (Choyce) the solution for the reduction in interface problems was to use fenestrations as small as 10 μm. There is some question as to whether there is degradation in the optical quality of the lens if this is done. Flat Fresnel optics lenses (Optical Radiation Corporation) will afford uniform thickness irrespective of the refractive error being corrected. Recall that in hyperopic lenses the center thickness is a barrier to permeability.

Intracorneal rings that run parallel to the limbus in a stromal tunnel have also emerged. They flatten the central cornea, invoking a myopic shift.

Epikeratophakia (Kaufman) involves cryolathing a donor cornea and suturing it to a deepithelialized recipient. This is especially useful in uniocular congenital aphakia and contact lens failure aphakia. Its easy reversibility is attractive. *Keratomilieusis* (Barraquer) similarly involves cryolathing an autolenticule of corneal tissue to correct for high myopia. Newer microkeratomes shave stroma similar to excimer photokeratectomy.

The common denominator in all of these procedures is surgical violation of the intact, healthy cornea. The use of lasers to achieve the same ends somehow seems more acceptable to the public and profession alike. Initially, traditional RK procedures were undertaken with the excimer laser. Soon, however, the central cornea became the object of interest.

Photorefractive keratectomy (PRK) with the excimer laser (L'esperance, Trokel, Marshall) involves sculpting the central cornea to flatten its radius of curvature. Using the argon fluoride 193 nm excimer laser, it was found that between 200 and 1000 mJ/cm/pulse a linear depth of tissue ablation was achievable (Aron-Rosa). The size of the optical zone and the depth of the ablation control the amount of myopic correction. Elliptical optical zones can correct for astigmatism. Hyperopic PRK involves ablation deeper in the peripheral zone. Other lasers, such as Raman-shifted Nd:YAG or pulsed visible 532 nm, 625 nm lasers have been tried for thermal vaporization or corneal stromal coagulation. Regression in their effect and more adjacent corneal damage seem to be the current limiting factors. The beauty of the excimer is the early absence of adjacent tissue injury.

The potential for harmonics of Nd:YAG or other tunable lasers to perform PRK is unknown. It is with great enthusiasm we await the new technology and salute the innovators.

Please see Part II: Problems and Part III: Solutions for typical examination questions pertaining to the material in this chapter.

APPENDIX A: ABBREVIATIONS

A	accommodation
AA	accommodative amplitude
AC	accommodative convergence
AR	antireflection
BD	base down
BI	base in
BO	base out
BU	base up
CAB	cellulose acetate butyrate
CCC	corrective combined cylinder
cyl	cylinder
D	diopter
DBL	distance between lenses
DK	diffusion solubility constant
EDL	effective diameter of the lens
EE	eye error
EOG	electrooculogram
ERG	electroretinogram
EXCIMER	excited dimer
FP	far point
H	horizontal
HIG	high index glass
HIP	high index plastic
IOL	intraocular lens
IR	infrared
K	keratometry readings
MA	meter angles
MVA	minimum visual angle
NP	near point
OC	optical center
OD	left eye
OS	right eye
OU	both eyes
P.D.	prism diopter
PD	pupillary distance
PRK	photorefractive keratectomy
RK	radial keratotomy
SL	standard lens
sph	sphere
SRK	Sanders, Retzlaff, and Kraft
UV	ultraviolet
VA	visual acuity
V	vertical
YAG	yttrium-aluminum-garnet

APPENDIX B: EQUATIONS

Accommodation through a telescope:

$$A_T = A_N \times M_A^2$$

Accommodative convergence/accommodation ratio (heterophoria method):

$$\frac{\text{AC}}{\text{A}} = PD + \frac{\text{P.D.}_{\text{N}} - \text{P.D.}_{\text{D}}}{\text{D}}$$

Angle of stereoacuity:

$$\theta = \frac{PD \times x}{\text{distance}^2}$$

Angular magnification:

$$M_A = xD$$

Angular magnification of a Galilean telescope:

$$M_A = \frac{-D_E}{D_O}$$

Angular magnification of a simple magnifier:

$$M_A = \frac{\text{D}}{4}$$

Axial magnification:

$$M_{AX} = (\text{linear magnification})^2$$

Critical angle:

$$n \sin i_c = n' \sin 90°$$

Dark focus:

$$\text{D.F.} = \frac{\text{Dark retinoscopy} - 0.25\text{ D}}{0.64}$$

Frequency and wavelength formulae:

$$c = \lambda v$$

$$\lambda_M = \frac{\lambda}{n}$$

Induced prism:

$$p\text{P.D.} = h\,(cm) \times D\,(\text{diopters})$$

IOL power for emmetropia:

$$P = A + (-2.5 \times \text{Axial length}) + (-0.9 \times \text{Average } K)$$

Keratometry power reading:

$$K = \frac{0.3375}{r}$$

Linear magnification:

$$M = \frac{v}{\mu} = \frac{U}{V} = \frac{I}{O}$$

Measurement error:

$$\text{Error} = 2.5 \times \text{D\%}$$

Minimum visual angle:

$$\text{MVA} = \frac{1}{\text{Visual acuity}}$$

New IOL power:

$$D_{IOL} = P - \frac{R}{1.5}$$

Mirrors:

$$f_m = \frac{r_m}{2};\ D_m = \frac{2}{r_m}$$

Power of an intraocular lens implant:

$$D_{air} = \frac{n_{IOL} - n_{air}}{n_{IOL} - n_{AQ}}$$

Power of a smooth refracting surface:

$$D_s = \frac{n' - n}{r}$$

Prism diopter:

$$\text{P.D.} = 100 \tan \beta$$

Radius of curvature:

$$r = \frac{0.3375}{D}$$

Reflection at an interface:

$$R = \left(\frac{n' - n}{n' + n}\right)^2$$

Snell's law:

$$n \sin i = n' \sin \mathrm{r}$$

Spherical equivalent:

$$\text{S.E.} = \text{Sphere} + \frac{\text{Cylinder}}{2}$$

Total hyperopia:

$$H_T = \text{Latent} + \text{Manifest}$$

Total magnification:

$$M_T = M_1 \times M_2 \ldots \times M_n$$

Vergence formulae:

$$U + D = V; \frac{1}{\mu} + \frac{1}{f} = \frac{1}{v}$$

$$nU + D_s = n'V$$

$$nU + \frac{n' - n}{r} = n'V$$

Vertex power:

$$D_V = D_1 + D_2 + \frac{t}{n} D_1^2$$

Visual acuity:

$$\text{VA} = \frac{1}{\text{MVA}} \times \left(\frac{20}{20}\right)$$

Visual angle:

$$V_A = \frac{20}{x}$$

Values and constants

- U: Object vergence
- V: Image vergence
- u: Object distance
- v: Image distance
- D: Vergence of the system
- f: Focal length
- n: Index of refraction
- c: Velocity of light in a vacuum (3.00×10^{10} cm/sec)
- v: Frequency of light
- λ: Wavelength of light
- i: Incident angle
- i_c: Critical angle
- r: Snell's law reflected angle
- r: Radius of curvature
- M: Magnification
- t: Thickness factor
- I: Image size
- O: Object size
- β: Angle of deviation
- d: Deviation and distance
- γ: Apex angle
- p: Induced prism
- h: Distance from the optical center in cm
- R: Reflection
- M_A: Angular magnification
- A_T: Accommodation through a telescope
- A_N: Normal accommodation
- V_A: Visual angle
- VA: Visual acuity
- MVA: Minimum visual angle
- θ: Angle of stereoacuity
- *PD*: Interpupillary distance
- P.D.: Prism diopter
- AC: Accommodative convergence
- A: Accommodation
- P.D._N: Near deviation
- P.D._D: Distance deviation
- P: IOL power for emmetropia
- A: Surgeon-specific constant
- R: Desired refractive error

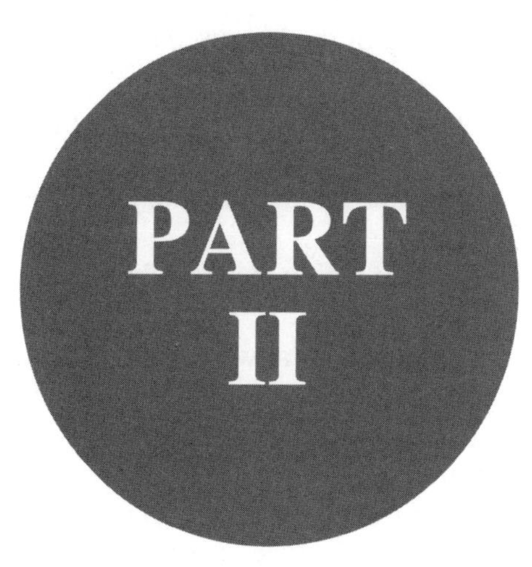

PROBLEMS

CHAPTER 1: THE BASICS

1-1. Which of the following is false?
A. Each photon has a defined wavelength
B. Infrared light is less phototoxic than UV light
C. Each wavelength has a corresponding quantum of energy
D. The longer the wavelength, the smaller the amount of energy per photon
E. UV light has a longer wavelength than visible light

1-2. Which of the following disorders has not been implicated to be the result of UV phototoxicity?
A. Pseudoexfoliation
B. Cataracts
C. Uveitis
D. Basal cell carcinoma
E. Pterygia

1-3. Chronic photoxicity can be induced by:
A. Superoxides
B. Ionized electrons
C. Free radicals
D. All of the above
E. None of the above

1-4. Prescribing UV filtered glasses is not recommended for:
A. Those with aphakia
B. Those taking photosensitizing drugs
C. Anisometropia of greater than 3.00 D
D. Cataract patients
E. Macular degeneration

1-5. The electric field of an advancing wavefront is:
A. Perpendicular to the magnetic field
B. In the same direction as the magnetic field
C. Opposite in direction to the magnetic field
D. Parallel to the optical axis
E. All of the above

1-6. The radius of curvature of a wavefront is a measure of the:
A. Luminance of a pencil of light
B. The arc of the lens used to produce it
C. Accommodative power of the optical system
D. Vergence of the advancing wavefront
E. Speed at which the wavefront is advancing

1-7. The vergence of a wavefront is zero when:
A. The distance from the source is infinite
B. It is parallel to the optical axis
C. The wavefront is converging to the source
D. The electric field is acted upon by a plus lens
E. None of the above

1-8. A diopter is the unit of:
A. Accommodative amplitude
B. Power of a lens
C. Divergence of a wavefront
D. Vergence at a specific distance from the source
E. All of the above

1-9. The radius of curvature is:
A. The radius of the circle needed to yield a vergence of zero
B. The accommodation required for an object of regard
C. Measured with the radiuscope
D. All of the above
E. None of the above

1-10. An object is 40 cm in front of a refracting surface of power +10.00 D. Which of the following is incorrect?
A. The object vergence is −2.50 D
B. The image is 13.3 cm to the right of the lens
C. The image is real
D. The image vergence is −7.50 D
E. The image is inverted

1-11. If parallel rays strike a +4.00 D lens, where will the image be?
A. 0.25 m to the left of the lens
B. 25 cm to the right of the lens
C. 2.5 cm to the left of the lens
D. 0.25 cm to the right of the lens
E. 4 cm to the left of the lens

1-12. An object point *O* is located 33 cm in

front of a lens of power +5.00 D. Which of the following statements does not correspond to this system?

A. The vergence of the incident rays is −3.00 D
B. The refracted vergence is +2.00 D
C. The image is located 50 cm to the right of the lens
D. The image is virtual
E. None of the above

1-13. An optically active surface alters the vergence:

A. By reflection
B. By refraction
C. Such that the emergent rays are more convergent
D. By diffraction
E. All of the above

1-14. The relationship $U + D = V$ holds true for:

A. All optical systems
B. Convergent lenses only
C. Mirrors only
D. All lenses and mirrors
E. Only the schematic eye

1-15. A plus lens always:

A. Adds vergence
B. Produces an image to the right of the lens
C. Reduces vergence
D. Produces an image to the left of the lens
E. None of the above

1-16. A minus lens always:

A. Adds vergence
B. Produces an image to the right of the lens
C. Reduces vergence
D. Produces an image to the left of the lens
E. None of the above

1-17. Spherical lenses:

A. Have different radii of curvature in two principal meridians
B. Have the same power in all meridians
C. Have an astigmatic focus when configured as a meniscus lens
D. Always add vergence power
E. All of the above

1-18. What is the focal length of a plus lens whose image is 25 cm behind the lens for an object at 60 cm in front of the lens?

A. $\frac{5}{3}$ m
B. $\frac{3}{5}$ m
C. $\frac{3}{7}$ m
D. $\frac{3}{17}$ m
E. 35 cm

1-19. Light that encounters a more dense medium might emerge?

A. With a greater vergence
B. Reflected or refracted
C. With the same wavelength
D. With the same frequency
E. All of the above

1-20. What is the frequency of yellow light of wavelength 589 nm?

A. 5.1×10^{16} seconds
B. 5.1×10 Hz
C. 2.0×10^{-17} Hz
D. -2.0×10^{-17} Hz
E. None of the above

1-21. Light of wavelength 460 nm encounters the interface of a new medium with an index of refraction of 1.24. Find the reduced wavelength in the new medium:

A. 570 nm
B. 371 nm
C. 270 nm
D. 652 nm
E. 460 nm

1-22. The power of light in a different medium is called:

A. Reduced vergence
B. Corrected vergence
C. Normalized vergence
D. All of the above
E. None of the above

1-23. Refraction:

A. Occurs only at high speeds
B. Is the unaltered transmission of light rays between media
C. Is a function of the incident angle
D. All of the above
E. None of the above

1-24. Snell's law is the relationship between the:

A. Incident angle and the radius of curvature of the medium
B. Incident and reflected media

C. Incident and reflected rays
D. Incident and refracted angles
E. None of the above

1-25. As light travels from one medium to a:
A. More dense medium, it is refracted away from the normal
B. More dense medium, it is refracted toward the normal
C. More dense medium, it not refracted but reflected
D. Less dense medium, it is refracted toward the normal
E. None of the above

1-26. A beam of light perpendicular to the interface between two media is:
A. Reflected but not refracted
B. Refracted toward the normal if going from a less to more dense-medium
C. Refracted away from the normal if going from a more to less dense medium
D. Transmitted at a higher speed if emerging from the more dense medium
E. None of the above

1-27. Calculate the angle of refraction of light traveling from air into a sheet of plastic (n = 1.42) at an incident angle of 50° to the normal (sin 33° = 0.545; sin 40° = 0.643; sin 50° = 0.767; sin 83° = 0.993):
A. 33° from the normal
B. 3.3° from the interface
C. 57° from the normal
D. 83° from the interface
E. None of the above

1-28. What would happen to light that is 25° incident to a sheet of glass (n = 1.5) immersed in a medium (n = 1.3) (sin 19° = 0.326; sin 21.5° = 0.366; sin 25° = 0.423)?
A. The angle of refraction is 21.5°
B. The angle of refraction is 19°
C. The light is reflected back into the glass at the second interface
D. The light is displaced but not deviated
E. None of the above

1-29. Light incident at 90° to a right angle prism (apex angle 30°) emerges at what angle from the perpendicular side of the prism (sin 11° = 0.191; sin 17° = 0.292; sin 30° = 0.50; sin 41° = 0.656; sin 73° = 0.956; sin 86° = 0.997)?
A. 41° to the interface
B. 86° to the interface
C. 73° to the normal
D. 17° to the normal
E. None of the above

1-30. Reflection occurs when light passes:
A. From a dense to a more dense medium
B. From a more dense to a less dense medium
C. At an angle equal to or greater than the critical angle
D. All of the above
E. None of the above

1-31. The critical angle can be altered by:
A. Increasing the radius of curvature
B. Contact lenses
C. Decreasing vergence
D. Increasing vergence
E. All of the above

1-32. The critical angle is important in all of the following phenomena except:
A. Fiberoptics
B. Gonioscopy
C. Retinoscopy
D. Reflecting prisms
E. Goldmann lens fundoscopy

1-33. What is the critical angle between an implant of refractive index 1.490 and aqueous of refractive index 1.333 (sin 27° = 0.454; sin 36° = 0.588; sin 63° = 0.891)?
A. 63°
B. 36°
C. 27°
D. This angle cannot be determined without knowing the incident angle
E. None of the above

1-34. When speaking of reflection:
A. Light is trapped in the same medium
B. The incident angle is slightly greater than the reflected angle
C. The reflected speed is greater
D. The wavelength decreases
E. None of the above

1-35. Which of the following is false?

A. A plus mirror adds positive vergence
B. A convex mirror adds negative vergence
C. A concave mirror adds positive vergence
D. A convex mirror adds positive vergence
E. A minus mirror adds negative vergence

1-36. Which of the following statements is true for mirrors?
A. The focal length equals half the radius of curvature
B. The focal length equals two times the radius of curvature
C. If the focal point is to the left of the mirror, the mirror is divergent
D. A plane mirror has different values for object and image vergence
E. None of the above

1-37. All of the following are true of a single smooth reflecting or refracting surface except:
A. It can be an interface between any two media of different indices of refraction
B. It obeys the laws of reflection
C. The use of different media demands the use of reduced vergence for refraction by the interface
D. It has the same sign convention as mirrors
E. The change in media does not affect the velocity

1-38. What is the refractive power of the back surface of a meniscus style implant of radius 15 mm in aqueous (n_{aq} = 1.333; n_{IOL} = 1.528)?
A. +191.00 D
B. +1.30 D
C. −13.00 D
D. −130.00 D
E. None of the above

1-39. Given an object 1 m to the left of a concave mirror (radius of curvature 20 cm) which of the following is applicable?
A. The power of the mirror is +5.00 D
B. The image is located 11 cm to the right of the mirror
C. The image is minified 9×
D. The image is erect
E. All of the above

1-40. If the interior surface of the cornea has a radius of 10 mm, which of the following is true of an object 50 cm away?
A. The magnification of the object is 100×
B. The reflecting power of the cornea is +100.00 D
C. The magnification of the object is 4×
D. The reflecting power of the cornea is −200.00 D
E. None of the above

1-41. Which of the following accurately describes the reflected image formed by the anterior corneal surface (D_m = −200 D) of an object 50 cm away?
A. Minified, erect, and virtual
B. Located 1.8 m to the left of the cornea
C. Magnified, erect, and real
D. Minified, inverted, and virtual
E. Magnified, inverted, and real

1-42. A mirror images an object 40 cm in front of it at 20 cm. What is its radius of curvature?
A. 11.4 cm to the right of the mirror
B. 45 cm
C. 8.9 cm to the left of the mirror
D. 11.4 cm to the left of the mirror
E. None of the above

1-43. What is the refracting power of a reflecting surface with a radius of curvature of 20 cm and an index of refraction greater than that of the air surrounding it by 0.50?
A. +7.50 D
B. +2.50 D
C. −0.10 D
D. +1.50 D
E. None of the above

1-44. Find the image vergence of an object placed 40 cm in front of the anterior lens–aqueous surface of radius of curvature 10 mm (n_{aq} = 1.33; n_{lens} = 1.50):
A. +9.12 D
B. −9.12 D
C. +10.28 D
D. −10.28 D
E. +8.13 D

1-45. Vergence formulae can determine all of the following except:
A. Incoming vergence
B. Outgoing vergence
C. Nature of the image (virtual, real, erect)
D. Magnification or minification of the system
E. Power of the lens

1-46. To define the optical system, which of the following is not a convention?
A. The direction of light is from right to left
B. The incoming rays are object rays
C. The outgoing rays are image rays
D. The object rays enter from the left
E. All of the above

1-47. A fish under water is to be speared. Should the fisherman looking into the water at the fish in front of him aim ahead of or behind, and above or below the fish?
A. Ahead, above
B. Ahead, below
C. Behind, above
D. Behind, below
E. The fish is exactly where he sees it

1-48. Consider a concave lens of -15.00 D. If the object distance is 20 cm behind the lens, describe the image nature and position:
A. The image is virtual and located 10 cm in front of the lens
B. The image is virtual and located 5 cm in front of the lens
C. The image is real and located 10 cm behind the lens
D. The image is virtual and located 20 cm in front of the lens
E. The image is real and located 5 cm behind the lens

1-49. Find the primary focal point for a lens with an object vergence of $+4.00$ D:
A. 25 cm behind the lens
B. 25 cm in front of the lens
C. 50 cm behind the lens
D. 50 cm in front of the lens
E. 4.0 mm behind the lens

1-50. Which of the following statements is not true for a plane mirror?
A. The power of the mirror is never zero
B. $U = V$
C. The image lies to the right and is virtual
D. The magnification is 1
E. None of the above

1-51. How far away from a plane mirror is the image of an object of vergence $+5.00$ D?
A. 2 m
B. 2 cm
C. 5 cm
D. 5 mm
E. None of the above

1-52. What is the radius of a 2× bar magnifier if it is made of plastic ($n = 1.49$)?
A. 3.11 m
B. 31.10 cm
C. 6.12 cm
D. 3.11 cm
E. None of the above

1-53. An observer is 1.5 m from a plane mirror. What is the difference between the observer's perceived magnification and the actual image magnification?
A. A factor of 1
B. A factor of 2
C. A factor of 4
D. A factor of 0.5
E. None of the above

1-54. The field of view of a plane mirror is:
A. Half the size of the mirror
B. The same size as the mirror
C. Twice the size of the mirror
D. Three times the size of the mirror
E. None of the above

1-55. Linear magnification:
A. Is calculated by dividing the object size by the image size
B. Is found by multiplying the image and object sizes
C. Is equal to the image height over the object height
D. Can also be called primary magnification
E. None of the above or more than one of the above

1-56. A $+3.00$ D lens is placed 20 cm from a -4.00 D lens. An object is placed 50 cm in front of the plus lens. Where is the final image?

A. 19 cm to the left of the minus lens
B. 16 cm to the right of the minus lens
C. 36 cm to the left of the minus lens
D. 1 cm to the right of the plus lens
E. 16 cm to the left of the minus lens

1-57. An object is placed 25 cm from a +2.50 D lens. A second −4.00 D lens is ⅛ m from the first. Where will the final image be?

A. 33.3 cm in front of the minus lens
B. 20 cm in front of the minus lens
C. 45 cm in front of the plus lens
D. 66.6 cm in front of the plus lens
E. 13.3 cm in front of the plus lens

1-58. An object is imaged by a +2.00 and a −3.00 D lens combination separated by 30 cm. If the final image is located 20 cm behind the second −3.00 D lens, where should the object be?

A. 23.0 cm in front of the plus lens
B. 0.125 m behind the plus lens
C. 2.86 m to the left of the plus lens
D. 2.86 cm to the left of the minus lens
E. 42.5 cm to the left of the plus lens

1-59. A multilens system can be:

A. Thought of as a thick lens if the spaces are minimal
B. Reduced using an optical bench to form two principal planes with two focal points
C. Depicted using ray diagrams
D. All of the above
E. None of the above

1-60. The back vertex power is:

A. A measurement taken from the back surface of the lens
B. The same as the anterior vertex power
C. Derived with the posterior surface facing the examiner
D. Equivalent to the lens effectivity
E. None of the above

1-61. When dealing with correcting spectacles, the power varies with:

A. The index of refraction of the lens material
B. The vertex distance
C. The optical center position relative to the visual axes
D. The front and back radii of curvature
E. All of the above

1-62. CAP:

A. Is an instrument used when measuring the vertex distance
B. Can be taken off to increase the vertex power
C. Means "clinically add plus"
D. Means "closer add plus"
E. Means "closer add power"

1-63. Consider an intraocular lens implant. The effective power is affected by the:

A. Difference in refractive indices
B. Change in vertex distance
C. Different incident angles
D. All of the above
E. None of the above

1-64. An object is placed 0.3 m from a +5.00 D lens. What power of lens could be placed at 0.2 m from the image to achieve the same effectivity?

A. +13.30 D
B. +1.67 D
C. +3.33 D
D. +6.43 D
E. None of the above

1-65. A posterior chamber intraocular lens implant power calculation reveals that a +12.50 D implant is required. What should this lens measure in air when packaged (n = 1.5 for the implant)?

A. +36.76 D
B. +16.63 D
C. +18.75 D
D. +8.33 D
E. +9.40 D

1-66. The reduced eye (n = ⁴⁄₃) has a single spherical surface of 60.00 D separating air from medium. If an object 50 cm long is placed 4 m from the eye, which of the following is true for this system?

A. The nodal point is 16.67 cm in front of the eye
B. The focal length is 5.55 cm
C. The retinal image is 2.08 cm high
D. The center of curvature is 12.00 cm from the vertex
E. None of the above

CHAPTER 2: LENS ABERRATIONS

2-1. Which of the following is not an important lens aberration for thick lenses?
- **A.** Astigmatism of oblique incidence
- **B.** Spherical
- **C.** Chromatic
- **D.** Diffraction
- **E.** Coma

2-2. A blur interval occurs when:
- **A.** Peripheral rays are subject to increased prismatic effect and too much power
- **B.** Parallel rays pass through the center of curvature of a spherical lens
- **C.** The retina is not on the radius of the sphere
- **D.** There is chromatic aberration
- **E.** None of the above

2-3. In spectacle correction with high power lenses, aspheric surfaces improve the spherical aberrations best for:
- **A.** Those with hyperopia
- **B.** Those with myopia
- **C.** Those with hyperopia and myopia
- **D.** Those with astigmatism
- **E.** None of the above

2-4. Spherical aberration occurs naturally, but three physiologic factors reduce its effect:
- **A.** Pupil size, pupillary distance, and radius of curvature of the peripheral cornea
- **B.** Index of refraction of the crystalline lens, index of refraction of the cornea, and the vertex distance
- **C.** Pupil size, radius of curvature of the peripheral cornea, and the index of refraction of the crystalline lens
- **D.** Pupillary distance, index of refraction of the cornea, and vertex distance
- **E.** None of the above

2-5. Coma relates to off axis peripheral rays causing:
- **A.** A blur spot of spherical dimensions on the image axis
- **B.** A spherical image deformity to axial portions of the image
- **C.** Blurred visual imagery
- **D.** Oblique distortion in the axial areas of the image
- **E.** None of the above

2-6. Astigmatism of oblique incidence results in:
- **A.** Image blur
- **B.** Astigmatic imagery
- **C.** Astigmatic interval in which the image is blurred
- **D.** Blur circles on the retina
- **E.** All of the above

2-7. The only advantageous aberration of the human eye is:
- **A.** Coma
- **B.** Chromatic
- **C.** Curvature of field
- **D.** Astigmatism of oblique incidence
- **E.** None of the above

2-8. Which of the following statements is false?
- **A.** Blue light is refracted more than red light
- **B.** Green light is the standard wavelength to calibrate the index of refraction
- **C.** In the emmetropic eye, the yellow portion of the spectrum is in best focus
- **D.** In the corrected myopic eye, green light would be in better focus than red
- **E.** Each wavelength has a different index of refraction

2-9. In addition to the ABCs of lens aberrations, which of the following problems are also associated with thick lenses?
- **A.** Visual field scotoma
- **B.** Magnification
- **C.** Minification
- **D.** Aberrant depth perception
- **E.** All of the above

CHAPTER 3: PRISMS

3-1. The effect of a plane parallel plate on light is:
- **A.** The ray emerging from the second

interface is undeviated and undisplaced from its initial path
B. The ray emerging from the second interface is displaced but undeviated from its initial path
C. The ray emerging from the second interface is displaced and deviated from its initial path
D. The ray emerging from the first interface is not reflected by the second
E. None of the above

3-2. A prism diopter is:
A. The power needed to regard an image at infinity
B. The apparent displacement of a ray (in meters) at 1 cm
C. The apparent displacement of the image (in meters) at 1 m
D. The apparent displacement of a ray (in centimeters) at 1 m
E. None of the above

3-3. A 6 P.D. prism will displace a ray how far at ⅓ m?
A. 6 cm
B. 4 cm
C. 2 cm
D. 18 cm
E. None of the above

3-4. To describe the orientation of the prism power we clinically use the:
A. Apex angle of the prism
B. Base of the prism
C. Degrees from the baseline of the apex
D. All of the above
E. None of the above

3-5. When presented with both a vertical and a horizontal prism at the same time, a single representative prism can be formed by:
A. Summing the individual components
B. Taking the difference between the different components
C. Vectorially adding the components of each separate prism
D. Vectorially subtracting the individual components
E. None of the above

3-6. What is the power of a prism that displaces an object 10 cm at a distance of 50 cm?
A. 20 P.D.
B. 0.2 P.D.
C. 10 P.D.
D. 50 P.D.
E. None of the above

3-7. How much will a 5 P.D. prism displace an object at 40 cm?
A. 2.5 cm
B. 12.5 cm
C. 0.8 mm
D. 2.0 cm
E. None of the above

3-8. Calculate the power of a prism that displaces an object 8 cm at a distance of 50 cm:
A. 4.00 P.D.
B. 0.0625 P.D.
C. 16.00 P.D.
D. 0.16 P.D.
E. None of the above

3-9. Two separate prisms are placed in front of the right eye. One prism is horizontal with 3 P.D. BO and the other is a BU prism of 4 P.D. Which of the following describes the resultant prismatic effect?
A. 7 P.D. BU
B. 5 P.D. BD and BO at 37°
C. −1 P.D. BO
D. 5 P.D. BO and BU at 37°
E. None of the above

3-10. The angle to place a combined prism can be determined with the help of all of the following except:
A. A protractor
B. A trial lens frame
C. A phoropter
D. Trigonometry
E. Stenopeic slit

3-11. The minimum angle of deviation is achieved:
A. At an inclination that yields equal deviation at both surfaces
B. When the angle is less than 10°
C. In any isosceles triangle
D. When the inclination is minimal
E. None of the above

3-12. Plastic prisms are calibrated in which position?

A. Frontal
B. Prentice
C. Inclined
D. Minimum deviation
E. Maximum deviation

3-13. When eye deviations are measured with plastic prisms, the:
A. Front surface should be held at the maximum deviation
B. Back surface should be held at the maximum deviation
C. Front surface should be held in the frontal position
D. Back surface should be held in the frontal position
E. None of the above

3-14. A plastic prism should be:
A. Parallel with the examiner
B. Parallel with the prism base
C. Parallel with the patient's forehead
D. Perpendicular to the prism base
E. None of the above

3-15. Glass prisms are calibrated in which position?
A. Frontal
B. Prentice
C. Inclined at 30°
D. Minimum deviation
E. Maximum deviation

3-16. For the measured deviation to correspond to the calibrated value for glass prisms:
A. The back surface of the prism must be parallel with the visual axis
B. The front surface of the prism must not be perpendicular to the visual axis
C. The front surface of the prism can face any way
D. Either surface of the prism must be perpendicular to the visual axis
E. The orientation doesn't affect the accuracy of the calibration

3-17. Which of the following statements is false?
A. You should never stack two prisms in the same direction for an additive effect
B. The combination of horizontal and vertical prisms is clinically useful for measuring deviations
C. When stacking prisms in the same direction, the emergent light from the first prism is not incident upon the second stacked prism at the correct angle of incidence
D. Prisms cannot be added to each eye separately
E. A loose prism can be used in conjunction with a rotary prism for measuring deviations

3-18. Other circular measurements that are interchangeable with the prism diopter include:
A. Radians and degrees
B. Radians and diopters
C. Radians and meter angles
D. Degrees and meter angles
E. None of the above

3-19. The angles expressed in prism diopters increase:
A. In a linear fashion
B. Slower than the tangents
C. Faster than the tangents when the angle is greater than 90°
D. All of the above
E. None of the above

3-20. The angle of deviation is approximately related to the prism diopter by the tangent to the prism diopter such that:
A. For small angles the ratio is 1° for every 1 P.D.
B. For small angles the ratio is 1° for every 2 P.D.
C. For small angles the ratio is 2° for every 1 P.D.
D. For small angles there is no relationship between the two
E. None of the above

3-21. What is the exact power of a prism whose angle of displacement is 10° ($\sin 10° = 0.1736$, $\tan 10° = 0.1763$)?
A. 20 P.D.
B. 10 P.D.
C. 1.0 P.D.
D. 5.0 P.D.
E. 17.63 P.D.

3-22. When one is grinding a prism, its power is verified using which of the following means?
A. Prismatic effect of decentration
B. Apex angle

C. Lensmeter measurement
D. Base width
E. All of the above

3-23. Which of the following statements is true?
A. At 90° the prismatic power approaches 200 P.D.
B. At 90° the light is refracted at an obtuse angle
C. At 90° the prism has infinite prism diopters
D. At 90° the light is reflected back upon itself
E. None of the above

3-24. A prism affects the image of a virtual object so as to:
A. Displace it toward the apex of the prism
B. Displace it toward the base of the prism
C. Invert it
D. Reverse it from left to right
E. None of the above

3-25. A prism displaces an object 100 cm at a distance of 1 m. Which of the following statements is not correct?
A. The angle of deviation is 45°
B. The true prismatic power is 90 P.D.
C. The approximation formula states 1° = 2 P.D. with an error of 10%
D. 45° is the cutoff angle for the approximation formula
E. None of the above

3-26. An object is placed 40 cm in front of a +3.00 D lens. The resultant image is displaced by a base down prism behind the lens. Which of the following statements is correct?
A. The image is 2 m from the lens
B. The image is real and behind the lens
C. Virtual images are displaced toward the base of the prism
D. The image is displaced toward the base of the prism
E. None of the above

3-27. Consider a patient with a prism in front of his eye:
A. Both the patient and the examiner see the eye displaced toward the apex
B. The patient sees the eye displaced toward the base
C. Only the examiner sees the eye displaced toward the base
D. The eye does not look displaced to either the patient or examiner
E. None of the above

3-28. A heterophoria or tropia is a:
A. Latent or manifest power deficiency
B. Chronic aberration
C. Latent or manifest deviation of the eye
D. All of the above
E. None of the above

3-29. Which of the following statements is true?
A. Esotropia is a temporal deviation
B. Exotropia is an eye deviated toward the nose
C. Hypertropia is too much deviation
D. Hypotropia is too little deviation
E. None of the above

3-30. If a base out prism is placed in front of an esotropic eye:
A. The deviation is shifted toward the nose
B. No change occurs within the system
C. The ray is focused toward the fovea of the deviated eye
D. The esotropia increases
E. None of the above

3-31. The correcting prism is always positioned such that:
A. The base is perpendicular to the fovea
B. The base points in the direction of the deviation
C. The apex points opposite the direction of the deviation
D. The apex points in the direction of the deviation
E. None of the above

3-32. If a pair of prism glasses is placed in front of straight eyes, the induced deviation:
A. Is pointed out by the direction of the apex of the prism required to correct it
B. Is equal and opposite in direction to

the prismatic effect of the prism being used to correct it

C. Is equal to half of the prismatic effect of the prism glasses

D. Is pointed out by the direction of the apex of the prism in the prism glasses

E. None of the above

3-33. The prismatic effect of lenses describes:

A. The results when a lens and a prism are combined in an optical system

B. Lenses as prisms of progressively increasing prismatic power outward from the optical center

C. The phenomenon that occurs when the incident angle to the lens equals the apex angle of the corresponding prism

D. The lens as a stack of prisms in the same direction

E. None of the above

3-34. A plus lens can be thought of as:

A. A lower BD and an upper BU prism

B. An outer BO and an inner BI prism

C. Two BU prisms, one on top of the other

D. An upper BD and a lower BU prism

E. Any of these answers is a possible structure for a plus lens

3-35. In the calculation of induced prism which of the following is not needed?

A. Interpupillary distance of the patient

B. Distrance between optical centers of the glass

C. Power of the lenses

D. All of the above are needed

E. None of the above are needed

3-36. Find the induced prismatic effect at the reading position 1 cm down and 0.2 cm in, if one wears a +5.00 D lens over both eyes:

A. The net vertical prism will be 5 p.d. *BU OD*

B. The horizontal prism *OS* will be 1 P.D. *BO*

C. The induced vertical prism in both eyes is different

D. The horizontal prism in both eyes is equal but opposite in direction

E. None of the above

3-37. An anisometropic person wears +5.00 D right eye and +2.00 D left. If he reads 8 mm beneath the optical centers, which of the following statements is correct?

A. A right hypodeviation is induced

B. The net effect is 5.60 P.D. *BD* OD

C. Neutralization can be achieved with a 2.4 P.D. *BU* OS

D. The correcting prism should be 5.6 P.D. *BD* OS

E. A left exodeviation is induced

3-38. Describe the induced horizontal deviation of a patient who reads 1.5 cm in from the optical centers of the following lenses:

OD: +4.00 +2.00 × 90

OS: −3.00

A. Corrected by a 9.00 P.D. *BI* OD

B. Net effect of 9.00 P.D. *BO* OS

C. 4.50 P.D. induced exophoria

D. No net effect

E. 4.50 P.D. induced esophoria

3-39. If one wears a +4.00 D sperical lens over both eyes,which of the following is true about the usual reading position (2 mm in, 8 mm down)?

A. No net vertical effect is present

B. A vertical effect of 6.4 P.D. BU OS

C. No net horizontal effect is present

D. A horizontal effect of 1.6 P.D. BI OD

E. No net vertical or horizontal effect is present

3-40. A patient has a right hyperdeviation. If we cover the left eye so that the right eye fixes the object of regard:

A. The left eye is hyperdeviated

B. The right eye is hypodeviated

C. The right eye is neutralized

D. The left eye is hypodeviated

E. None of the above

3-41. Which of the following statements is not true?

A. A hyperdeviation in one eye is equivalent to a hypodeviation in the other eye

B. A BU prism over one eye is the same as a BU prism over the other
C. A BO prism over one eye is the same as BU prism over the other eye
D. A BD prism over one eye is the same as a BU prism over the other eye
E. The above statements, if correct, do not apply to dissociated vertical deviations

3-42. A patient requires 3.2 P.D. *BU OS* to correct a left hypodeviation. Which statement is false?
A. Looking through the left lens only, everything is better focused than without the prism
B. A bifocal might pose special problems
C. Tilting the head would complicate the problem if the deviation was incomitant
D. Looking outside the optical centers of the lenses might increase the hypodeviation
E. None of the above

3-43. Anisometropia with induced hypodeviation might be treated by:
A. Single vision readers
B. Lens decentration
C. Ground-in prism of the appropriate amount
D. Lens slab-off to the more minus or less plus lens
E. All of the above

3-44. A right hyperdeviation induced by an anisometropic prescription in a straight-eyed patient can be partially compensated for by:
A. Bifocals
B. Dropping the optical centers of both lenses
C. Slabbing off the right lens
D. BU prism *OD*
E. All of the above

3-45. If 8 P.D. *BI* and 6 P.D. *BD* placed before the left eye are needed to correct a strabismic deviation, find the single prism needed to accomplish the same purpose (tan 37° = $\frac{6}{8}$, tan 53° = $\frac{8}{6}$):
A. 14 P.D. BI and BO at 180°
B. 2 P.D. BD at 90°
C. 16 P.D. BO and BD at 45°
D. 10 P.D. BI and BD at 37°
E. None of the above

3-46. A patient reads 1 cm below the optical centers of his single vision glasses (*OD*: $+2.00 + 3.00 \times 90$; *OS*: -1.00). What is the induced vertical deviation with the glasses?
A. A 1.00 P.D. right hyperdeviation
B. A 2.00 P.D. left hypodeviation
C. A 4.00 P.D. right hypodeviation
D. A 3.00 P.D. left hypodeviation
E. None of the above

3-47. What is the induced prismatic effect of an anisometropic person who reads 0.5 cm below the optical centers of her single vision glasses?

OD: $+4.00$ D

OS: -2.00 D -1.00×180

A. 2.50 P.D. *BD* OS
B. 1.50 P.D. *BU* OS
C. 1.00 P.D. *BU* OD
D. 1.50 P.D. *BU* OD
E. 0.50 P.D. *BD* OD

3-48. A patient wearing bifocals reads 10 mm below and 3 mm in from the optical centers. If the optical center of the bifocal segment coincides with this point, what will be the induced prism if the lens power is $+3.00$ D in both eyes with $+2.00$ D adds?
A. No net effect vertically
B. Net effect of 3.00 P.D. *BU OD*
C. Net effect of 0.90 P.D. *BO*
D. No net horizontal effect
E. None of the above

3-49. A patient has a pupillary distance of 58 mm and optical centers 74 mm apart. Which of the following statements accurately describes the system?
A. Decentration is 8 mm for each lens
B. The lenses are decentered 8 mm in total
C. Each lens is decentered 6 mm in total

D. The effect of decentration may be relieved by BO prism
E. None of the above

3-50. If one has an esodeviation or exodeviation, the direction of the correcting prism for the deviation:
A. Depends on which eye is turned
B. Is the same no matter which eye is turned
C. Must be corrected using prisms whose base points in the direction of the deviation
D. Base out prism over one eye is the same as base in prism over the other
E. None of the above

3-51. When an exodeviation is present:
A. Vertical fusional amplitude is required to maintain singular binocular vision
B. A blur interval exists in the affected field of view
C. BO prism neutralizes it
D. BI prism is always prescribed
E. None of the above

3-52. Which of the following statements is true?
A. Most people have less horizontal than vertical fusional amplitude
B. The induced deviation is in the direction of the base of the neutralizing or correcting prism
C. The magnitude of decentration is the sum of similar vertical prisms
D. Decentration is never beneficial
E. None of the above

3-53. The power of a cylinder is:
A. Along its axis
B. In the meridian 90° to any tangent
C. Constant
D. In the meridian 90° to its axis
E. None of the above

3-54. For the cylinder +2.00 × 180:
A. Its maximum power is at 90°
B. The distance correction has all its power at 180°
C. There is no power at 45° to the axis
D. For near there is an additional diopter in every direction
E. None of the above

3-55. An anisometropic person wears +3.00 D right eye and +4.00 D left eye. What is the induced horizontal prism looking 2 mm inside the optical centers to read?
A. 5.6 P.D. BI
B. 0.8 P.D. BO
C. 0.2 P.D. BI
D. 1.4 P.D. BO
E. None of the above

3-56. One can ignore the power of the add for induced deviations if:
A. It is less than +6.00 D and the same style
B. It is equally set at the same height and is the same style and power in both eyes
C. It is on the 90° axis
D. It is equal in magnitude and opposite in direction to the distance power
E. One can never ignore the power of the add

3-57. If the measuring prism is in the same direction as the induced prismatic effect of the spectacle correction, the amount of measuring prism will be:
A. Greater than the true deviation
B. Less than the true deviation
C. The opposite sign of the true deviation
D. Equal to the true deviation
E. Dependent on the style of prism used

3-58. Calculate the induced vertical prism of the following lenses in the reading position 8 mm beneath the distance optical centers:

OD: +4.00 sphere

OS: +1.00 sphere

Add +2.50 *OU*

A. 1.00 P.D. BU OD
B. 2.40 P.D. BU OD
C. 4.00 P.D. BU OS
D. No net effect
E. None of the above

3-59. A patient wears bifocals with −2.50 D lenses and an add of+1.00 *OD* and

+2.00 *OS.* Calculate the induced prismatic effect if the patient reads 8 mm below and 2 mm in from their optical centers:

A. 1.6 P.D. *BD OD,* 0.4 P.D. *BI OD*
B. 0.4 P.D. *BD OD,* 0.8 P.D. *BO OS*
C. 0.8 P.D. *BD OD,* 0.2 P.D. *BO OD*
D. 0.8 P.D. *BD OD,* 0.4 P.D. *BI OS*
E. None of the above

3-60. A patient wears +3.00 D bifocals with +2.50 D adds in both eyes. The segment optical centers are at different heights such that *OD* is a round top lens 1.0 cm below the patient's distance optical center and *OS* is a flat top 0.5 cm below the distance optical center. Which of the following is true?

A. The patient will view through the OC of the flat top segment 0.5 cm above the distance OC *OS.*
B. There is no net horizontal effect
C. The net vertical effect is equal to 1.25 P.D. *BD OD*
D. The net horizontal effect is equal to 1.0 P.D. *BO OD*
E. None of the above

3-61. What single correcting prism placed in front of the right eye would compensate for both the horizontal and vertical induced prism of the following lenses when reading is done 5 mm down and 3 mm in from the optical centers? (*OD* +3.00 +1.00 × 90; *OS* −2.00+1.00 × 180)

A. 2.06 P.D. BD and BI at 29°
B. 1.17 P.D. BD and BI at 59°
C. 2.69 P.D. BD and BI at 48°
D. 2.09 P.D. BD and BI at 17°
E. 1.56 P.D. BD and BI at 50°

3-62. An anisometropic bifocal wearer reads 8 mm below and 2 mm in from the optical centers of the lenses. What prism will correct the induced deviation? (*OD* +3.00; *OS* +1.00; add +2.00 *OU*)?

A. 3.35 BD and BI at 17° OS
B. 1.89 BD and BI at 32° OD
C. 1.79 BU and BI at 27° OS
D. 3.26 BU and BI at 11° OS
E. None of the above

3-63. Calculate the induced vertical deviation at the reading position (0.8 cm down) for *OD:* +4.00 +2.00 × 135 and *OS:* +1.00 + 4.00 × 45:

A. 6.4 P.D. right hyperdeviation
B. 1.6 P.D. left esophoria
C. 2.4 P.D. left hypodeviation
D. 4.0 P.D. right hypodeviation
E. 1.6 P.D. right hyperdeviation

3-64. Calculate the horizontal prismatic effects of decentered −5.00 D lenses for a patient with a pupillary distance of 56 mm when the distance between optical centers is 68 mm:

A. There is no induced horizontal deviation
B. 6.0. P.D. BI prism is induced
C. 6.0 P.D. BO prism is induced
D. A 6 P.D. exophoria is induced
E. None of the above

3-65. A patient with a 30 P.D. exotropia wears the following glasses centered properly: *OD*: −10.00, *OS*: plano. What will the exotropia measure at distance through the glasses?

A. With the right eye fixing, 30 P.D.
B. With the right eye fixing, 25% less
C. With the left eye fixing, no exotropia
D. With the left eye fixing, 2.5% more
E. None of the above

3-66. What is the actual amount of exotropia if a −16.00 D spectacle-corrected myopia measures 25 P.D.?

A. 21.25 P.D.
B. 35 P.D.
C. 15 P.D.
D. 40.6 P.D.
E. None of the above

3-67. An esotropic person measures 30 P.D. wearing +15.00 D glasses. Which of the following is true?

A. The induced error in measurement is 37.5 P.D.
B. The true amount of esotropia is 41.25 P.D.
C. The induced error measures less for myopia
D. Without spectacle correction the patient has an esotropia of 12 P.D.
E. None of the above

3-68. When measuring the primary versus secondary deviation, the fixing eye becomes:
- **A.** The eye without the prism
- **B.** The eye with the prism
- **C.** The eye with the paretic muscle
- **D.** The eye without the paretic muscle
- **E.** None of the above

3-69. Image jump is the sudden shift in the image position when:
- **A.** The visual axis rotates 180° in the segment
- **B.** The visual axis descends from the distance optical center to the bifocal segment optical center
- **C.** The visual axis descends to the reading position in any lens
- **D.** All of the above
- **E.** None of the above

3-70. Which form of bifocal has the least image jump?
- **A.** Progressive bifocals
- **B.** Anisometropes
- **C.** Flat-top or executive style bifocals
- **D.** Round top bifocals
- **E.** None of the above

3-71. In a minus lens with flat top or executive lenses:
- **A.** Only jump is minimized
- **B.** Only displacement is minimized
- **C.** Jump is maximized and displacement is minimized
- **D.** Both jump and displacement are minimized
- **E.** None of the above

3-72. Which of the following cannot occur with a rotary prism?
- **A.** The maximum is in the apex-to-apex position
- **B.** The minimum is in the base-to-base position
- **C.** Variable powers are achieved over a range of base-to-apex positions
- **D.** These prisms are used to measure eye deviations
- **E.** None of the above

3-73. The principle behind the Press-On Fresnel Prism is that:
- **A.** The power is related to the prism size
- **B.** The apex angle is the same for all prisms of the same material
- **C.** The apex angle is related to the power of the prism
- **D.** The prismatic effect is related to the prism size
- **E.** None of the above

3-74. The smaller the prism, the:
- **A.** Smaller the apex angle
- **B.** Larger the size of the base
- **C.** Lighter the prism
- **D.** Greater the power
- **E.** None of the above

3-75. The Fresnel Press-On Prism has several disadvantages. Which of the following is not among them?
- **A.** Reduced visual acuity due to reflection
- **B.** Reduced visual acuity due to scatter at the interface
- **C.** Peeling
- **D.** Spherical aberration
- **E.** Discoloration

3-76. Which of the following is a possible use for the Fresnel Press-On Prism?
- **A.** Static incomitant deviations
- **B.** Nystagmus
- **C.** Visual field defects
- **D.** All of the above
- **E.** None of the above

3-77. Prisms of increasing apex angle stacked on top of one another yield an optical system equivalent to:
- **A.** A plus cylinder
- **B.** A minus cylinder
- **C.** A compound lens
- **D.** A spherical lens
- **E.** None of the above

CHAPTER 4: VISUAL IMAGERY

4-1. Which of the following does not apply to the human eye?
- **A.** There are many indices of refraction
- **B.** There are many refractive interfaces

C. The eye can be considered to be a condensed thin lens
D. The eye is a multilens system
E. None of the above

4-2. Which of the following corresponds to the anterior, posterior corneal, and total air-cornea interface values, in that order?
A. +48.80 D, −5.90 D, +42.90 D
B. +47.80 D, +5.90 D, +53.70 D
C. −5.90 D, +47.80 D, +41.90 D
D. +5.90 D, +48.80 D, +54.70 D
E. None of the above

4-3. The anterior air-cornea interface is:
A. Less powerful than the lens
B. Only a reflecting surface
C. Only a refracting surface
D. Both a reflecting and a refracting surface
E. None of the above

4-4. The cornea is:
A. An advantage when performing gonioscopy
B. A stronger refracting than reflecting surface
C. A mirror equal to +260.00 D
D. All of the above
E. None of the above

4-5. What percentage of light incident upon the air-cornea interface ($n = 1.376$) is reflected?
A. 15.8%
B. 7.9%
C. 2.5%
D. 21.8%
E. 17.7%

4-6. Where is the focal point of a cornea as a mirror whose radius of curvature is 7.7 mm?
A. 12.9 mm in front of the cornea
B. 2.60 mm behind the cornea
C. 2.60 mm in front of the cornea
D. 3.85 mm behind the cornea
E. None of the above

4-7. The Purkinje-Sanson images include all of the following except:
A. The reflection from the anterior surface of the cornea
B. The reflection from the posterior surface of the cornea
C. The reflection of the pupil
D. The reflection from the anterior lens surface
E. The reflection from the posterior lens surface

4-8. The posterior corneal surface and the anterior lens surface are convex mirrors whose images are:
A. Inverted
B. Real
C. Minified
D. All of the above
E. None of the above

4-9. The posterior lens surface is a concave mirror whose image is:
A. Smaller
B. Erect
C. Virtual
D. Magnified
E. None of the above

4-10. Which of the following is not the true value for the specified index of refraction?
A. Aqueous: 1.336
B. Lens: 1.46
C. Vitreous: 1.336
D. Cornea: 1.37
E. All of the above are true

4-11. Given the following constants, which of the following statements is true ($n_L = 1.42$, $n_{aq} = 1.336$, $n_v = 1.336$, $r_{LA} = 10.2$ mm, $r_{LP} = 6.0$ mm)? (L = lens, aq = aqueous, v = vitreous, A = anterior, and P = posterior)
A. The power of the anterior lens surface is +14.00 D
B. The power of the posterior lens surface is +8.24 D
C. The difference between the lens surface powers is 5.24 D
D. The total lens surface power as a combination thin lens is +22.24 D
E. All of the above are true

4-12. Which of the following statements is true?
A. The anterior surface of the cornea is a concave mirror
B. The image formed by the anterior corneal surface reflection is minified

C. The posterior corneal surface forms a reflected real image
D. The posterior corneal surface contributes BO prismatic effects
E. None of the above

4-13. If a scotoma is found to measure 30 mm on a Goldmann perimeter (330 mm), what is the corresponding size of the retinal lesion?
A. 1.54 mm
B. 15.4 mm
C. 18.7 mm
D. 1.87 mm
E. None of the above

4-14. A nonseeing area or a scotoma is found to measure 40 mm on a Goldmann perimeter (330 mm). What is the corresponding retinal lesion?
A. 20.6 mm
B. 10.3 mm
C. 2.06 mm
D. 1.03 mm
E. None of the above

4-15. A schematic eye views an object 6 cm tall at a distance of 15 cm. What is the image size on the retina?
A. 6.8 mm
B. 42.5 cm
C. 53 mm
D. 40 cm
E. 43.4 cm

4-16. A scotoma measures 15 cm on a Goldmann perimeter (330 cm). What is the corresponding size of the retinal lesion?
A. 291 nm
B. 17.05 mm
C. 0.77 mm
D. 1.29 mm
E. None of the above

4-17. The power of an eye is +6.00 D stronger than the emmetropic schematic eye but has the same axial length. Which of the following is true?
A. The focal point will be 1.9 mm anterior to the focal point of the emmetropic eye
B. The focal point is 1.51 cm from the corneal plane of the schematic eye
C. This condition is refractive myopia
D. There is an excess of power relative to the length of the eye
E. All of the above

4-18. Axial myopia occurs when:
A. The refractive powers of the eye are less than needed
B. The refractive powers of the eye are greater than needed
C. The eye is too short with normal refractive powers
D. The eye is too long with normal refractive powers
E. None of the above

4-19. If an object moves in one direction, the image follows in the same direction because:
A. The focal point is always changing
B. The signs are the same
C. It must obey the formula $U + D = V$
D. All of the above
E. None of the above

4-20. What power must theoretically be added to compensate for a 5 mm axial lengthening of the schematic eye?
A. −45.50 D
B. −14.54 D
C. −4.54 D
D. −20.00 D
E. None of the above

4-21. Where is the focal point if the power of the schematic eye is +55.00 D?
A. 1.1 mm anterior to the retina
B. 1.81 mm past the retina
C. 0.71 mm anterior to the retina
D. 1.81 cm from the cornea
E. None of the above

4-22. If the power of the lens remains the same, a change in object position will always result in a:
A. Change in image distance in the same direction relative to the light
B. An increase in v equal to the decrease in u
C. Change in image size
D. All of the above
E. None of the above or more than one of the above

4-23. Which of the following statements is true?
- **A.** Image movement is dioptrically related to object movement
- **B.** Object movement is linearly related to image distance
- **C.** If the power of the lens is made more plus, the image is pushed away from the light
- **D.** If the power of the lens is made more minus, the image is pulled toward the light
- **E.** None of the above

4-24. To correct a myopic eye, one could:
- **A.** Move the object closer
- **B.** Place a minus lens in front of the eye
- **C.** Push the image with the light onto the retina
- **D.** All of the above
- **E.** None of the above

4-25. The far point is the:
- **A.** Retina
- **B.** Point imaged by the unaccommodated eye on the retina
- **C.** Blind spot
- **D.** Point coincident with the blur interval
- **E.** None of the above

4-26. If the correcting lens has its secondary focal point coinciding with the far point, the image is:
- **A.** Out of focus
- **B.** In focus
- **C.** Two far planes
- **D.** Coincident with the blind spot
- **E.** None of the above

4-27. Accommodation is:
- **A.** Age dependent
- **B.** Susceptible to fatigue
- **C.** Closely related to convergence
- **D.** All of the above
- **E.** None of the above

4-28. Using maximum accommodation we can find:
- **A.** A near point
- **B.** A point beyond which a clear image cannot be maintained on the retina
- **C.** The amplitude of accommodation
- **D.** The interval of clear vision
- **E.** All of the above

4-29. In myopia the near point would be represented dioptrically by:
- **A.** The amount of myopia plus the accommodative amplitude
- **B.** The accommodative amplitude minus the myopia
- **C.** Only the accommodative amplitude
- **D.** The accommodative amplitude minus the far point
- **E.** None of the above

4-30. Which of the following statements is incorrect?
- **A.** Proximal to the near point the chromatic interval would be similar to that of unaccommodated myopia
- **B.** Distal to the near point the chromatic interval would be similar to corrected hyperopia
- **C.** Proximal to the near point the color blue would be in better focus than the color red
- **D.** Distal to the near point the color red is in better focus than blue
- **E.** None of the above

4-31. A hyperopic patient uses some accommodative amplitude to bring an image into focus. This leaves the patient:
- **A.** Able to focus closer than an emmetropic or myopic counterpoint
- **B.** Unable to focus at any other distance
- **C.** Unable to focus on as near a point as a myopic counterpart
- **D.** Able to overcome the blur circle and focus at all distances
- **E.** None of the above

4-32. Hyperopic persons have a near point dioptrically represented by:
- **A.** The accommodative amplitude plus the hyperopia
- **B.** The accommodative amplitude plus the near point
- **C.** The accommodative amplitude only
- **D.** The accommodative amplitude minus the hyperopia

E. The accommodative amplitude plus the far point

4-33. Which of the following statements is not true about emmetropic persons?

A. Their far point is at infinity
B. Their near point is related dioptrically to their accommodative amplitude
C. They have neither a near nor a far point
D. They have normal accommodation
E. None of the above are true

4-34. What is the interval of clear vision for an uncorrected −5.00 D myope with 8.00 D of accommodative amplitude?

A. 7.69 to 25 cm
B. 20 to 25 cm
C. 7.69 to 20 cm
D. There is no interval of clear vision
E. There is an interval of clear vision but it is not listed

4-35. An uncorrected −5.00 D myope with 8.00 D of accommodative amplitude cannot be said to have a:

A. Far point at 20 cm
B. Near point at 7.69 cm
C. Interval of clear vision between 7.69 and 20 cm
D. Range of accommodation of approximately 12.00 D
E. Life

4-36. Which of the following is false if an uncorrected +4.00 D hyperopic eye has a 6.00 D accommodative amplitude?

A. The far point is 20 cm behind the eye
B. With accommodation, the far point is infinity
C. The near point is 50 cm
D. The interval of clear vision is 50 cm to infinity
E. There is +2.00 D of accommodative amplitude in reserve at distance

4-37. What can be said of +4.00 D uncorrected hyperopia with an accommodative amplitude of 10.00 D?

A. The far point is 25 cm behind the eye
B. The near point is 10 cm
C. The interval of clear vision is 10 cm to infinity
D. A book at 15 cm is readable
E. All of the above

CHAPTER 5: ASTIGMATISM

5-1. In some eyes the power in one meridian is stronger than the other. This can be explained by the fact that:

A. Two meridians 90° apart have different vertex distances
B. Two meridians 90° apart have different accommodative amplitudes
C. Two meridians 90° apart have different radii of curvature
D. The two meridians are 90° apart
E. None of the above

5-2. Toric surfaces can occur:

A. In hyperopia only
B. In the cornea
C. In the retina
D. In prisms
E. None of the above

5-3. The cylinder:

A. Is the most complicated spherocylinder
B. Has its greatest power normal to its axis
C. Never has power at 90°
D. All of the above
E. None of the above

5-4. The power meridian of a cylinder:

A. Is always at 90°
B. Is always rotating
C. Is the same for all cylinders
D. Depends on the cylinder radius of curvature
E. None of the above

5-5. A power cross is used to:

A. Multiply the powers of two different astigmatic eyes
B. Calculate the power of a prism combination
C. Depict the power of a spherocylinder
D. Place the power on the axis meridian
E. None of the above

5-6. For the cylindrical lens +5.00 @ 135°, which of the following is applicable?
- **A.** The axis is 135°
- **B.** The power is at 45°
- **C.** The axis is 45°
- **D.** It has +10.00 net power
- **E.** None of the above

5-7. Cylinder notation convention is not along:
- **A.** The power meridian
- **B.** The axis of the cylinder
- **C.** The two principal meridians
- **D.** The radius of the cylinder
- **E.** None of the above

5-8. Which of the following conventions applies to cylinder notation?
- **A.** The axis is never the same for both eyes
- **B.** The power is the average of the two eyes
- **C.** The scale ranges between 0° and 180° with reference to the left ear
- **D.** 0° is used to mean 0° and 180°
- **E.** None of the above

5-9. If we took multiple small cross-sections of a cylinder, we would find that:
- **A.** Each segment has its own point focus that transcribes a focal line
- **B.** Each segment has a point focus that creates a sphere of clear vision
- **C.** Peripheral rays converge to form a single focal point for the cylinder
- **D.** Kilroy was there
- **E.** None of the above

5-10. The following power cross represents which spherocylinder?

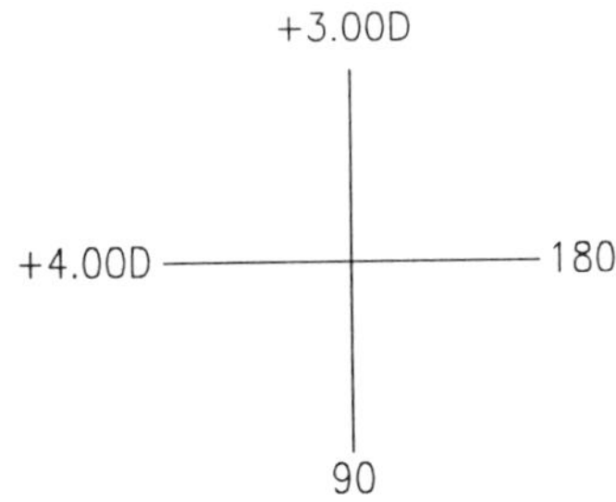

- **A.** +3.00 = +1.00 × 90
- **B.** +3.00 × 90 = +4.00 × 180
- **C.** −1.00 = +3.00 × 180
- **D.** +4.00 = −1.00 × 90
- **E.** None of the above

5-11. The Maddox rod is a device that:
- **A.** Clinically measures accommodative amplitude
- **B.** Is made of a high plus cylinder of red or white plastic
- **C.** Clinically determines the far point
- **D.** Corrects simple astigmatism
- **E.** None of the above

5-12. A spherocylinder has:
- **A.** Two focal points
- **B.** Two principal meridians parallel to one another
- **C.** Two meridians with the same radii of curvature
- **D.** A toric surface
- **E.** None of the above

5-13. The conoid of Sturm:
- **A.** Is a complex conical image space
- **B.** Is a series of focal lines that converge to form an image
- **C.** Is a combination of two oblique cylinders
- **D.** Is bound by the focal sphere of the spherocylinder
- **E.** All of the above

5-14. The orientation of the focal lines of a spherocylinder:
- **A.** Is in the direction of the power meridian
- **B.** Is in the direction of the cylinder axes
- **C.** Depends on the power meridians of each cylindrical component
- **D.** Can be changed with any change in the power of the cylinder
- **E.** None of the above

5-15. The interval of Sturm:
- **A.** Is the range of powers needed to obtain two focal lines
- **B.** Is the range of distances that separate the focal lines from different spherocylinders
- **C.** Is the distance separating the focal lines
- **D.** Is used to estimate the conoid of Sturm
- **E.** None of the above

5-16. A high plus cylinder has a power +180 D. If a light source is held 5 cm in front of the cylinder, which of the following statements is true?
- **A.** The image vergence is 11% greater than the object vergence
- **B.** The image is located 6.25 cm to the left of the cylinder
- **C.** The image is inverted
- **D.** The image is virtual
- **E.** None of the above

5-17. Which of the following describes the image in the axis meridian of a +2.00 D cylinder if the object is 40 cm in front of the cylinder?
- **A.** The image is real
- **B.** The image is not visualized
- **C.** The image is parallel to the cylinder axis
- **D.** The image is at the object
- **E.** All of the above

5-18. The circle of least confusion is:
- **A.** Dioptrically midway between the two focal lines
- **B.** Where the vertical and the horizontal dimensions of the blurred image are approximately equal
- **C.** A circle where the image is least blurred
- **D.** All of the above
- **E.** None of the above

5-19. The circle of least confusion is described by:
- **A.** The spherical equivalent of the spherocylindrical lens
- **B.** The radius of the sphere
- **C.** The cylindrical power of the spherocylindrical lens
- **D.** All of the above
- **E.** None of the above

5-20. The spherical equivalent can be calculated as follows:
- **A.** Add the sphere to the cylinder
- **B.** Multiply the sphere and cylinder
- **C.** Add the sphere to two times the cylinder
- **D.** Add one half the sphere to the cylinder
- **E.** None of the above

5-21. For any combination of sphere and cylinder;
- **A.** The circle of least confusion is the same
- **B.** The net sphere is the same
- **C.** If the spherical equivalent is the same, the circle of least confusion will be in the same place
- **D.** All of the above
- **E.** None of the above

5-22. The size of the blur circle:
- **A.** Depends on the combination of sphere and cylinder
- **B.** Depends on the difference between sphere and cylinder
- **C.** Depends on the interval size
- **D.** Is constant
- **E.** None of the above

5-23. A spherocylinder can be thought of as:
- **A.** A combination of a sphere and a cylinder at right angles to each other
- **B.** An axial combination of two spheres of different powers
- **C.** A combination of two cylinders of different powers
- **D.** A combination of a sphere and a cylinder with equivalent powers
- **E.** None of the above

5-24. Contact lenses should always be dealt with in:
- **A.** Spherocylinder form
- **B.** Plus cylinder form
- **C.** Minus cylinder form
- **D.** Combined cylinder form
- **E.** None of the above

5-25. Which of the following steps is not involved in converting from plus to minus cylinder form?
- **A.** Add the sphere to the cylinder to yield a new sphere
- **B.** Change the sign of the cylinder
- **C.** Divide the cylinder by two
- **D.** Change the axis by 90°
- **E.** All of the above are steps in this conversion

5-26. Which of the following is true for the following plus cylinder?

$$+2.00 = +1.00 \times 90$$

- **A.** The spherical equivalent is +2.00

B. The sphere is less than the cylinder
C. The minus cylinder form is $+2.00 = -1.00 \times 180$
D. The sphere in minus cylinder form is $+3.00$
E. None of the above

5-27. Which of the following is correct for the following minus cylinder?

$$+2.00 = -3.00 \times 45$$

A. The plus cylinder form is $-1.00 = +3.00 \times 135$
B. The plus cylinder form is $+5.00 = +3.00 \times 135$
C. The spherical equivalent is -2.00 D
D. The power is in the 90° axis
E. None of the above

5-28. Which of the following is not equivalent to $+2.00 \times 180 = +3.00 \times 90$?
A. $+3.00 = -1.00 \times 180$
B. $+3.00 = +1.00 \times 180$
C. $+2.00 = +1.00 \times 90$
D. All of the above
E. None of the above

5-29. Which of the following is equivalent to $+4.00 \times 90 = +2.00 \times 180$?
A. $+4.00 = -2.00 \times 180$
B. $+6.00 = -2.00 \times 90$
C. $+2.00 = +1.00 \times 180$
D. $+4.00 = +2.00 \times 90$
E. None of the above

5-30. Which of the following interconversions should be used if prescribing contact lenses for a patient with the following prescription?

$$+1.00 \times 90 = +3.00 \times 180$$

A. $+1.00 = +2.00 \times 90$
B. $+4.00 = -1.00 \times 180$
C. $+3.00 = -2.00 \times 90$
D. $+3.00 = +1.00 \times 90$
E. None of the above

5-31. Which of the following are equivalent interconversions?
A. $+1.00 = +1.50 \times 90$ and $+2.50 = -1.00 \times 180$
B. $+4.25 = -1.75 \times 15$ and $+2.50 = -1.75 \times 105$
C. $+1.50 = -2.75 \times 45$ and $-1.25 = +2.75 \times 135$
D. $+3.00 = -4.00 \times 70$ and $-1.00 = +4.00 \times 150$
E. All of the above

5-32. Which of the following is an equivalent form of writing the combined cylinder $+2.00 \times 180$ and $+3.00 \times 90$?
A. $+3.00 - 1.00 \times 180$
B. $+2.00 + 1.00 \times 180$
C. $+3.00 + 1.00 \times 90$
D. $+2.00 - 1.00 \times 90$
E. $+1.00 + 3.00 \times 90$

5-33. Which of the following is not involved in the conversion from a combined cylinder to a spherocylinder?
A. Add an equal cylinder at 90° to one of the cylinders in the combination
B. The sum in the resulting meridian is a sphere
C. If a sphere of equal magnitude but opposite sign is placed in the same meridian, the net effect is zero
D. All of the above
E. None of the above

5-34. The combined cylinder is $+2.00 \times 90 = -1.00 \times 180$ and an object is at infinity. Which of the following is true?
A. The vertical focal line is at 50 cm to the left of the lens
B. The horizontal focal line is 1 m to the right of the lens
C. The circle of least confusion is 50 cm to the right of the lens
D. The interval of Sturm is between the focal lines
E. None of the above

5-35. Convert the following minus cylinder to its combined cylinder form:

$$+3.00 = +3.00 \times 45$$

A. $+3.00 \times 135 = +3.00 \times 45$
B. $+6.00 \times 135 = +6.00 \times 45$
C. $+6.00 \times 90 = +3.00 \times 180$
D. $+3.00 \times 135 = +6.00 \times 45$
E. None of the above

5-36. Refraction reveals $-3.00 = +6.00 \times 160$. The cylinder is to be reduced by 50% and rotated to 180°. What is the resultant prescription?

A. $+3.00 -6.00 \times 180$
B. $-2.00 +4.00 \times 180$
C. $-1.50 +3.00 \times 180$
D. $+2.00 -4.00 \times 180$
E. None of the above

5-37. A postoperative aphakic person has *K* readings of 48 @ 70/40 @ 160 six weeks after cataract surgery. Which of the following statements is true?

A. The curvature is greater vertically
B. The astigmatism is against the rule
C. The 160° meridian has the steepest *K*
D. The 12 o'clock suture could be tightened to correct the astigmatism
E. All of the above

5-38. A $+1.00 \times 180$ cylinder is added to a $+2.00 \times 180 = +3.00 \times 90$ combined cylinder. The resultant combined cylinder has which of the following properties?

A. The interval of Sturm is between the local lines
B. The interval of Sturm has collapsed
C. This is a cylinder with crossed focal lines
D. The cylinder and the sphere are at right angles to one another
E. None of the above

5-39. Which of the following statements is correct for the following combined cylinder and an object at infinity?

$$+3.00 \times 180 = +4.00 \times 90$$

A. The interval of Sturm lies between 25 and 33 cm
B. The horizontal focal line is parallel to $+3.00 \times 180$
C. The circle of least confusion is 28.5 cm from the cylinder
D. The vertical focal line is at 25 cm
E. All of the above

5-40. Which of the following statements is true for an object at infinity and the spherocylinder

$$+2.00 = +3.00 \times 90?$$

A. The horizontal focal line is 20 cm from the spherocylinder
B. The vertical focal line is 50 cm from the spherocylinder
C. The circle of least confusion lies at 35 cm from the spherocylinder
D. The circle of least confusion is outside the interval of Sturm
E. None of the above

5-41. The combined cylinder $+4.00 \times 90 = -2.00 \times 180$:

A. Has its interval of Sturm from 25 to 50 cm
B. The vertical focal line is to the right of the lens
C. The circle of least confusion is located between the focal lines
D. The horizontal focal line is to the right of the lens
E. None of the above

5-42. What is the effect of an additional cylinder of $+1.00 \times 90$ to the combined cylinder $+3.00 \times 180 = +2.00 \times 90$?

A. The vertical focal line is moved toward the light
B. The resultant combined cylinder is a sphere
C. The interval of Sturm is collapsed
D. All of the above
E. None of the above

5-43. Refraction in the spectacle plane 12 mm from the cornea is $-10.50 +1.50 \times 90$. What is the refraction at the cornea?

A. $-9.33 +1.20 \times 90$
B. $+8.13 -3.48 \times 180$
C. $-8.13 -4.65 \times 90$
D. $-8.13 +3.48 \times 90$
E. $-12.78 +4.65 \times 90$

5-44. One focal line behind the retina and the other in front of the retina is:

A. Simple hyperopic astigmatism
B. Simple myopic astigmatism

C. Compound hyperopic astigmatism
D. Compound myopic astigmatism
E. Mixed astigmatism

5-45. One focal line on the retina and the other behind the retina is:
A. Simple hyperopic astigmatism
B. Simple myopic astigmatism
C. Compound hyperopic astigmatism
D. Compound myopic astigmatism
E. Mixed astigmatism

5-46. If the eye error is +cyl × 180, what is the type of astigmatism?
A. Simple hyperopic
B. Simple myopic
C. Compound hyperopic
D. Compound myopic
E. Mixed

5-47. If the eye error is −cyl × 180 and −cyl × 90, what type of astigmatism is present?
A. Simple hyperopic
B. Simple myopic
C. Compound hyperopic
D. Compound myopic
E. Mixed

5-48. An eye error of +cyl × 180 and −cyl × 90 is what type of astigmatism?
A. Simple hyperopic
B. Simple myopic
C. Compound hyperopic
D. Compound myopic
E. Mixed

5-49. If the correcting combined cylinder lens is placed in the corneal plane, it will be:
A. Equal in magnitude and the same sign as the eye error
B. Equal in magnitude and opposite in sign to the eye error
C. Smaller and of the same sign as the eye error
D. Larger and of the opposite sign to the eye error
E. None of the above

5-50. When sphere is added, what is the impact on astigmatic focal lines?
A. Both lines move an equal amount dioptrically
B. Both lines move different amounts dioptrically
C. The interval of Sturm changes linearly
D. The circle of least confusion does not change
E. Both the lines and the interval of Sturm change or move in a linear fashion.

5-51. What type of astigmatism is corrected by a +2.00 = −1.00 × 90 spherocylindrical lens at the corneal plane?
A. Compound hyperopic
B. Compound myopic
C. Mixed
D. Simple hyperopic
E. Simple myopic

5-52. A patient has mixed astigmatism. Which of the following might correct the eye error?
A. +4.00 = −3.00 × 90
B. +2.00 × 90 = +3.00 × 180
C. +4.00 × 180 = +1.00 × 90
D. −3.00 × 180 = +1.00 × 90
E. All of the above

5-53. What type of astigmatism is corrected by −4.00 = +2.00 × 90?
A. Compound hyperopic
B. Compound myopic
C. Mixed
D. Simple hyperopic
E. Simple myopic

5-54. To selectively move one focal line:
A. A cylinder with its axis parallel to the line is used
B. A plus lens will move the focal line away from the light
C. A minus cylinder will move the focal line toward the light
D. A cylinder with its power meridian parallel to the line is used
E. None of the above

5-55. Which of the following does not occur in plus cylinder refracting technique?
A. All astigmatism is converted to simple hyperopic astigmatism
B. The sphere is adjusted so that the anterior focal line is proximal to the retina
C. A plus cylinder then moves the

posterior focal line toward the light and onto the retina
D. The astigmatic interval is collapsed
E. A point focus is created

5-56. Minus cylinder refracting technique requires that:
A. Sphere is adjusted to obtain compound hyperopic astigmatism
B. The anterior focal line is pushed with the light
C. Minus cylinder is used in one meridian and plus cylinder at 90°
D. Streak retinoscopy is of minimal use
E. None of the above

5-57. In an astigmatic eye there is not a single far point. Which of the following best characterizes astigmatic imagery?
A. With correction stigmatic imagery is always achieved
B. Two far point planes coincident with the correcting cylinder focal planes exist
C. Two far point planes exist corresponding to the eye error in the two principal meridians
D. There are only ever two astigmatic far point planes
E. All of the above

5-58. To obtain conjugacy between the far point planes and the retina, the correcting spherocylindrical lens can be placed:
A. Where the circle of least confusion between the secondary focal lines of the lens is coincident with the far point of the eye
B. Where the secondary focal lines of the lens are perpendicular with the far point of the eye
C. Where the secondary focal lines of the correcting spherocylinder are coincident with the far point planes of the eye
D. Where the secondary focal lines are separated by an equal interval of Sturm to the distance between the far point planes
E. None of the above

5-59. If the power of a spectacle lens in combined form is $+3.00 \times 180 = +2.00 \times 90$ and it corrects an eye error of $-3.22 \times 180 = -2.08 \times 90$, what is the vertex distance?
A. 12 mm
B. 22 mm
C. 20 mm
D. 8 mm
E. 4 cm

5-60. Symmetrical astigmatism exists when:
A. The correcting cylinders of both eyes are of the same power and axes
B. The axes of the two correcting cylinders are mirror images of each other
C. The axes of the correcting cylinders sum 90°
D. All of the above
E. None of the above

5-61. Regular astigmatism exists when the toricity of the cornea in the visual axis presents a:
A. Radius of curvature equal to that of the schematic eye
B. Uniform refractive surface with repeatable results
C. Nonuniform refractive surface by keratometry readings at other than perpendicularity
D. A refractive surface altered by rapid blinking
E. None of the above

5-62. Irregular astigmatism occurs when a different astigmatic error is obtained with:
A. A slight deviation from the periphery of the visual axis
B. A slight rotation, less than 45°, of the visual axis in keratometry
C. Small excursions from the very central portion of the visual axis
D. Great deviations from the center to the periphery of the visual axis
E. None of the above

5-63. In the case of irregular astigmatism:
A. A single spherocylindrical correction will correct most of the pupillary aperture

B. A contact lens may smooth out the surface yielding regular astigmatism
C. A contact lens of high water content will reduce greatly the amount of astigmatism
D. All of the above
E. None of the above

5-64. Keratoconus is a degenerative process affecting the corneal thickness resulting in:
A. Deviation of the central ray in an irregular manner due to diffractive properties of the cornea
B. Asymmetric splitting of rays due to reduced transmittive properties of the cornea
C. A temporary change in the index of refraction of the cornea that upsets the balancing forces of the eye
D. The outbowing of the central cornea in an irregular fashion
E. All of the above

5-65. Irregular astigmatism is often mistakenly diagnosed when:
A. The two prinicpal meridians are of different powers
B. The toric surface comprises one irregular and one regular meridian
C. The astigmatism cannot be corrected with spectacle correction
D. The two principal meridians are not normal to each other
E. None of the above

5-66. If keratometry shows that the two principal meridians are not normal to each other then:
A. Two different areas of the visual axis are being tested
B. Two zones of the cornea are being tested
C. Irregular astigmatism may be present
D. You made a mistake
E. All of the above

5-67. With the rule astigmatism occurs when the axis of the correcting cylinder is:
A. At 90° when using plus cylinders
B. At 180° when using plus cylinders
C. At 90° when using minus cylinders
D. Perpendicular to the visual axis
E. None of the above

5-68. Against the rule astigmatism is:
A. Corrected at 180° to with the rule astigmatism
B. Is better tolerated than with the rule astigmatism
C. Can be corrected with a minus cylinder at 90°
D. Can be corrected with a plus cylinder at 90°
E. None of the above

5-69. Which group of people is most likely to get against the rule astigmatism?
A. Newborns
B. Infants
C. Young adults
D. Adults under 40 years
E. All of them are equally likely

5-70. What power of spectacle lens at a vertex distance of 10 mm is required to correct an eye error of $+4.00 \times 180 = +6.00 \times 90$?
A. $-4.17 \times 180 = -6.38 \times 90$
B. $+4.17 \times 90 = +6.38 \times 180$
C. $-3.85 \times 180 = -6.38 \times 90$
D. $+3.85 \times 90 = -5.38 \times 180$
E. $-4.17 \times 90 = -6.38 \times 180$

5-71. An eye error of $-2.00 \times 90 = +4.00 \times 180$ is what type of astigmatism?
A. Compound hyperopic
B. Compound myopic
C. With the rule
D. Against the rule
E. Irregular

5-72. An eye error of $-1.00 \times 90 = -2.00 \times 180$ is what type of astigmatism?
A. Compound myopic
B. With the rule
C. Simple hyperopic
D. Mixed
E. Against the rule

5-73. Once the anterior focal line is on the retina, plus cylinder axis 180 will bring the posterior focal line toward the light onto the retina:
A. This is with the rule astigmatism
B. +cyl × 180 translates to a cor-

recting cylinder of +cly × 90 and therefore is with the rule

C. +cly × 180 translates to a correcting cylinder of −cyl × 180 and is therefore with the rule

D. All of the above

E. None of the above

5-74. Whenever a lens is tilted, the amount of induced sphere and cylinder is:

A. Proportional to the sphere portion of the spherocylinder

B. Inversely related to the cylinder power

C. Related to the power of the lens

D. Inversely proportional to the amount of tilt

E. None of the above

5-75. Tilting a minus lens induces a:

A. Large amount of minus sphere and a small amount of minus cylinder at axis 90

B. Small amount of minus sphere and a smaller amount of minus cylinder at axis 180

C. Small amount of minus sphere and a larger amount of minus cylinder at axis 180

D. Large amount of minus sphere and a large amount of minus cylinder at axis 90

E. The same amount of minus sphere and minus cylinder at axis 90

5-76. Keratometry yields *K* readings of 40.00 D horizontally and 46.00 D vertically. Which of the following statements is not applicable to this example?

A. The eye error is +6.00 × 180

B. The correcting cylinder is −6.00 × 180

C. The plus cylinder form for the correcting cylinder is +6.00 × 90

D. This is against the rule astigmatism

E. None of the above

5-77. Tilting a plus lens induces a:

A. Large amount of sphere and a large amount of plus cylinder at axis 180

B. Small amount of plus sphere and a larger amount of plus cylinder at axis 180

C. Small amount of plus sphere and a small amount of plus cylinder at axis 90

D. Small amount of plus sphere and a small amount of plus cylinder at axis 180

E. Large amount of plus sphere and a small amount of plus cylinder at axis 180

5-78. If a plus lens is tilted, which of the following will be true?

A. Plus cylinder at 90° is produced

B. Minus cylinder at 180° is produced

C. This is against the rule astigmatism

D. All of the above

E. None of the above

5-79. An intraocular lens implant can tilt. The amount of tilt can be estimated by:

A. The distance separating Purkinje-Sanson images III and IV

B. The distance separating Purkinje-Sanson images I and II

C. The distance separating Purkinje-Sanson images II and III

D. All of the above

E. None of the above

5-80. A spectacle-corrected myopic patient increases the pantoscopic tilt of her glasses by raising her temples. What is the resultant induced refractive error?

A. Simple myopic astigmatism

B. Against the rule astigmatism

C. Corrected by plus cylinder at 90°

D. All of the above

E. None of the above

5-81. A patient is wearing spectacle correction of +3.00 = +4.00 × 90. Keratometry reveals *K* readings of 42.00 D horizontally and 44.00 D vertically. Which of the following is not true about this patient?

A. The total astigmatic error can be corrected with a regular hard contact lens

B. +2.00 D of the astigmatic error can be attributed to the cornea

C. +2.00 D of the astigmatic error is lenticular
D. A little more of the astigmatism can be attributed to the cornea if vertex distance is corrected for
E. All of the above are true

5-82. A bitoric hard contact lens:
A. Corrects irregular astigmatism
B. Corrects lenticular astigmatism
C. Corrects corneal astigmatism
D. Corrects oblique astigmatism
E. All of the above

5-83. A suture at 12 o'clock whose tension is too tight will:
A. Reduce the chord diameter horizontally
B. Increase the chord diameter vertically
C. Reduce the radius of curvature vertically
D. Reduce the power meridian in the axis of the tight suture
E. None of the above

5-84. A loose suture will:
A. Cause plus cylinder astigmatism at 90° to the axis of the suture
B. Increase the power in the meridian
C. Shorten the chord diameter
D. Decrease the radius of curvature along the meridian
E. None of the above

5-85. A patient has *K* readings of 40.00 D horizontally and 36.00 D vertically. Which of the following is correct?
A. This patient has with the rule astigmatism
B. The horizontal cylinder is +40.00 × 180
C. The eye error is +4.00 × 180
D. The correcting combined cylinder is +4.00 × 180
E. None of the above

5-86. A patient has *K* readings of 42.00 D horizontally and 45.00 D vertically. Which of the following is correct?
A. The eye error is −3.00 × 180
B. The correcting combined cylinder is −3.00 × 180
C. The patient has mixed astigmatism
D. The patient has against the rule astigmatism
E. None of the above

5-87. A patient's spectacle correction is +3.00 = +6.00 × 90. *K* readings reveal 42.00 D horizontally by 47.00 D vertically.
A. The total astigmatic error is 5.00 D
B. The cornea contributes +3.00 D
C. There is +2.00 D of lenticular astigmatism
D. The astigmatism is with the rule
E. All of the above

5-88. The rationale behind inducing astigmatism in pseudophakic patients includes which of the following principles?
A. It reduces distortion
B. It enables near and distance vision without spectacle correction
C. It restores complete distance vision in conjunction with reading lenses
D. It restores near vision with the use of soft toric lenses
E. None of the above

5-89. A pseudophakic person (with an IOL implant) complains of poor vision postoperatively. Eight interrupted 10-0 nylon sutures were used for closure, and the wound is well healed. *K* readings are 38.00 D horizontally and 48.00 D vertically.
A. This patient has an eye error of +10.00 × 180
B. This is against the rule astigmatism
C. Sutures are too loose at 12 o'clock
D. The plus cylinder needed for correction is +10.00 × 180
E. All of the above

5-90. The postoperative *K* readings in pseudophakia are 44.00 D at 120° by 34.00 D at 30°. What is the implication?
A. The suture is too loose at 120°
B. The suture should be cut at 30°
C. The suture is not contributing to the astigmatism

D. The suture should be removed at 75°
E. None of the above

5-91. If the axis of astigmatism is different from the correcting cylinder axis, then:
A. The resultant is a cylinder of different power
B. Two cylinders at oblique axes form a new resultant cylinder at a new axis
C. The power of the new optical system remains the same
D. The axis of the resultant is the same but the power is reduced
E. The new axis is the bisector of the obliquely crossed cylinders

5-92. When obliquely crossed cylinders (such as the eye error and correcting cylinder axes) of equal power and different sign are crossed the:
A. New axis is perpendicular to the bisector of the original axes
B. New axis is 45° from the correcting cylinder axis
C. New axis is perpendicular to the correcting cylinder axis
D. New axis is 45° from the eye error axis
E. New axis is not related to the original axes

5-93. When the spherical equivalent is zero:
A. You are dealing with a cross cylinder
B. The circle of least confusion of the optical system will differ depending on the eye it is in front of
C. The power of the system is zero
D. All of the above
E. None of the above

5-94. Subjective refinement of the cylinder power is performed:
A. Using the Jackson cross cylinder with the stenopeic slit
B. Before refinement of the axis
C. Only with cycloplegic refraction
D. Using a cross cylinder and rotary prism
E. None of the above

5-95. If the circle of least confusion is on the retina:
A. Objective refraction can be refined
B. Subjective refraction can be refined
C. This could be mixed astigmatism
D. This could be emmetropia
E. All of the above

5-96. The markings on the cross cylinder denote:
A. Power crosses
B. The axes
C. The perpendicular focal lines that are affected by the cross cylinder
D. All of the above
E. None of the above

5-97. If a correcting minus cylinder is oriented parallel to the posterior focal line:
A. Vision diminishes
B. It pushes the focal line with the light
C. The interval of Sturm increases
D. The circle of least confusion enlarges
E. All of the above

5-98. At the endpoint of cross cylinder refinement of the axis and power with the cross cylinder still in place:
A. The astigmatism is completely eliminated
B. The astigmatism induced by the cross cylinder is completely neutralized
C. The residual astigmatism is corneal
D. The residual astigmatism is from the cross cylinder
E. None of the above

5-99. When the cross cylinder is "flipped" at the endpoint of subjective refinement of the axis and power:
A. The remaining focal lines remain the same
B. The circle of least confusion increases in size
C. The circle of least confusion remains on the retina
D. The interval of Sturm is shortened

E. Accommodation is stimulated changing the interval of Sturm

5-100. During power refinement of the correcting cylinder during cross cylinder testing:

A. The circle of least confusion is always maintained on the retina
B. The focal lines are always in the same position
C. The interval of Sturm is lengthened but never shortened
D. All of the above
E. None of the above

5-101. Adding +0.50 D of cylinder shifts the circle of least confusion by an amount equal to:

A. The sphere portion of the spherocylinder
B. The cylinder portion of the spherocylinder
C. The spherical equivalent
D. The spherical equivalent plus one half of the cylinder
E. None of the above

5-102. The power of the cross cylinder selected for use:

A. Depends on the visual acuity of the patient
B. Produces better vision in the patient as it is decreased
C. Determines how precise the refinement will be
D. All of the above
E. None of the above or more than one of the above

5-103. During axis refinement, the cross cylinder is placed such that:

A. The two axes are both perpendicular to the correcting cylinder
B. The two axes straddle the eye error axis
C. The two axes are both parallel to the eye error axis
D. The two axes straddle the correcting cylinder axis
E. None of the above

5-104. The end point of axis refinement occurs when the eye error axis and the correcting cylinder axis are:

A. Crossed
B. Coincident
C. Parallel but distinguishable
D. Perpendicular
E. None of the above

5-105. If the correcting cylinder is not at the correct axis relative to the eye error, two oblique cylinders exist. Which of the following statements is true in this case?

A. Their new axis is 45° to the correcting cylinder axis
B. If the plus axis position is the same as the induced minus axis, the resultant cylinder is less
C. If minus cylinders are used, the correcting cylinder is rotated toward the plus axis of the cross cylinder
D. All of the above
E. None of the above

5-106. When one is using plus cylinders, the correcting cylinder is:

A. Always rotated toward 180°
B. Rotated toward the plus axis of the cross cylinder in the better position
C. Rotated away from the plus axis of the eye error axis
D. Rotated 45° to the new axis
E. None of the above

5-107. The number of degrees the cross cylinder is rotated at each choice during axis refinement depends on:

A. The amount of cylinder present
B. The strength of the cross cylinder
C. The axis of the eye error
D. The direction the cross cylinder is perceived better
E. All of the above

5-108. Which of the following is a cross cylinder?

A. $+2.00 = +4.00 \times 90$
B. $+6.00 = -8.00 \times 180$
C. $-2.50 = +5.00 \times 180$
D. $-3.00 = -6.00 \times 90$
E. $+2.00 = +2.00 \times 180$

5-109. If the power is refined before refinement of the axis, the result is:

A. Equivalent to the opposite cylinder transposition
B. The best power for the incorrect axis
C. The maximum power of the spherocylinder
D. All of the above
E. None of the above

5-110. The astigmatic clock is based on:
A. The angle in minutes of arc the cylinder is rotated to correct the astigmatism
B. The position of the two focal lines described as hands of a clock
C. The axis of the astigmatism in the correcting cylinder
D. The angular subtense separating the correcting and eye error axes
E. None of the above

5-111. In the interval of Sturm, if the vertical focal line is closest to the retina, the:
A. Vertical aspects of an extended object are distorted.
B. Vertical aspects of an extended object are blurred
C. Vertical aspects of an extended object are in best focus
D. Horizontal aspects of an extended object are better focused than the vertical aspects
E. Horizontal aspects are properly positioned to be imaged further

5-112. When an astigmatic person looks at six equally dark lines in the configuration of a clock, the sharpest line corresponds to:
A. The axis of the focal line nearest the retina
B. The eye error axis
C. The axis to position the cross cylinder
D. The correcting cylinder axis in plus cylinder form
E. None of the above

5-113. The sharpest line during astigmatic clock testing corresponds to the:
A. Anterior focal line
B. Posterior focal line
C. Eye error axis
D. Cross cylinder axis
E. None of the above

5-114. Fogging involves:
A. Converting all types of astigmatism to simple hyperopic
B. Maintaining enough plus sphere to bring both focal lines onto the retina
C. Controlling any rotation of the cylinder
D. Stopping any stimulus to accommodation
E. None of the above

5-115. During astigmatic clock testing the sharpest line is the:
A. Anterior focal line parallel to the posterior focal line
B. Anterior focal line coincident with the posterior focal line
C. Anterior focal line perpendicular to the posterior focal line
D. Posterior focal line perpendicular to the anterior focal line
E. None of the above

5-116. For each clock hour between 1 and 6 o'clock:
A. 1.00 D of correcting power is needed
B. 30° of correcting minus cylinder is added
C. 45° of correcting plus cylinder is added
D. The cylinder should be rotated 90° clockwise
E. None of the above

5-117. The double click method:
A. Should be used in conjunction with any minus cylinder
B. Should be used after the astigmatic clock test to check accuracy
C. Adds 90° to the results of the astigmatic dial test
D. Subtracts 45° from the results of the astigmatic clock test
E. Allows the use of plus cylinders for techniques best suited to minus cylinders

5-118. To prevent the stimulation of accommodation:

A. The posterior focal line is kept slightly behind the retina
B. A fog of about 20/40 should be maintained at all times
C. A fog is maintained at 20/300
D. The anterior focal line is kept in front of the retina
E. None of the above

5-119. Which of the following statements is correct?
A. Postoperative corneal astigmatism is caused by a slight tilt (under 10°) in the intraocular lens
B. An IOL tilted about the horizontal meridian induces plus cylinder axis 180
C. Irregular astigmatism cannot be precipitated by surgery and does not contribute to the postoperative corneal astigmatism
D. Disparity between keratometric astigmatism and refractive astigmatism is often caused by high ametropia in pseudophakia
E. None of the above

5-120. The change in spherical power of the lens for a given tilt is approximately:
A. An increase by half of the induced cylinder
B. A decrease by half of the induced cylinder
C. An increase equal to two times the induced cylinder
D. A decrease equal to two times the induced cylinder
E. None of the above

CHAPTER 6: MAGNIFICATION

6-1. Meridional magnification is when an object appears all of the following except:
A. Taller
B. Wider
C. More oval
D. Deeper
E. Narrower

6-2. Which of the following statements is not true
A. Linear magnification means that the image appears larger
B. Linear minification means that the image appears smaller
C. Lateral magnification is the same as linear magnification
D. Axial magnification is the same as meridional magnification
E. Axial magnification deals with depth perception

6-3. Linear magnification can be calculated by:
A. Using the vertex distance
B. Using image and object distance
C. Dividing the power of the eye by the meridional magnification
D. All of the above
E. None of the above

6-4. Linear magnification of the image compared to the object is measured relative to the distance:
A. Between the eye and the image
B. Away from the optical axis of the image and object
C. Between the image and the object
D. Away from the tangent to the image of the retina
E. Along the optical axis

6-5. Axial magnification is measured relative to the distance:
A. Along the optical axis
B. Away from the retina
C. Between the eye and the image
D. Between the image and the object
E. None of the above

6-6. An object subtends an angle at the nodal point such that the tangent of this angle is equal to:
A. Image size over the object distance from the nodal point
B. Object size over the object distance from the nodal point
C. Image size over object size
D. Image distance from the nodal point over the object size
E. None of the above

6-7. An object is 20 cm tall and is located 40

cm from the observer. The image produced is 10 cm from the eye. Which of the following statements is true?

A. The image is 5 cm high
B. The linear magnification is 4×
C. The axial magnification is 16×
D. All of the above
E. None of the above

6-8. Angular magnification compares:

A. The image size to the angle subtended without the optical system
B. The object size to the image distance
C. The object size to the angle subtended with the optical system
D. The angle subtended with the optical system to that without the optical system
E. None of the above

6-9. Simple magnification describes the power of a magnifier and a reference distance that has been standardized with few exceptions to:

A. 1 m
B. ½ m
C. ⅓ m
D. ¼ m
E. None of the above

6-10. What is the difference in simple magnification if the standard reference distance is changed from 25 to 30 cm for an emmetropic eye?

A. 15×
B. 18×
C. 3×
D. 33×
E. None of the above

6-11. Calculate the magnification of a +28.00 D hand-held magnifier if the object must be at *f* to be in focus:

A. 11.2×
B. 7.0×
C. 4.2×
D. 2.8×
E. None of the above

6-12. An object's magnification is calculated for viewing at 40 cm. By how much would the image appear smaller or larger if it were brought 15 cm closer?

A. It would appear smaller by 3/8
B. It would appear larger by 8/3
C. It would appear larger by 8/5
D. It would appear smaller by 5/8
E. None of the above

6-13. What is the magnification of an aphakic eye with an anterior focal point of 22 mm?

A. 10×
B. 11.4×
C. 5×
D. 12.5×
E. Need more information to calculate the answer

6-14. If we increase the reference distance for simple magnifiers from 25 to 50 cm, what will happen to the perceived image size?

A. It appears 2× larger
B. No change would occur
C. It appears smaller by half
D. It appears 3× larger
E. It appears smaller by one third

6-15. When comparing the magnification of the appearance of the optic nerve of a myopic eye with an anterior focal point of 15 mm to an emmetropic eye, which of the following is true?

A. The magnification of the myopic eye is 16.67×
B. This myopic eye magnifies 67% more than the emmetropic eye
C. The image of the emmetropic eye will be 11.13% larger than that of the myopic eye
D. The magnification of the myopic eye is 66.67×
E. None of the above

6-16. Consider an aphakic eye with an anterior focal point of 20 mm. What is the apparent magnification at a distance of 50 cm when compared to the standard reference distance?

A. 50× smaller
B. 12.5× smaller
C. 4× smaller
D. 6.25× smaller
E. 10× smaller

6-17. The Galilean telescope has:

A. A plus objective lens and a minus eyepiece

B. A minus objective lens and a plus eyepiece
C. A plus objective lens and a plus eyepiece
D. A minus objective lens and a minus eyepiece
E. As long as the focal points are coincident the sign of the objective and eyepiece lens is irrelevant

6-18. The lenses of a Galilean telescope are placed such that the secondary focal point of the objective lens is:
A. In front of the primary focal point of the second lens
B. Behind the primary focal point of the second lens
C. Coincident with the secondary focal point of the eyepiece
D. Imaged by the eyepiece lens
E. None of the above

6-19. With a Galilean telescope the real image of the first lens becomes the virtual image for the second. This results in:
A. Parallel rays emergent from the eyepiece
B. The image on the retina is larger
C. The image on the retina is inverted
D. All of the above
E. None of the above

6-20. The magnification of a telescope can be calculated by dividing the power of the eyepiece by the:
A. Angular magnification and changing the sign
B. Angle subtended by the eyepiece
C. Power of the objective lens and changing the sign
D. Object size
E. None of the above

6-21. The separation of the lenses of a Galilean telescope:
A. Is the sum of the focal lengths of the two lenses
B. Is the product of the focal lengths of the two lenses
C. Is the difference of the focal lengths of the two lenses
D. Is the quotient of the focal lengths of the two lenses
E. Is the average of the focal lengths of the two lenses

6-22. Which of the following statements is true?
A. If the angular magnification is positive, the perceived image is upright
B. If the angular magnification is positive, the real image is upright
C. If the angular magnification is positive, the perceived image is inverted
D. If the angular magnification is negative, the perceived image is upright
E. If the angular magnification is negative, the real image is inverted

6-23. In the astronomical telescope:
A. The power of the eyepiece is minus
B. The perceived image is erect
C. The separation of the lenses will be the sum of the focal lengths
D. All of the above
E. None of the above

6-24. Which of the following is not a property of the astronomical telescope?
A. The eyepiece is positive
B. The image is inverted when perceived
C. The secondary focal point of the objective lens coincides with the primary focal point of the eyepiece
D. The emergent rays are parallel
E. The separation is the difference of the focal lengths

6-25. A Galilean telescope has an eyepiece with a 5 mm focal length and an objective lens of +5.00 D. Describe the image produced on the retina:
A. The image is larger and perceived upright
B. The image is the same size but inverted
C. The image is perceived inverted but larger
D. The image is upright and smaller
E. None of the above

6-26. A monocular aphakic patient corrected with a contact lens still complains of an image size disparity. You decide to decrease the image size further by prescribing a spectacle lens/contact lens combination. You overplus the contact lens by 3.00 D. The glasses are at a vertex distance of 10 mm. Which of the following is true?

A. The appropriate spectacle power is −3.10 D
B. The image is magnified by 3%
C. The vertex distance is ignored when considering the magnification
D. The system is equivalent to a Galilean telescope
E. All of the above

6-27. Consider a telescope with a +40.00 D objective lens and a −120.00 D eyepiece lens. Which of the following statements accurately describes this system?

A. The magnification of this telescope is 4×
B. The separation of the telescope is 16.7 cm
C. The perceived image is upright
D. All of the above
E. None of the above

6-28. As an object is brought closer for viewing with a telescope, the object vergence is more:

A. Difficult to calculate
B. Divergent
C. Convergent
D. Dependent on the power of the lenses
E. Magnified

6-29. Viewing a near object through a telescope has certain accommodative demands. These include:

A. More accommodation to overcome the increased vergence demands by the telescope
B. More convergence of the visual axes to compensate for the telescope simulating a closer object distance
C. Less accommodation is required, since the object appears larger
D. All of the above
E. None of the above

6-30. What is the accommodation required through a 4× Galilean telescope if the object is 25 cm away?

A. 18.00 D
B. 25.00 D
C. 50.00 D
D. 64.00 D
E. None of the above

6-31. A 4× telescope requires accommodation for an object at 50 cm. What is needed to eliminate the accommodative demand?

A. A +18.00 D lens in front of the objective lens
B. A −18.00 D lens behind the objective lens
C. A +2.00 D lens in front of the eyepiece
D. A −2.00 D lens in front of the objective lens
E. None of the above

6-32. What magnification of telescope has a 36.00 D accommodative demand viewing an object at 25 cm?

A. 1×
B. 2×
C. 3×
D. 4×
E. 5×

6-33. How much closer must an object be held when viewed by a 5× monocular add when compared to a 5× loupe focused at 25 cm?

A. 30 mm
B. 30 cm
C. 25 mm
D. 20 cm
E. 20 mm

6-34. A patient finds that he can read newsprint with +8.00 D readers and a 3× hand-held magnifier. What single magnifier would be required to yield equivalent magnification?

A. 6×
B. 5×
C. 1×
D. 11×
E. 24×

6-35. When dealing with multiple lens systems, the total magnification is:

A. The sum of each component magnifier
B. The average of all the component magnifiers
C. The product of each component magnifier

D. The product of each component magnifier divided by the number of component magnifiers used
E. None of the above

6-36. When one is correcting ametropia, one is dealing with:
A. A system that resembles a telescope but cannot be treated as one
B. Two lenses of the same power and sign
C. Lenses where the secondary focal point of the first lens is coincident with the primary focal point of the second lens
D. The secondary focal point of the first lens falls on the retina
E. None of the above

6-37. An object at 40 cm is viewed through a 5× Galilean telescope with an eyepiece of −40.00 D and objective lens of +8.00 D. Describe the magnification of the system if a +2.50 D lens is placed in front of the objective lens:
A. The difference in magnification is 3.81×
B. The new magnification is 3.81×
C. The accommodation needed for this telescope is +27.50 D
D. The magnification is decreased to 1.19×
E. None of the above

6-38. A 4× telescope views an object at ⅛ m but accidentally incorporates a +3.00 D lens into the eyepiece lens instead of the objective. What would be the accommodative requirements?
A. +16.00 D
B. +48.00 D
C. +33.00 D
D. +9.00 D
E. None of the above

6-39. Consider the aphakic person whose spectacle correction equals +12.00 D at a vertex distance 10 mm. Which of the following is not true for this patient?
A. The far point of the eye is 8.33 cm
B. The correct vertex distance adds 5 mm (for the lens plane to the cornea) to the spectacle vertex distance
C. The eye error is equivalent to an eyepiece power of −14.64 D
D. The magnification is 1.22×
E. The optic disk of 1.5 mm would appear 1.83 mm when examined without correction

6-40. As the vertex distance decreases:
A. The power of the eyepiece always increases more than that of the objective lens
B. The power of the eyepiece always decreases more than that of the objective lens
C. The magnification always increases
D. The magnification always decreases
E. None of the above

6-41. A spectacle-corrected aphakic person can be considered a telescopic system where there is:
A. A plus eye error or eyepiece power
B. A minus spectacle or objective lens power
C. Magnification greater than 1×
D. A reverse Galilean telescope
E. None of the above

6-42. Consider a spectacle-corrected +5.00 × 45 astigmatic person with a 10 mm vertex distance. All of the following are correct except:
A. A +5.25 × 45 lens would be required at the corneal plane
B. The far point plane of the eye is 20 cm from the spectacle plane
C. The 135° meridian would appear smaller than the 45° meridian
D. Without correction there is blur but no distortion
E. Less distortion would be experienced with a contact lens

6-43. Aniseikonia is:
A. The perception of image distortion between two principal meridians
B. Based on image magnification or minification between the eyes or from normal seeing
C. Related to image disparity between a normal and an astigmatic eye
D. Often worse with smaller vertex distances
E. None of the above

6-44. Which of the following is true of a +14.00 D spectacle-corrected aphakic eye at a vertex distance of 7 mm?

A. The far point of the eye is at 7.14 mm
B. The total vertex distance for calculations is 1.9 cm
C. The eyepiece power is equal to 14×
D. The image is magnified by 20%
E. None of the above

6-45. What is the magnification of a −12.00 D spectacle correction at vertex distance of 10 mm?
A. 31% minification
B. 43% minification
C. 15% minification
D. 18% magnification
E. 44% magnification

6-46. Which of the following may be used to describe a +5.00 × 45 astigmat with a vertex distance of 9 mm?
A. The far point plane is 11.1 cm from the eye
B. The image is minified 7.5% in the 135° meridian
C. The image is magnified by 7.5% in the 135° meridian
D. The 45° meridian is magnified 7.5%
E. All of the above

6-47. In normal seeing an object of regard falls on corresponding retinal elements and is:
A. Fused peripherally by anomalous retinal correspondence
B. Diverged to produce a scatter, which is then imaged on the retina
C. Convergent, producing a virtual image
D. Fused centrally into single binocular vision
E. None of the above

6-48. Diplopia occurs when:
A. The image from each eye falls on noncorresponding retinal points
B. Is distorted equally by both eyes
C. Is fused at all retinal points except the macula
D. Different objects of regard fall on noncorresponding retinal points
E. None of the above

6-49. In young children suffering from an eye deviation, visual adaption to diplopia and visual confusion can occur by:
A. Suppression
B. Normal retinal correspondence
C. Ocular dominance
D. Inhibition of the medial geniculate
E. None of the above

6-50. If the amount of image disparity and aniseikonia is:
A. Small, adjustment is difficult
B. Small, the occipital cortex is rigid
C. Large, the visually mature patient sees double
D. Large, adjustment is easily achieved
E. None of the above

6-51. Which of the following methods is a valid approach to eliminating or reducing an image size disparity within binocular single vision?
A. The placement of a balance lens over the eye with the larger image
B. An intraocular lens impant in aphakia
C. Placement of an iseikonic lens over an aphakic eye
D. Switching from contact lenses to spectacles
E. None of the above

6-52. One way of reducing some of the image disparity in monocular aphakia is to:
A. Underplus the aphakic contact lens and overcorrect with plus glasses
B. Overplus the contact lens and overcorrect with minus glasses
C. Undercorrect with minus cylinders in the bifocal correction
D. Create a Galilean telescopic effect with iseikonic spectacles
E. None of the above

6-53. Knapp's rule states that if the correcting lens is placed at the primary focal point:
A. Emergent rays are convergent
B. The image will remain the same size for all axial lengths
C. Longer axial lengths increase the retinal image size
D. Shorter axial lengths decrease the retinal image size
E. None of the above

6-54. Clinically it is hard to determine the exact:

A. Axial and refractive component to the refractive error
B. Amount of refractive error due to corneal astigmatism
C. Direction of the posterior focal line
D. Fusion occurring centrally versus peripherally
E. All of the above

6-55. The myopic person who converts to contact lenses:
A. Uses less accommodation
B. Needs to use more accommodation
C. Experiences no change in accommodation demands
D. May be able to delay entry into bifocals
E. None of the above

6-56. What is the accommodative demand on a +6.00 D spectacle-corrected hyperopic person viewing an object at 25 cm compared to a contact lens–corrected counterpart if the spectacle vertex distance is 10 mm?
A. 23% less with glasses
B. 21% more with glasses
C. 19% more with glasses
D. 17% less with glasses
E. None of the above

6-57. +6.00 D and −15.00 D lenses are used to make a Galilean telescope. Which of the following statements is true for an object at 5 cm?
A. The image is real and to the right of the objective lens
B. Total magnification is 1%
C. The image of a near object is coincident with that for far
D. The image is inside the telescope
E. None of the above

6-58. Describe the above system with an object at infinity:
A. The image vergence is positive
B. The image rays emerge parallel
C. The image is located 3.3 mm from the objective lens
D. All of the above
E. None of the above

6-59. Calculate the accommodative demands a +7.00 D hyperopic person would avoid by using contact lenses instead of spectacles for an object at 40 cm (vertex distance is 8 mm):
A. 10.3% will be avoided
B. 11.0% will be avoided
C. 12.4% will be avoided
D. 88.8% will be avoided
E. None of the above

6-60. Compare the accommodative demands of a ±5.00 D spectacle-corrected hyperopic person and myopic person (vertex 10 mm) for an object of 25 cm relative to correction in the corneal plane with contact lenses:
A. The normal accommodative demand is +4.00 D
B. Spectacle-corrected myopia requires 9.4% less accommodation than contact lens–corrected myopia
C. Myope has a far point plane 20 cm to the left of the lens
D. Spectacle-corrected hyperopia requires 19.625% more accommodation than contact lens–corrected myopia
E. All of the above

6-61. The myopic person who wears spectacles can remove them and:
A. See very clearly at the near point with a small amount of accommodation
B. See very clearly at the far point with a small amount of accommodation
C. Eliminate any minification
D. Create a reverse Galilean telescopic effect
E. None of the above

6-62. Magnification, minification, and distortion are all:
A. Related to the correcting lens
B. Related to the ametropia
C. More severe in myopia than in hyperopia
D. Much more intense in small children than elders
E. None of the above

6-63. Which of the following statements is true?
A. An astigmatic person who is uncor-

rected experiences a great deal of distortion
- **B.** An astigmatic person has no blurring of near vision
- **C.** The amount of monocular distortion is pronounced
- **D.** The amount of distortion manifested binocularly is minimal
- **E.** None of the above

6-64. What will rotating the correcting cylinder toward 90° or 180° accomplish?
- **A.** It eliminates oblique cylinder forms and creates a more tolerable form of distortion
- **B.** It corrects all residual refractive error in the horizontal and vertical plane
- **C.** It simulates the use of contact lenses
- **D.** All of the above
- **E.** None of the above

6-65. Distortion can be reduced by:
- **A.** Using plus posterior toric lenses
- **B.** Using minimal angular deviation
- **C.** Using minimal vertex distance
- **D.** All of the above
- **E.** None of the above

CHAPTER 7: RETINOSCOPY

7-1. Streak retinoscopy:
- **A.** Can also be called skiascopy
- **B.** Deals with light reflexes and shadows as they emerge from the eye
- **C.** Gives an estimate to work with in later refinement of the sphere
- **D.** Gives an estimate to work with in later refinement of the cylinder power and axis
- **E.** All of the above

7-2. Which of the following is not true about the far point?
- **A.** In unaccommodated myopia it is in front of the eye
- **B.** Its position varies with the amount of myopia
- **C.** In the emmetropic eye it is on the retina
- **D.** In the hyperopic eye it is behind the eye
- **E.** All of the above are true

7-3. In astigmatism:
- **A.** Of the simple myopic form, the far point is in front of the eye
- **B.** Two far points exist; both are always behind the eye
- **C.** Two far line planes exist that are always perpendicular to one another
- **D.** Two far points of varying position exist
- **E.** None of the above

7-4. If the retina is illuminated with a light source, such as a retinoscope, it then becomes:
- **A.** Irresponsive to any incoming object rays
- **B.** An object whose image will be formed at the far point
- **C.** An object and image that are coincident
- **D.** A far point
- **E.** None of the above

7-5. One can simulate eye errors by:
- **A.** Placing objects inside the near point
- **B.** By placing minus sphere in front of the eye
- **C.** By placing plus sphere in front of the eye
- **D.** Displacing the far point
- **E.** All of the above

7-6. Retinoscopy is based on the:
- **A.** Direction of movement of light reflexes
- **B.** Sphere causing a simulated eye error
- **C.** Direction of movement of the far point
- **D.** Precipitated response to a stimulus
- **E.** None of the above

7-7. The basis of retinoscopy and the retinoscope involves:
- **A.** Detection of movement at far points or planes
- **B.** Different far point magnifications
- **C.** Shadows of reflecting rays which may be directly neutralized by lenses

D. Discrimination between simple and compound astigmatism
E. None of the above

7-8. The key point in retinoscopy is:
A. The point when the far point is on the retina
B. When the direction of the light reflex is reversed
C. When the light reflex passes the far point
D. The focal point
E. None of the above

7-9. As the streak from the retinoscope descends, the retina is illuminated, and it becomes imaged at the far point plane:
A. This streak image is now an object for the examiner to follow
B. This streak now casts a shadow for the examiner to follow
C. The perceived image and the direction the retinoscope is moving are opposite
D. The result is an against motion
E. None of the above

7-10. Which of the following statements is correct?
A. The weak myopic eye with less than 1.50 D of myopia yields a with response
B. The myopic eye greater than −1.50 D minifies the image of the streak on the retina of the examiner
C. The myopic eye greater than −1.50 D yields a with response
D. When the far point is at the peephole of the retinoscope, with movement is seen
E. None of the above

7-11. When the light of the retinoscope fills the examiner's pupil, this corresponds to:
A. The inverse of the eye error, which should be corrected
B. The point at which the most movement is seen
C. The far point of the hyperopic eye
D. The point beyond which with motion becomes against motion
E. None of the above

7-12. The working lens:
A. Is a lens of −1.50 D
B. Redefines emmetropia for retinoscopy
C. Makes all patients hyperopic
D. Produces only against motions
E. All of the above

7-13. If neutrality has been achieved and the examiner moves forward:
A. The far point is now at the retina
B. The far point is now in front of the examiner
C. An against movement can be seen
D. A with response can been seen
E. None of the above

7-14. Which of the following statements is not true?
A. Against motion is more easily neutralized than with motion
B. With motion is faster and closer to neutrality
C. Myopic eyes of −1.50 D display an against motion when no correction is in place
D. It is easier to add minus sphere to convert myopia to hyperopia and neutralize with motion
E. None of the above

7-15. With a (sleeve-up) streak retinoscope:
A. Emergent light is divergent in the sleeve-down position
B. In the sleeve-up position, the condensing lens position is varied such that emergent light is convergent
C. Emergent light in the sleeve-down position reverses against to with motion or vice versa
D. All of the above
E. None of the above

7-16. A refractionist performs streak retinoscopy at 50 cm without the working lens. The retinoscope sleeve is adjusted for a plano-mirror effect. If the patient has −2.00 D myopia, what type of motion would the examiner see?
A. With motion
B. Against motion
C. Phases shift at 90° to each other

D. No motion
E. A skew of the reflex to the intercept

7-17. If the eye is astigmatic:
A. Two bands of equal motion exist
B. Two bands of unequal motion exist
C. Two bands of opposite motion exist at 180° to each other
D. A with and an against motion can always be seen
E. None of the above

7-18. When using plus cylinders in streak retinoscopy of an astigmatic eye:
A. Two far lines exist for some types of astigmatism
B. Simple astigmatism is converted to compound astigmatism
C. One band will be appoaching neutrality faster than the other
D. The first band to neutralize corresponds to the cylindrical component
E. None of the above

7-19. When using plus cylinder streak retinoscopy, the second band:
A. Remains at 90° to the first
B. Is the standard to which the axis of the minus cylinder is aligned
C. Is straddled by the corrective cylinders
D. All of the above
E. None of the above

7-20. There are five descriptive phenomena that aid in the refinement of the cylinder axis. Which of the following is not among them?
A. The streak is thinnest when on axis
B. A skew is seen when moving away from the correct axis
C. A break in the reflex relative to intercept is seen if off axis
D. Dropping the sleeve points away from the axis
E. None of the above

7-21. Streak retinoscopy with minus cylinder technique can use:
A. The double click method
B. Both spheres and cylinders for neutralization of the two meridians
C. Only spheres for neutralization of the two meridians
D. All of the above
E. None of the above

7-22. If one were to use only spheres to neutralize the two principal meridians:
A. Nothing would happen; retinoscopy needs cylinders
B. A power cross is formed that must be converted to axis notation
C. The recording is in direct axis notation
D. Neutralization is a blur interval induced by spherical aberration
E. None of the above

7-23. The two major sources of inaccuracy in retinoscopy are:
A. Irregular reflexes and the loss of accommodative control
B. Examiner accommodation and the irregularity of reflexes
C. Subjectivity of measurements and the loss of accommodative control
D. Varying intensities of the light source and the subjectivity of measurements
E. None of the above

7-24. Retinoscopy is usually performed
A. One eye at a time with the other covered
B. Both eyes at the same time
C. One eye scoped and the other focusing on a small accommodative target
D. One eye fogged and the other scoped
E. With both eyes occluded

7-25. Irregular astigmatism can give rise to a:
A. Wider range of neutrality
B. Irregular intervals of myopia and hyperopia
C. Scissors type reflexes
D. All of the above
E. None of the above

CHAPTER 8: REFRACTION

8-1. Refining the sphere can be achieved by:
A. Adding a +0.25 D sphere in a mon-

ocular fashion and asking the patient to rate the change as better or worse
B. Performing the duochrome test
C. Binocular balancing with plus sphere
D. Vectographic techniques with stereo glasses
E. All of the above

8-2. When performing subjective sphere refinement, better means:
A. You should keep adding plus until no further improvement is noted
B. You should add minus until no further improvement is noted
C. The patient's refractive error has been corrected
D. The patient is accommodating
E. None of the above

8-3. When a patient states visual acuity is better but it does not measure better when plus is added, the examiner should check for:
A. A bias from magnification
B. Accommodation with a Galilean telescopic effect
C. Astigmatism with a shifting circle of least confusion
D. Further improvement with plus cylinder axis 180°
E. None of the above

8-4. If the patient states that the visual acuity is worse with additional plus sphere, the examiner should add:
A. Minus sphere and check for a reverse Galilean telescopic effect
B. A larger amount of plus sphere and ask if better or worse
C. Minus sphere to compensate for any accommodation
D. More plus sphere until vision is completely blurred and then quickly add the same net minus sphere
E. None of the above

8-5. The endpoint is achieved when:
A. Vision can no longer be corrected to 6/6 without −0.50 D
B. Visual acuity is reduced by adding any more plus
C. Minification occurs with the cross cylinder in the minus position
D. All of the above
E. None of the above

8-6. Chromatic aberration by the crystalline lens results in:
A. Yellow being refracted more than blue
B. Blue and green being refracted more than red
C. Yellow being absorbed more than red or blue
D. A chromatic interval that bridges the retina for 3.50 to 4.25 D
E. None of the above

8-7. Clinically, during duochrome testing:
A. A blue-green split filter is used
B. Vision is preferentially reduced for red light
C. A chromatic interval of +0.75 D exists that must be compensated for with minus sphere
D. Yellow holds the emmetropic position
E. All of the above

8-8. In aphakia and pseudophakia the duochrome test is:
A. Of no value
B. Of little value because the green is always dimmer
C. Of little value because the blue is always brighter
D. Affected by the paucity of red cones
E. Excellent for refining the final sphere

8-9. Which of the following statements is true of duochrome testing?
A. The patient is fogged to 20/80
B. Once fogged, a patient should claim the green side is clearest
C. The final step is when the green side is worse than the red side
D. It is not valid with protanopia
E. None of the above

8-10. Binocular balancing is most useful when:
A. Visual acuity is equal in both eyes
B. Cycloplegia is not present
C. The red side is equal to the green side

D. The power of sphere is less than ±3.00 D
E. None of the above

8-11. Binocular balancing is best accomplished by:
A. Prism balancing with 6 P.D. BU in front of one eye
B. Polarizing lenses and vectographic slides
C. Crossing cylinders for equal blur
D. 4 P.D. prism refinement with horizontal prism before each eye
E. All of the above are good methods of binocular balancing

8-12. In prism dissociation for binocular balancing:
A. The patient is binocularly fogged
B. A vertical Risley prism before the dominant eye is used
C. A single line is presented that is horizontally diplopic
D. Plus sphere is added until vision is equally clear and no further
E. None of the above

8-13. A 40-year-old woman complains of difficulty seeing at near. The examination reveals that the patient is wearing *OD* +3.00; *OS* +5.50. Uncorrected vision in both eyes is 20/200. With +5.50 D for each eye, vision is 20/20. When +0.75 D is added, J_2 is seen and vertical and horizontal orthophoria are present. If the patient requires precise near and far vision at the same time, what would you prescribe?
A. Bifocals
B. Full distance correction in single vision glasses
C. Full near correction with contact lenses
D. Full distance and half near correction
E. Any of the above

8-14. A 41-year-old man complains of poor vision. On examination his vision without correction is 20/50 *OD* and 20/40 *OS*. With +1.50 *OD* and with +1.00 *OS* acuity is 20/20. He will not accept more plus. At near he is J_5 without correction, J_3 with +1.50, +1.00, and J_2 with +2.00, +1.50. Cycloplegic refraction reveals +2.50, +2.00. He has an 8 P.D. exophoria and 4 P.D. right hyperphoria. He spends half of his day with a computer. What is your management?
A. +1.75 *OD*, +1.25 *OS*, 2.0 P.D. *BI OD*, 2 P.D. *BI OS*
B. +1.00 *OD*, +0.50 *OS*, 1.0 P.D. *BD OD*, 1 P.D. *BU OS*
C. +2.00 *OD*, +1.50 *OS*, 1.0 P.D. *BD OD*, 1 P.D. *BU OS*
D. +1.50 *OD*, +1.00 *OS*, 0.5 P.D. *BD OD*, 0.5 P.D. *BU OS*
E. +2.00 *OD*, +1.50 *OS*, 1.0 P.D. *BU OD*, 1 P.D. *BD OS*

8-15. A 48-year-old refugee taxi driver never wore glasses in his country of origin. He failed his driver's test for immigration purposes. He is very motivated to undertake whatever is necessary to meet government requirements for driving. What is most likely to succeed given the following information?

Without correction: *OD* 20/60, *OS* 20/60
Manifest: *OD* +0.50 +4.00 × 60 – 20/40
OS +0.50 +3.50 × 45 – 20/30
Cyclo: *OD* +1.00 +4.00 × 60 – 20/30
OS +1.00 +3.50 × 45 – 20/30

A. Glasses: *OD* +0.50 +4.00 × 60 and *OS* +0.50 +3.50 × 45, +1.75 add
B. Glasses: OD +1.50 +2.00 × 60 and *OS* +1.50 +1.50 × 45, +1.75 add
C. Contact lenses with +1.75 half glasses for reading
D. Astigmatic keratotomy with glasses for reading
E. Bifocal contact lenses

8-16. A 40-year-old woman is having difficulty seeing at both distance and near. During refraction the following observations are made: The accommodative amplitude is +5.00 D.

Without correction: *OD* 6/15, *OS* 6/15
+1.00D both eyes: *OD* 6/6, *OS* 6/6

+1.75D both eyes: *OD* 6/6, *OS* 6/6
+2.00D both eyes: *OD* 6/7.5, *OS* 6/7.5
Cycloplegia: +2.50 both eyes *OD* 6/6, *OS* 6/6

What prescription is indicated for comfortable close work at 40 cm with clear distance vision?

A. *OD* +2.50, *OS* +2.50
B. *OD* +1.75, *OS* +1.75, +0.75 add
C. *OD* +1.00, *OS* +1.00, +1.50 add
D. *OD* +1.75, *OS* +1.75
E. *OD* +1.00, *OS* +1.00

8-17. A postoperative cataract patient refracts to 6/6 *OU* with the following:

OD: −4.50 +4.00 × 60
OS: +1.50 +2.00 × 180
+2.50 add J_2 at 40 cm

The mode of correction to attempt first with this patient is:

A. Full spectacle correction as bifocals
B. Reduced cylinder *OD* with axis rotation toward 180°
C. Soft toric contact lenses to correct the anisometropia with bifocal overcorrection
D. Soft toric contact lenses with readers or half glasses
E. Bifocal hard contact lenses

8-18. A 2-year-old is esotropic. The deviation measures 30 P.D. esotropia at distance and 45 P.D. esotropia at near. With +3.00 D lenses the deviation at near measures 30 P.D. Cycloplegic refractive error is +2.00 *OU*. Which of the following is appropriate to prescribe?

A. +1.75 D *OU*
B. There is too little hyperopia to account for the esotropia; surgery should be performed first
C. +2.00 D *OU* +1.50 add
D. +2.00 D *OU* +2.25 add
E. +2.00 D *OU* +3.00 add

8-19. A patient with nuclear cataracts is wearing *OD* −2.00 +0.50 × 180 (20/60) and *OS* −2.50 (20/60) with an add of +2.25 J_2. She refracts to *OD* −4.00 +0.50 × 180 (20/25+) and *OS* −4.50 (20/25+). What do you prescribe?

A. *OD* −4.00 +0.50 × 180; *OS* −4.50; add +2.25 *OU*
B. *OD* −4.00 +0.50 × 180; *OS* −4.50; add +3.25 *OU*
C. Distance glasses only
D. *OD* −3.00 +0.50 × 180; *OS* −3.50; add +2.25 *OU*
E. There is no sense in changing glasses with cataracts present

8-20. A 38-year-old woman works for a local accounting firm that you retain professionally. She wears no correction but complains of easy fatigue, blur at distance, and occasional diplopia. She measures:

Without correction: *OD* 20/50; *OS* 20/50
−1.25 *OU*: *OD* 20/20; *OS* 20/20
Distance: 12 P.D. exophoria
Near at ⅓ m: 6 P.D. exophoria

What prescription would be most appropriate?

A. −1.25 *OU* glasses
B. −1.25 *OU* +1.25 add
C. −1.50 *OU,* 3 P.D. BI *OU*
D. −1.50 *OU,* 1.5 P.D. BI *OU*
E. −1.25 *OU* contacts

8-21. Light rays passing through the pupil but missing the IOL:

A. Are internally reflected
B. Emerge at reduced speed
C. Produce a poorly focused secondary image
D. Produce no image, merely a blur
E. None of the above

8-22. A patient has the following refraction to manifest and cycloplegic sequences:

OD +2.00
OS +5.00

Which of the following is beneficial to alter the spectacles and reduce the aniseikonia?

A. Alter the lens shape
B. Reduce the distance between the lenses

C. Increase the effective diameter of the lens
D. Alter the frame size
E. Alter the temple configuration

8-23. A 40-year-old man has difficulty reading with his current prescription. The patient's uncorrected vision is 20/20 in both eyes. The present prescription is +2.00 D in both eyes. With +2.50 D, the patient is blurred to 20/100, but once he relaxes his accommodation he is able to regain 20/20 acuity. When tested with cycloplegia he accepts *OD* +3.75; *OS* +4.00, but vision is again initially blurred and then cleared to 20/20 with the cycloplegic homatropine. Which of the following is an appropriate management?
A. Full correction is required
B. Gradually increase the concave power of the lens
C. Prescribe glasses halfway between full correction and present correction
D. Prescribe bifocals with a +0.25 D add
E. None of the above

CHAPTER 9: VISION TESTING

9-1. Which of the following is most sensitive to test for early optic neuropathy?
A. Snellen visual acuity
B. Central visual fields with threshold testing
C. Color vision with pseudoisochromatic plates
D. Stereoacuity with Titmus testing
E. Contrast sensitivity with sine gratings

9-2. Testing central visual acuity in uncooperative patients is best with:
A. Snellen fraction interferometry
B. Minimum discernible EOG
C. Stereoacuity ERG
D. Vernier acuity callipers
E. None of the above

9-3. Which of the following is true for the Snellen optotype?
A. Each stroke width represents 5′ of arc
B. To identify it the eye must resolve a visual angle of 1′
C. Each gap width represents 2′ of arc
D. At 20 feet the letter subtends 8′ of arc at the eye's nodal point
E. None of the above

9-4. If the visual angle is 2′ of arc, which of the following statement(s) is (are) true?
A. This corresponds to 0.2 vision
B. This patient can see at 40 feet what the normal patient can see at 20 feet
C. This patient has better than normal vision
D. The Snellen fraction would be 6/12
E. All of the above

9-5. If the letter originally subtending 1′ of arc is moved 15 feet toward the eye, the new angle subtended at the nodal point of the eye is:
A. 15″
B. 4′
C. 3′
D. 5′
E. 30″

9-6. What is the visual acuity of a patient who can discriminate 1′ of arc at a distance of 5 feet?
A. 20/20
B. 20/40
C. 20/60
D. 20/80
E. 20/100

9-7. What does a visual acuity of 20/100 mean?
A. The patient can resolve at 100 feet what the average patient can resolve at 20 feet
B. The Snellen letter must be held five times as far to subtend 1′ of arc
C. The minimum visual angle is 4′ of arc
D. The interval of Sturm lies between 20 and 100 cm
E. None of the above

9-8. A 45-year-old patient has 20/100 vision. The visual angle:
A. Is constant at 3′ of arc
B. Is constant to age 65 years

C. Has been the same throughout his lifetime
D. Is equal to 5′ of arc
E. None of the above

9-9. Glare occurs when patients are sensitive to bright lights and reflected light. Patients often are found to have:
A. Media opacities
B. Corneal astigmatism
C. Posterior subcapsular cataracts
D. Lens aberrations
E. All of the above

9-10. Which statement is true?
A. Opacities decrease axial magnification
B. In bright light the pupil is smaller and glare is less of a problem
C. Lens opacities often degrade immediate paraxial rays
D. Glare testing is of limited value in the evaluation of cataracts
E. Glare at night is made worse by antireflective coatings

9-11. Contrast sensitivity is:
A. Distortion due to the glare of monochromatic light
B. The ability to detect slight changes in luminance in regions without sharp contours
C. Calculated using the difference of luminance from object to image
D. Specific to diseases of the optic nerve
E. Measured with a vectographic projector and polarized glasses

9-12. Testing contrast sensitivity can be done:
A. In chart form
B. In projected form
C. Subjectively
D. In oscilloscope form
E. All of the above

9-13. Which of the following principles does a diffractive bifocal implant use to establish two distinct orders of diffraction?
A. Concentric rings of varying spherical power
B. Diffractive rays emerge from an intraocular lens with a larger depth of focus
C. Multislope diffractive rings on the back of an implant
D. Fresnel optics on a convex-plano optic
E. None of the above

9-14. When using refractive or diffractive lenses, one must be concerned with whether the light defocused:
A. By the unused portion of the lens degrades the contrast of the one focused on the object of regard
B. Is interfering with emerging rays
C. Can later be imaged on the retina
D. Reduces the amount of glare reaching the other eye
E. None of the above

9-15. Stereopsis is all of the following except
A. The ability of the visual system to appreciate depth
B. Expressed in terms of stereoacuity
C. A binocular phenomenon
D. Normal with the monofixation syndrome
E. Reduced with optic neuritis

9-16. Stereopsis within the confines of single binocular vision can be perceived only if an axial or horizontal disparity in the object of regard:
A. Can be appreciated within Panum's fusional space
B. Can be imaged inside Panum's fusional space
C. Is partially imaged in Panum's fusional space
D. Is surrounded by Panum's fusional space
E. Is independent of Panum's fusional space

9-17. When we speak of stereoacuity, fine stereopsis is a function of:
A. The different amounts of distortion that each eye suffers
B. The perspective difference of the images of an object presented to each eye
C. The amount of pupil dilation of each eye
D. All of the above
E. None of the above

9-18. The image disparity generated by angle θ at the nodal point can be fused if:
- **A.** The image disparity still falls on corresponding retinal points
- **B.** The angle θ is small with respect to the retinal image size
- **C.** The depth of the object lies outside of Panum's fusional space
- **D.** The tangent of θ is equal in magnitude to the depth of the object
- **E.** None of the above

9-19. Which of the following statements is not true?
- **A.** As the distance away from the eye increases, the stereoacuity decreases
- **B.** As the depth of the object increases, the angle it subtends increases
- **C.** The larger the pupillary distance, the greater the stereoacuity
- **D.** The smaller the pupil, the greater the stereoacuity
- **E.** All of the above are true

9-20. Some materials have their molecular structure so arranged that, as light passes through them, only those with:
- **A.** Electric fields oriented parallel to the direction of transmission are transmitted
- **B.** Electric fields perpendicular to the direction of the light are stopped
- **C.** Magnetic fields in the same direction as transmission are allowed to emerge
- **D.** Helical fields are eliminated
- **E.** None of the above

9-21. Which of the following materials has no polarizing properties?
- **A.** Water
- **B.** Glass
- **C.** Plastic
- **D.** Mirrors
- **E.** All of the above can have polarizing properties

9-22. Which of the following statements is incorrect regarding the Haidinger brush entoptic test?
- **A.** The test is clinically determined by rotating a polarizing filter in a uniform blue field
- **B.** The test is used to determine macular position
- **C.** The test is used to determine macular function
- **D.** All of the above
- **E.** None of the above

9-23. Placing a horizontal polarizing filter over one eye and a vertical polarizing filter over the other enables the examiner to:
- **A.** Perform stereotesting
- **B.** Perform sphere refinement
- **C.** Selectively project polarized objects to either eye
- **D.** Determine the fixing eye penalization
- **E.** All of the above

9-24. In the perifoveal region:
- **A.** There is a rich capillary network
- **B.** A red blood cell column is queued in single file interrupted by white blood cells
- **C.** The photoreceptors are relatively dark adapted beneath the blood column
- **D.** All of the above
- **E.** None of the above

9-25. Using the blue field entoptoscope, the presence of white spots is presumed evidence of:
- **A.** Relative blue receptor loss
- **B.** An intact capillary network
- **C.** Macular pucker that scatters light, creating white spots
- **D.** Perifoveal edema
- **E.** None of the above

9-26. If two light waves are of equal magnitude and in phase, the interaction is called:
- **A.** Constructive interference
- **B.** Destructive interference
- **C.** Birefringence
- **D.** Coherence
- **E.** Spatial cohesion

9-27. Which of the following, when combined with a monochromatic light

source, will produce two wavefronts that will interfere with each other?
- **A.** Stenopeic slit
- **B.** Parallel plate of glass
- **C.** Prism
- **D.** Bifocals
- **E.** Pinhole

9-28. Which of the following statements is not true about interference patterns?
- **A.** A bright band indicates constructive interference
- **B.** A dark band indicates that the minima of one wave are equal to the maxima of the other wave
- **C.** The pattern of interference rings is from diffraction at the aperture edges
- **D.** Coherence is a measure of how well the two light beams interfere
- **E.** All of the above are true

9-29. Which of the following is true of the potential acuity meter?
- **A.** It magnifies a visual acuity chart on the retina by a factor of 3×
- **B.** It focuses the acuity chart on the retina with an optometer
- **C.** It cannot be used to determine a Snellen fraction visual acuity
- **D.** It has an aerial aperture equal to 0.1 nm
- **E.** None of the above or more than one of the above

9-30. Uncorrected visual acuity is standardized in all of the following except:
- **A.** Military service
- **B.** Aviation
- **C.** Law enforcement
- **D.** Firefighting
- **E.** None of the above

9-31. Visual maturity is reached at age:
- **A.** 1 to 2 years
- **B.** 2 to 4 years
- **C.** 4 to 6 years
- **D.** 6 to 10 years
- **E.** 10 years and up

9-32. For a 3-year-old emmetropic eye, the normal visual acuity is:
- **A.** 20/10
- **B.** 20/20
- **C.** 20/30
- **D.** 20/80
- **E.** 20/200

CHAPTER 10: ACCOMMODATION AND CONVERGENCE

10-1. Accommodation is:
- **A.** Stimulated by blurred retinal imagery
- **B.** Contributed to by coma induced blur
- **C.** Directly proportional to the near point
- **D.** Always accompanied by convergence
- **E.** None of the above

10-2. Bitemporal retinal disparity may affect:
- **A.** The orientation of the visual axes
- **B.** The effectivity of the perifoveal area
- **C.** The range of accommodation that is possible for the optical system
- **D.** Retinal correspondence of the fovea
- **E.** None of the above

10-3. The near response is a synkinetic triad made up of:
- **A.** Chromatic aberration, coma, and convergence
- **B.** Convergence, accommodation, and astigmatism
- **C.** Accommodation, chromatic aberration, and coma
- **D.** Accommodation, convergence, and miosis
- **E.** Accommodation, convergence, and pupillary dissociation

10-4. Each part of the synkinetic triad can occur:
- **A.** Independently of the other two under controlled conditions
- **B.** Only in conjunction with each other
- **C.** Despite the addition of prisms

D. Despite adding plus lenses
E. None of the above

10-5. Accommodation causes the movement of the following ocular structures, except the:
A. Iris
B. Cornea
C. Lens
D. Vitreous
E. Retina

10-6. Structural changes during accommodation do not include;
A. Contraction of the ciliary muscle
B. Relaxation of the zonules of the lens
C. Increase in the anteroposterior diameter of the lens
D. Increase in the radii of curvature of the anterior and posterior surfaces
E. All of the above

10-7. Which of the following statements is not correct?
A. The increased convexity of both lens surfaces results in an increase in plus power to the lens
B. Relaxation of the zonules decreases the effectivity of the lens
C. An anterior shift in lens position may provoke angle closure in a susceptible patient
D. Miosis decreases spherical aberration
E. Miosis increases depth of field

10-8. Accommodation decreases with age because:
A. The lens oxygen demands can no longer be met
B. The lens proteins are structurally altered and become more rigid and less deformable
C. The rods and cones lose Styles-Crawford type II effectivity as their ability to trap light declines
D. All of the above
E. None of the above

10-9. When the zonular tension is decreased, there tends to be a:
A. Shift toward hyperopia
B. An increase in spherical aberration
C. A shift toward myopia
D. A decrease in spherical aberration
E. None of the above

10-10. Presbyopia is:
A. The result of less zonular tension from reduced elasticity
B. The reduction of accommodation with age
C. The change in the index of refraction of the crystalline lens as a consequence of too much photopic exposure
D. Any increase in hyperopia occurring after visual maturity
E. All of the above

10-11. The accommodative amplitude change for every 4 years between the ages of 40 and 48 is:
A. −1.00 D
B. +2.00 D
C. −1.50 D
D. +3.00 D
E. None of the above

10-12. Which of the following statements is true?
A. With the distance correction in place, the far point is at infinity
B. In emmetropia the near point can be directly converted to accommodative amplitude
C. If the eye is overplussed, the refractive error will affect both the far and near points but the difference will always equal the amplitude
D. All of the above
E. None of the above or more than one of the above

10-13. The Prince rule:
A. Measures accommodative convergence on a ruler
B. Uses +3.00 D lenses
C. Uses lenses to push the far and near points farther apart to facilitate measurement
D. States that minus lenses stimulate

accommodation less effectively than an object moving closer
E. None of the above or more than one of the above

10-14. Which of the following holds true for the amplitude of accommodation?
A. Half the amplitude should always remain in reserve
B. Corrective lenses are prescribed to maintain half the amplitude in reserve
C. If less than half remains in reserve, fatigue will occur
D. Recession of the near point can occur with only one fourth of the amplitude remaining in reserve
E. All of the above

10-15. A −3.00 D myopic person has an accommodative amplitude of +5.00 D. What is the interval of clear vision without correction?
A. 10 to 25 cm
B. 12.5 to 33 cm
C. 12.5 to 25 cm
D. 20 to 33 cm
E. 20 to 25 cm

10-16. Cycloplegia is an important refractive tool best used in the identification of:
A. Latent hyperopia
B. Pseudohyperopia
C. Anisometropia
D. Accommodative insufficiency
E. All of the above

10-17. The basis of action of cycloplegics is their:
A. Inhibition of the postganglionic response associated with acetylcholine
B. Blockade of acetylcholinesterase such that the acetylcholine is not removed
C. Alteration of the receptors involved in norepinephrine binding
D. Stimulation of the postganglionic cells
E. None of the above

10-18. Cycloplegics are absorbed into the nasal mucosa and hence have:
A. Cholinergic side effects
B. Similar effects to the administration of atropine
C. Great effects on the respiratory functions of the individual
D. Sympathomimetic side effects
E. None of the above

10-19. Distribution and dosage of cycloplegics depends on:
A. Body weight
B. Surface area
C. Method of administration
D. All of the above
E. None of the above

10-20. A 44-year-old patient is +4.00 D hyperopic. His accommodative amplitude measures 4.00 D. His current glasses are +2.00 D. What would one prescribe to make him comfortable for work at 50 cm?
A. +2.00 D single vision glasses
B. +4.00 single vision glasses
C. +3.75 D and +2.25 D add bifocals
D. +2.00 D and +4.00 D add bifocals
E. None of the above

10-21. A 40-year-old has a manifest refraction of +6.50 (6/6) and cycloplegic refraction of +7.00 D. His accommodative amplitude is +3.00 D. His current glasses are +2.00 D. What should you prescribe for work at 40 cm?
A. +3.00 D single vision reading glasses
B. +4.00 D and +2.50 D add bifocals
C. +7.00 D single vision reading glasses
D. +6.50 D and +1.50 D add bifocals
E. +4.50 and +1.00 add bifocals

10-22. Which of the following is a common side effect of atropine 1%?
A. Nausea
B. Headaches
C. Nose bleeds
D. Shivers
E. All of the above

10-23. The time for maximum cycloplegia in the shorter acting agents is crucial:
A. To reduce the side effects
B. If residual accommodation is to be effectively reduced
C. To make up for the lack of exposure
D. If mydriasis is desired
E. None of the above

10-24. A −4.00 D myopic patient has an accommodative amplitude of +5.00 D. What is the interval of clear vision without correction?
A. 11.1 to 25 cm
B. 20 to 25 cm
C. 11.1 to 20 cm
D. 11.1 cm to infinity
E. None of the above

10-25. A patient has a 15 P.D. esophoria at distance and 20 P.D. esophoria at ⅓ m. Find the AC/A ratio by the clinical method:
A. 5/33
B. 35/3
C. 3/5
D. 33/5
E. 5/3

10-26. Using the following information, at 1.0 m = 10 P.D. esotropia and at 20 m = 25 P.D. esotropia, calculate the AC/A ratio:
A. 25/4
B. 35/10
C. 35/4
D. 10/25
E. 10/4

10-27. The total accommodative convergence found by the heterophoria method is:
A. The distance deviation plus the normal convergence
B. The tonic deviation minus the normal accommodation
C. The normal accommodative convergence plus the overshoot or undershoot of convergence
D. The overshoot of convergence minus the distance deviation
E. None of the above

10-28. The heterophoria method of AC/A determination yields:
A. Lower values than the lens gradient method
B. The same values as the lens gradient method
C. More accurate values than the lens gradient method
D. Higher values than the lens gradient method
E. None of the above

10-29. In determining the AC/A ratio by the heterophoria method, a patient is found to be more exodeviated at near. The exodeviation:
A. Represents an overshoot of divergence
B. Must be added to the normal convergence
C. Must be subtracted from the normal accommodation
D. Must be subtracted from the normal convergence
E. None of the above

10-30. A patient has a pupillary distance of 5 cm, a near deviation of 15 P.D. esophoria, and a far deviation of 10 P.D. esophoria. If her accommodation is +6.00 D, calculate the AC/A ratio using the heterophoria method:
A. 15.83:1
B. 5.83:1
C. 6.67:1
D. 9.16:1
E. 5.26:1

10-31. A presbyopic patient has a range of accommodation from 2 m to ⅔ m. He goes without distance glasses. What glasses are necessary to allow him to see clearly and comfortably at 40 cm?
A. +3.00 D for reading
B. −0.50 +2.00 add bifocals
C. −2.00 D single vision glasses
D. −1.50 +1.00 add bifocals
E. None of the above

10-32. A patient wearing a −25.00 D spectacle lens is still 2.00 D myopic. How can the residual myopia be corrected with the −25.00 D lens?

A. By moving the lens toward the eye 37 mm
B. By moving the lens away from the eye 37 mm
C. By moving the lens 3 mm closer to the eye
D. By moving the lens 3 mm farther away from the eye
E. None of the above

10-33. The clinical method:
A. Ignores the pupillary distance
B. It is not numerically accurate enough for AC/A studies
C. Reflects the same abnormalities as the heterophoria method
D. All of the above
E. None of the above

CHAPTER 11: PRESCRIBING

11-1. Which of the following does not result in acquired hyperopia?
A. A retroorbital tumor
B. Diabetes insipidus
C. Sulfonamides
D. Lens subluxation
E. Central serous chorioretinopathy

11-2. The basis of orthokeratology in the correction of myopia is:
A. Peripheral corneal flattening with central steepening
B. Central and peripheral steepening
C. Central flattening alone
D. Central steepening alone
E. Peripheral and central flattening

11-3. Astigmatism can be acquired by:
A. Ptosis
B. Pterygia
C. Keratoplasty
D. Lid tumors
E. All of the above

11-4. Manifest hyperopia is that amount of hyperopia that can be accepted by the patient while maintaining 20/20 visual acuity:
A. With correction of less than +1.50 D
B. With under 1 P.D. of manifest heterophoria
C. With accommodation maximally stimulated with minus lenses
D. Without cycloplegia
E. None of the above

11-5. The absolute part of the manifest hyperopia is that portion that cannot be compensated for by:
A. Changing the size of the pupil
B. Adjusting the power of the eye with cycloplegia
C. Increasing the accommodative range
D. the available accommodative amplitude
E. None of the above

11-6. Latent hyperopia is:
A. Compensated for by the accommodative amplitude
B. Exposed with cycloplegia
C. Uncompensated for by accommodative insufficiency
D. Uncorrectable except under cycloplegia
E. None of the above

11-7. Total hyperopia is equal to:
A. The difference between the sum of the latent plus manifest and the facultative
B. The average of the latent and the manifest components
C. The sum of the facultative, absolute, and latent components
D. The sum of the facultative, absolute, and manifest components
E. None of the above

11-8. Certain factors must be considered before deciding on the amount of correction for hyperopia. Which of the following is not among them?
A. Visual needs
B. Amplitude of accommodation
C. Gender
D. Occupation
E. Height

11-9. No correction is necessary if a hyperopic patient:
A. Is old

B. Is asymptomatic
C. Has a small amplitude of accommodation
D. Has recently acquired the hyperopia
E. Does not drive

11-10. A patient during refraction reveals the following: vision without correction 20/50; with +2.00 D he obtains 20/20; he accepts up to +5.00 D and still maintains 20/20; under cycloplegia with cyclopentalate 1% his refractive error is +8.00 with 20/20 vision. Which of the following is true about this patient?
A. The absolute hyperopia is +3.00 D
B. The facultative hyperopia is +3.00 D
C. The latent hyperopia is +4.00 D
D. The total hyperopia is +10.00 D
E. All of the above

11-11. If a patient is young with an exophoria:
A. Only the absolute hyperopia need be corrected
B. Only the facultative hyperopia need be corrected
C. Only the latent hyperopia need be corrected
D. All of the manifest hyperopia should be corrected
E. All of the hyperopia should be corrected

11-12. Correction to preserve half the amplitude of accommodation is important when a hyperopic patient has:
A. Accommodative insufficiency
B. Presbyopia
C. Orthophoria
D. Esophoria
E. All of the above

11-13. Which of the following is not true of hyperopia?
A. If a patient is exophoric, a balance between accommodative reserve and motility control is attempted
B. The prepresbyopic patient can delay the use of bifocals by avoiding contact lenses
C. The total hyperopia of the prepresbyopic patient should be corrected before bifocals are prescribed
D. In the young anisometropic patient the difference between the two eyes is prescribed to balance the accommodative demand
E. All of the above are true

11-14. Those with hyperopia:
A. Readily accept plus during refraction
B. Tolerate overcorrection more easily than undercorrection
C. Accept bifocals more easily than those with myopia
D. Tolerate undercorrection more easily than overcorrection
E. Are generally psychopaths

11-15. Myopia is:
A. A nonprogressive disease
B. Frequently associated with exodeviations
C. Rarely fully corrected
D. Seldom axial in origin
E. Always associated with an astigmatic component

11-16. Factors contributing to the progression of myopia include:
A. Accommodation
B. Convergence
C. The synkinetic triad
D. UV exposure
E. All of the above

11-17. Night myopia is an anomalous myopia similar to:
A. Acquired myopia
B. Accommodative myopia
C. Instrument myopia
D. All of the above
E. None of the above

11-18. A laser speckle optometer is used to measure the amount of night myopia. It:
A. Creates reflected laser light from a granular surface whose direction of motion varies with the refractive error
B. Has speckles that are out of focus and require accommodation to be

focused at the photoreceptors

C. Creates speckles by using a prism to scatter the light coming from the laser and redirecting them to the retina

D. Converges all light onto the photoreceptors during scotopic conditions only

E. None of the above

11-19. The movement of the speckles when using a laser speckle optometer:

A. Is always in the direction of the incoming laser beam

B. Reflects the movement of photons as energy is emitted by stimulated emission

C. Is with in hyperopia

D. Is with in myopia

E. None of the above

11-20. Dark retinoscopy and laser speckle optometry converge on the concept of:

A. One-way motion of light

B. A true resting state between distance and near

C. Spherical aberration

D. Absolute darkness

E. None of the above

11-21. Under scotopic conditions one tends to:

A. Overaccommodate for distance and near

B. Underaccommodate for near only

C. Underaccommodate for distance only

D. Overaccommodate for near only

E. None of the above

11-22. Which of the following statements is true regarding radial keratotomy?

A. The Japanese were the first to approach it from the epithelial side

B. The procedure involves radial, partial-thickness incisions designed to flatten the central cornea

C. Modified radial keratotomy involves incisions on the endothelial side of the cornea

D. Radial keratotomy is quite unpredictable for most myopic patients less than -5.00 D

E. None of the above

11-23. Keratomileusis involves:

A. YAG laser treatment of the autolenticule

B. The removal and lathing of a lamellar autolenticule that is flattened and then replaced

C. The sculpting of the central cornea with the use of ultraviolet light

D. No risk and predictable results

E. None of the above

11-24. A 3-year-old astigmatic child cyclopleges to *OD*: $-1.50 +3.00 \times 90$; *OS*: $-1.00 +2.00 \times 90$. Which of the following is true?

A. Accommodation is stimulated by full correction

B. Accommodative insufficiency will accompany full correction

C. Partial correction of half the cylinder is prescribed

D. No correction is indicated until visual maturity has been achieved

E. None of the above

11-25. Corrected astigmatic children have little problem with distortion because:

A. Their eyes are still visually immature

B. They use little to no accommodation

C. They rarely suffer spherical aberration

D. The retinal adaption time is rapid

E. None of the above

11-26. The practitioner must be wary of changing the axis of the correcting cylinder in:

A. Children having not yet reached visual maturity

B. Prepresbyopic persons

C. Asymptomatic adults having achieved adaption

D. Those with acquired astigmatism

E. All of the above

11-27. A 35-year-old engineer is wearing *OD*: $+0.50 +3.00 \times 95$; *OS*: $+0.75 +3.00 \times 85$. His new refraction is

OD: +0.50 +3.00 × 130; *OS*: +0.75 +3.00 × 60. It is appropriate to:
A. Fully recorrect at the new axis
B. Rotate any correction toward 90°
C. Rotate any correction toward 180°
D. Overminus so that accommodation compensates for the change in axis
E. No change should be given

11-28. In a presbyopic undercorrected myope the only way to test if full correction for distance will precipitate problems at near is to:
A. Perform dark retinoscopy and give the full value obtained
B. Measure the amount of distortion and prescribe only 10%
C. Place a trial lens in front of one eye and see if a monofit is acceptable
D. Perform retinoscopy at near
E. None of the above

11-29. If a previously undercorrected astigmatic patient does not tolerate full correction, and distortion proves to be the problem:
A. Reduce the power of the cylinder
B. Prescribe contact lenses
C. Correct at the minimum vertex distance
D. Rotate the cylinder axis toward 180, 90, or the old axis, whichever is most acceptable
E. All of the above

11-30. Which of the following statements is not true?
A. Intersecting curvilinear keratotomy procedures reduce corneal astigmatism predictably
B. If the astigmatism is all corneal, one can prescribe soft torics for correction
C. Elliptical excimer photokeratectomy may reduce myopic astigmatism
D. Bilateral amblyopia should be identified before any treatment
E. All of the above are true

11-31. Important issues to consider when correcting presbyopia include:
A. Accommodative range and amplitude
B. Image jump and displacement
C. Induced anisophoria
D. Contact lenses and the altered accommodative demand
E. All of the above

11-32. Which of the following is not common practice in prescribing for presbyopia?
A. Undercorrection is better than overcorrection
B. Bifocals are tried if any distance correction is required
C. Cervical disk disease sufferers should use trifocals
D. The induced prismatic effect in anisometropia can best be handled with slab-off prism or single vision readers
E. None of the above

11-33. When measuring high plus or minus bifocal lenses for presbyopia:
A. The glasses must be reversed from their normal position in the lensmeter
B. A new reading in the segment should be performed
C. A new measurement for the distance front vertex power should be taken
D. All of the above
E. None of the above

11-34. When nuclear sclerosis produces myopia:
A. The reading distance becomes closer
B. The patient adjusts to the proximity and magnification of the new reading distance
C. If the myopia is corrected for distance, a boost of the add is better tolerated
D. All of the above
E. None of the above

11-35. Convergence is:
A. A disconjugate eye movement to maintain the object of regard on corresponding retinal points
B. A discrete form of accommodation that pushes the focal point behind the retina

C. A form of binocular eye movement that follows the direction of accommodation and bisects the cross cylinder axis
D. Made up of slow and fast components that have the same drives and perform the same tasks
E. None of the above

11-36. Based on Sheard's criteria, how much of the phoria is measurable as the horizontal fusional amplitude?
A. Less than half
B. All
C. One fourth
D. More than twice
E. None of the above

11-37. High adds:
A. Are better tolerated by monocular patients
B. Increase the convergence demands of binocular patients
C. Can be coupled with prisms
D. All of the above
E. None of the above

11-38. Amblyopia is:
A. Common in young anisometropic persons
B. More common in myopia than hyperopia
C. Always treated by occlusion therapy
D. A progressive disease even after treatment of the cause
E. None of the above

11-39. In anisometropic adults the desired amount of correction is the amount of correction needed to:
A. Form an image on the retina
B. Correct 50% of the anisometropia
C. Maintain the 50% reserve of accommodative amplitude
D. Maintain fusion and single binocular vision
E. None of the above or all of the above

11-40. Nonpresbyopic adults can avert any induced anisophoria by:
A. Accommodating more with one eye than the other
B. Wearing bifocals to correct their anisometropia
C. Using the optical centers of their distance correction
D. Overcorrection in the reading segment of the lens
E. None of the above

11-41. Prism therapy:
A. Should be given only to symptomatic patients
B. Should involve the exact amount of prism needed to control symptoms
C. With decentration is efficacious with high myopia and hyperopia
D. May be used to shift the null point in nystagmus patients when a head turn is present
E. All of the above

11-42. What prism is required to induce an exophoria?
A. Base out
B. Base in
C. Base up
D. Base down
E. None of the above

11-43. A postoperative strabismus patient complains of persistent diplopia 4 weeks after the surgery. He has a 10 P.D. esotropia which increases to 12 P.D. at near. There is no lateral incomitance. He is not capable of fusion or suppression. He is out of sick leave at work. What do you prescribe?
A. The least amount of BO prism to enable him to fuse
B. 12 P.D. BI prism to enable fusion at near
C. 6 P.D. BO prism to allow half the horizontal fusional amplitude to be held in reserve
D. 10 P.D. BO prism to allow fusion at distance
E. Any prism prescribed at this stage will impair the success of the final outcome

11-44. Occasionally incomitant strabismus can be treated with:
A. Surgery
B. Orthoptics
C. Prisms for primary and downgaze
D. Fresnel prisms
E. All of the above

11-45. Which of the following statements is false?
A. Cyclovertical disorders cannot be corrected with prisms
B. Combined horizontal and vertical prisms add vectorially
C. A double Maddox rod test is useful to examine incomitant strabismus (it is useful for superior oblique palsies, etc.)
D. Patients "eat up" prism as their fusional amplitudes are relaxed
E. None of the above

11-46. When binocular aphakia is spectacle corrected:
A. A larger portion of the visual field of each eye now covers a smaller retinal area
B. A larger blur interval spans the retina
C. Images are less distorted because of the magnification
D. Peripheral astigmatism results in an increased depth of focus
E. None of the above

11-47. The size of a refractive scotoma depends on the:
A. Color of the test object and tint of the lens
B. Position of the examiner relative to the scotoma
C. Angle between the most peripheral ray and the central ray
D. Power, vertex distance, and size of the lens
E. None of the above

11-48. Through a high plus lens the scotoma corresponding to the blind splot
A. Appears larger and closer to fixation
B. Appears to be meridionally magnified
C. Appears to have doubled in size
D. Is smaller and displaced away from fixation
E. None of the above

11-49. The induced prismatic effects of a bilateral spectacle-corrected aphakic person trying to read inside the distance optical centers:
A. Can diminish the amount of convergence needed
B. Can be improved by segment decentration
C. Are favorable and predictable
D. May require stronger than normal adds in the bifocal segments
E. None of the above

11-50. Plus aspheric lenses afford all of the following advantages except:
A. Weight reduction
B. Cosmetic superiority
C. The patient's eyes are not magnified
D. They can be set in modern frames
E. All of the above are advantages

11-51. Each millimeter of anterior displacement of an intraocular lens is equal to a change in implant power equal to:
A. 1.00 D
B. 2.00 D
C. 4.00 D
D. The two values are not related
E. The relationship is exponential and not linear

11-52. Each millimeter error in axial length results in a refractive error of:
A. 1.00 D
B. 2.00 D
C. 4.00 D
D. The two are exponentially related
E. None of the above

11-53. The important factors in accurately predicting the correct implant power include:
A. The position of the lens implant
B. The type of lens implant selected
C. The surgeon
D. The *K* readings
E. All of the above

11-54. To improve the predictability of implant power selection, the anterior chamber depth factor estimates:
A. The depth from the anterior corneal surface to the back of the lens
B. The depth from corneal to lens epithelium
C. The distance from the iris to the principal plane of the IOL

D. The depth of the postoperative endothelium to implant distance
E. None of the above

11-55. To achieve a refractive error of −2.00 D postoperatively, what strength of IOL is required if the SRK formula predicts +15.00 D for emmetropia?
A. +15.00 D
B. +13.67 D
C. +16.33 D
D. +17.00 D
E. +13.00 D

11-56. To achieve a refractive error of −4.50 D postoperatively, what strength of IOL is required if the SRK formula predicts +22.00 D for emmetropia?
A. +25.00 D
B. +17.00 D
C. +26.50 D
D. +17.50 D
E. +19.00 D

11-57. A +17.00 D IOL is planned for a posterior chamber implant with an *A* constant of 118.7. The posterior capsule ruptures and inadequate fixation for a posterior chamber lens is present. An anterior chamber lens with an *A* constant of 116.2 is selected. What power for emmetropia should be used?
A. +19.50 D
B. +14.50 D
C. +13.60 D
D. +17.00 D
E. +17.34 D

11-58. Occasionally conversion from a posterior chamber IOL to an anterior chamber IOL is necessary. The only important factor in selecting the implant power is:
A. The *A* constant
B. The *K* readings
C. The axial length
D. The lens shape
E. None of the above

11-59. Which factor most significantly contributes to the IOL power and the *A* constant?
A. Size of the implant
B. Shape factor
C. Asphericity
D. Age of the patient
E. None of the above

11-60. Biconvex implants are currently favored because they:
A. Minimize spherical aberrations
B. Cause less image degradation when decentered
C. Reduce posterior capsular opacification rates
D. All of the above
E. None of the above

11-61. When converting from a meniscus to a biconvex lens, the *A* constant usually requires a change of:
A. +1.00 D
B. +1.50 D
C. +2.00 D
D. +2.50 D
E. None of the above

11-62. What power of IOL is required to achieve a refractive error of −4.00 D postoperatively if the SRK formula predicts +16.00 D for emmetropia?
A. +18.67 D
B. +13.33 D
C. +16.38
D. +15.63
E. None of the above

11-63. A +16.50 D IOL is planned for a posterior chamber implant with an *A* constant of 118. The posterior capsule ruptures and inadequate fixation for a posterior chamber lens is present. If the power for emmetropia for an anterior chamber lens is +12.50, what would the *A* constant for the anterior chamber lens be?
A. 112.5
B. 116.7
C. 122
D. 156
E. 114

11-64. If an IOL of +18.00 D is predicted for a postoperative refractive error of −4.50 D, what would the SRK formula predict for emmetropia?
A. +18.00 D
B. +21.00 D
C. +15.00 D

D. +14.66 D
E. None of the above

11-65. A preoperative cataract patient measures the following:

$OD: -\frac{12.00 +2.00 \times 90}{20/100}$

$OS: -\frac{7.00 +1.00 \times 90}{20/30}$

Axial length: *OD* = 26.00 mm
OS = 24.50 mm
Modified SRK II: *OD* + 8.00 D for emmetropia
OS + 11.00 D for emmetropia

The measurements are repeated by another technician and give exactly the same results. Which of the following is the most reasonable course of action?

A. Implant a +10.00 D IOL for −3.00 D of postoperative myopia
B. Postoperatively fix *OS* with a soft toric contact and shoot for emmetropia *OD*
C. Implant a +12.50 D IOL for −4.50 D of postoperative myopia
D. Preoperatively fit with contacts and shoot for emmetropia *OD* with a +8.00 D IOL
E. Preoperatively fit with contacts and do not implant an IOL

11-66. Attempts have been made to produce bifocal contact lenses by diffractive and refractive means by having:

A. Concentric distance and near bands
B. Fresnel optics
C. Simultaneous distance and near perception
D. Asphericity
E. All of the above

11-67. Preoperatively a patient comfortably wears −1.00 +4.00 × 90. Postoperatively the refraction is plano. The patient complains of distortion despite 6/6 vision. Cortical adaption has:

A. Ceased temporarily
B. Been lost forever
C. Occurred to correct the astigmatism but is no longer necessary
D. Occurred to correct the distortion but is no longer necessary
E. None of the above

11-68. Diffraction:

A. Is the limiting factor in most ophthalmic optics
B. Means to break apart
C. Is the reflective bending that occurs as light hits a curved surface
D. Always causes a ring scotoma to be produced
E. None of the above or all of the above

11-69. The size of the pupil that has the highest resolving power is:

A. 1 mm
B. 2.5 mm
C. 3 mm
D. 4 mm
E. This value is individual dependent

11-70. A patient wearing her "best" correction improves with a pinhole. This may mean:

A. The correction is not the best possible
B. Irregular astigmatism is present
C. The pupil is dilated
D. All of the above
E. None of the above

11-71. A patient wearing his "best' correction reduces acuity with a pinhole. This may mean:

A. Media opacities of a focal nature exist
B. Retinal pathology exists
C. The pupil is dilated
D. Mixed astigmatism is present
E. None of the above or all of the above

11-72. When the pinhole is used as a screening process, it can determine:

A. The immediate size of the pupil
B. If the reduced acuity is due to spherical or astigmatic aberrations
C. If the reduced acuity is on a refractive basis
D. The diffractive limit of the system

E. None of the above or all of the above

11-73. When using a pinhole, which of the following is a true statement?
A. Diffraction will reduce a 20/20 emmetropic patient's visual acuity to 20/25
B. Those with high hyperopia and high myopia will experience the greatest improvement
C. The response to movement of the pinhole in hyperopia can be augmented if prisms are also used
D. A with motion when moving a pinhole while the patient fixes an accommodative target means the patient is hyperopic
E. None of the above

11-74. The most accurate method of measuring the power of an IOL once implanted is currently:
A. Ultrasonography
B. Postoperative refractions
C. Anterior chamber depth
D. Slit-lamp photography
E. None of the above

11-75. With the slit-lamp beam illuminating a rectangular diffusing target mounted 10 mm anterior to the center of the reflecting mirror, which of the following can be visualized with the biomicroscope?
A. Purkinje-Sanson image I
B. Purkinje-Sanson image III
C. Posterior IOL image
D. Anterior corneal image
E. All of the above

11-76. When measuring the power of an IOL within the eye using the reflected image from the anterior IOL surface one must take into account:
A. The patient's fixation
B. The index of refraction of the crystalline lens
C. The magnifying effect of the cornea
D. The tilt of the IOL with respect to the optical axis
E. None of the above

11-77. An error of 0.50 D in the *K* readings results in an error in the computed lens power equal to:
A. 0.10 D
B. 0.25 D
C. 0.50 D
D. 1.00 D
E. 1.50 D

11-78. What amount of error is induced by an error of 0.5 mm in the anterior chamber depth?
A. 0.50 D
B. 1.00 D
C. 1.50 D
D. 2.00 D
E. No error is induced

11-79. If the magnification ratio of the reflected image is off by 15%, what is the error in the computed lens power equal to?
A. 0.50 D
B. 2.00 D
C. 1.00 D
D. 1.50 D
E. 0.15 D

11-80. Decentration of an IOL is clinically significant if it is greater than:
A. 0.5 mm
B. 1 mm
C. 1.5 mm
D. 2 mm
E. 2.5 mm

11-81. Which shape of IOL causes the greatest amount of astigmatism with decentration?
A. Meniscus and convexo-plane lenses
B. Biconvex and aspheric lenses
C. Plano-convex and meniscus lenses
D. Aspheric and meniscus lenses
E. Plano-convex and convexo-plane lenses

11-82. The main optical considerations for determining the optimal size of a capsulotomy is:
A. Refraction
B. Reflection
C. Size disparity

D. Diffraction
E. None of the above

11-83. How should the optimal posterior capsulotomy relate to the diameter of the pupil in scotopic conditions?
A. It should always be equal in value
B. It should always be less than the diameter
C. It should equal or exceed
D. It must exceed the diameter by 150%
E. None of the above

11-84. What is the typical scotopic pupil diameter following extracapsular cataract extraction with a posterior chamber lens?
A. Between 2 and 3.4 mm
B. Between 1.5 and 4.3 mm
C. Between 3.9 and 5 mm
D. 2.6 mm
E. 5.5 mm

11-85. Preoperative cataract evaluation reveals *A*-scan biometry results that suggest to achieve emmetropia requires the insertion of a +27.00 D IOL based on an axial length of 20 mm. The nonaffected contralateral eye would require a +22.00 D IOL based on an axial length of +22.5 mm. Which of the following is indicated?
A. Insert a +27.00 D IOL to shoot for emmetropia
B. Repeat the measurements
C. Insert a +25.00 D IOL to slightly undercorrect in case the result is off a bit
D. If the results concur with the refractive error, proceed with the patient's desire for −2.00 D of postoperative myopia
E. Order a CAT scan to verify the axial length disparity

11-86. Two years after cataract surgery a patient's best corrected vision is 20/100 in the operated eye. The posterior capsule is opacified. The optimal posterior capsulotomy should:
A. Exceed the scoptopic pupil and extend beyond the border of the IOL
B. Equal the photopic pupil
C. Equal the IOL border
D. Equal 2 mm in all cases
E. Equal or exceed the scotopic pupil and remain within the border of the IOL

CHAPTER 12: MATERIALS

12-1. Glass is:
A. Amorphorous
B. Organic
C. Ionically bound
D. A crystal lattice structure
E. All of the above

12-2. Glass:
A. Has a definite melting point
B. Can be annealed or softened
C. For optical grade lenses is made of natural raw materials
D. Can be made from a combination of sulfides
E. None of the above

12-3. Crown glass:
A. Is the name given to all optical grade lenses
B. Has an index of refraction equal to 1.523
C. Weighs 50% less than plastic
D. Is naturally impact resistant
E. None of the above

12-4. High index glass:
A. Has greater vergence for the same radius of curvature
B. Is brittle and not easy to work with
C. Has an index of refraction that cannot be brought above 1.709
D. Has greater color dispersion than other materials
E. All of the above

12-5. Photochromic glass:
A. Changes color on absorption of UV light
B. Uses the chemical dissociation of silver chloride on absorption of UV light to change color
C. Darkens at a speed that is inversely proportional to the temperature of the glass

D. All of the above
E. None of the above

12-6. A person with −10.00 D myopia is getting new frames and lenses. She requests an opinion about what would best suit her needs functionally and cosmetically. All of the following are true except:
A. Smaller, rounder frames reduce the rings and edge thickness
B. High index materials reduce lens thickness
C. Antireflection coatings reduce glare and make the lenses easier to keep clean
D. Tinting the edges of the lenses can reduce the appearance of edge thickness
E. There are minimum center thickness standards for safety reasons

12-7. With photochromic glass incorporating silver chloride one can:
A. Integrate a tint
B. Put a UV coat on the back that will not inhibit the dissociation process
C. Perform antireflection treatment without affecting the chemical nature of the glass
D. Trap the darkened state permanently under special conditions
E. All of the above

12-8. Composite technology:
A. Combines several different oxides to form a sheet of high index glass which is bonded to a CR-39 core
B. Binds a central plastic polymer to an outer glass lens without the use of bonding agents
C. Creates a weave of different oxides and plastics that is lighter and more stable than those which use glass fibers
D. All of the above
C. None of the above

12-9. Plastics are:
A. Organic polymers
B. Randomly structured
C. Melted at a definite temperature
D. All of the above
E. None of the above

12-10. CR-39:
A. Makes up 50% of all lenses dispensed
B. Has an index of refraction equal to 1.567
C. Has a relatively low color dispersion
D. Is very difficult to mold in the lab
E. None of the above

12-11. High index plastics (HIP) make lenses:
A. With flatter curves
B. Thinner
C. With an index of refraction around 1.600
D. Lighter
E. All of the above

12-12. Which of the following statements is correct?
A. All HIPs filter all UV < 380 nm
B. The surface is softer than CR-39, so scratch coating is necessary
C. There is considerably more reflection in HIPs necessitating more AR coating
D. HIPs need wash coating
E. All of the above

12-13. Polycarbonate "of old" had among its disadvantages:
A. A brittle nature making it prone to cracking
B. It was too coarse, adversely impairing visual quality
C. It would flex and warp when mounted in a tight frame
D. A chronic instability that altered color dispersion
E. None of the above

12-14. The "new" polycarbonate:
A. Can be cast in glass molds
B. Is more flexible, allowing for easier pliability
C. No longer requires special edge cutting and scratch coating
D. Has a center thickness of approximately 2 mm
E. All of the above

12-15. Which of the following is not true for polycarbonates?

A. Edge thickness is a problem in myopia
B. Aspheric lenses increase the curvature from the center to the periphery of the lens
C. By reducing the curvature, the lens thickness is reduced
D. If the lens thickness is reduced, the field increases
E. All of the above are not true

12-16. Newer aspheric lenses:
A. Flatten a lens
B. Reduce oblique astigmatism
C. Are available in larger lenses
D. Approach a flat front surface
E. All of the above

12-17. The residual myopic halo rings can be reduced by:
A. Coloring the edges with Cruxite
B. Selecting darker frames
C. Polishing the edges with a light pink
D. All of the above
E. None of the above

12-18. Special high index glass for x-ray protection:
A. Has an index of refraction equal to 2.0
B. Is only used for safety goggles
C. A minimum center thickness must be maintained with or without side shields
D. All of the above
E. None of the above

12-19. The standards for impact resistance vary:
A. According to the end use of the lens
B. For center thickness according to the material
C. In different countries
D. All of the above
E. None of the above

12-20. In the United States the standard test for impact resistance involves:
A. Dropping a 16 oz steel ball of ⅝ inch diameter from a height of 50 inches without breaking the lens to be considered safe for casual dress wear
B. Dropping a 32 oz, 1 inch steel ball from a height of 50 inches without breaking the lens to be considered safe for casual dress wear
C. Dropping a ½ oz, ½ inch diameter steel ball from a height of 50 inches without breaking the lens to be classified as impact resistant
D. All of the above
E. None of the above

12-21. Which of the following standards is not currently used to ensure consumer protection?
A. Heat hardened crown must have a center thickness of at least 2 mm
B. Chemically hardened lenses can have a minimum center thickness of only 1.5 mm
C. Industrial safety crown must be 3 mm thick in the center
D. Industrial safety crown must have an edge thickness equal to 2.5 mm
E. None of the above

12-22. Which of the following is not a true step in the heat tempering of glass?
A. The glass is heated between its annealing and softening point
B. The finished weight is quickly quenched, which cools the inside faster than the outside of the lens
C. The result of the cooling is the compression of the outside surface into a toughened shell
D. The inside remains under internal stress, which is a problem when the lens is scratched
E. None of the above or all of the above

12-23. With heat tempered lenses:
A. Breakage results in multiple similar, small, smooth-edged pieces
B. Breakage results in splinters and shards
C. A deep scratch has little effect on impact resistance
D. Once tempered they are as impact resistant as polycarbonate
E. None of the above

12-24. A heat treated lens:
A. Cannot be reworked in the lab

B. Is left with slightly different indices of refraction in different regions.
C. Is able to polarize light, which can be detected before the lens is worked on
D. All of the above
E. None of the above

12-25. Chemical tempering:
A. Cannot meet minimum center thickness requirements
B. Rarely maintains its impact resistance with scratching
C. Is cheaper with a shorter turnaround time in the lab
D. Involves the exchange of smaller sodium ions on the lens surface with larger potassium or lithium ions
E. None of the above

12-26. Chemical tempering can be used for which of the following lenses?
A. Aspheric plastics
B. HIPs
C. Photochromics
D. Polycarbonates
E. None of the above require tempering

12-27. Tints can be:
A. Deposited on a lens surface in a vacuum
B. Integrated into the material during its manufacture
C. Fused or cemented as a layer to white glass
D. All of the above
E. None of the above

12-28. An integrated tint will have the depth of color of the tint vary with the:
A. Distance from the center of the lens
B. Thickness of the lens
C. Degree of anisometropia
D. All of the above
E. None of the above

12-29. The fusion of an equitint or graduated tint layer to the surface of glass distributes the color:
A. As desired irrespective of the prescription
B. Evenly
C. Centrally spreading peripherally
D. Such that the periphery receives the most color
E. None of the above

12-30. Which of the following statements is true with respect to metals and metallic compounds?
A. They can be deposited on the surface of glass by a vacuum deposition process
B. They can be finished with gold, silver, zinc, or chromium
C. Special equipment is required to deposit on plastic lenses
D. They alter the reflected light rather than the absorption spectrum
E. All of the above

12-31. Plastic lenses in a heated immersion bath can be surface dyed according to:
A. The surface characteristics
B. The index of refraction of the lens
C. The power of the lens
D. The temperature of the dye bath
E. None of the above

12-32. Which of the following statements is not true:
A. Ultraviolet filtration can be achieved by an integrated chromophore that absorbs UV light
B. Infrared tints can use ferrous oxides and other absorptive lens materials
C. Tinted lenses cannot adversely affect color matching traffic lights and signals
D. Ultraviolet filtration can be achieved by dipping the lens in a heated, colored bath
E. None of the above are false

12-33. A plastic IOL is marked +18.00 D. What should its power be marked if it were made of crown glass with the same thickness and surface curvature?
A. +21.38 D
B. +15.15 D
C. +18.20 D
D. +18.00 D
E. None of the above

12-34. Which of the following is the true per-

centage of incident light reflected for each given material?
A. Crown glass (n = 1.523) = 3.9%
B. CR-39 (n = 1.490) = 4.3%
C. Index 7 (n = 1.70) = 7%
D. All of the above
E. None of the above

12-35. If reflected light from the first surface is 180° out of phase with the reflected light from the second surface:
A. Constructive interference would double the reflection
B. Destructive interference would eliminate all reflection
C. The amount of reflection would be reduced an amount dependent upon the distance separating the two surfaces
D. The amount of reflection would be increased depending upon the distance separating the two surfaces
E. None of the above

12-36. Which of the following is not a step in the application of a multilayer AR coating to a lens?
A. The lens must be cleaned with an ultrasonic cleaner until the lenses are particle free
B. The lens must be cooled to improve the coating adherence
C. Any moisture is removed and an electron beam gun evaporates sodium or lithium metals as a series of proprietary coatings
D. The material to be deposited is held in a copper crucible, soaked in water, and vaporized with the electron beam
E. The vacuum chamber transports the vapor to the lens, which accepts the deposit

12-37. Certain lens materials cannot undergo AR coating because of the elevated temperature. They include:
A. HIPs
B. High index glass
C. Polarized lenses
D. Bifocals
E. None of the above

12-38. AR coatings can be predictably stripped chemically from:
A. Polycarbonate
B. HIPs
C. CR-39
D. All of the above
E. None of the above

12-39. Antiscratch coating:
A. Should be applied after AR coating
B. Is deposited onto the surface of the lens in a vacuum
C. Is not permanent and should be replenished every 6 months
D. Should be put on after the washcoat
E. None of the above

12-40. Glazing is the process of:
A. Mounting lenses into frames
B. Antiglare coating the lens
C. Tinting the lens
D. Anticondensation coating the lens
E. None of the above

12-41. Organic frame materials expand when heated. This can be safely accomplished by:
A. A bath of hard rock salt
B. A hot water bath
C. A hot air blower
D. A 3M oven
E. None of the above

12-42. If a lens is off-axis by a few degrees, an attempt to heat the frame and rotate the lens is recommended except in the case of:
A. Bifocals
B. High plus lenses
C. High minus lenses
D. All of the above
E. None of the above

12-43. The effective diameter of the lens:
A. Is the narrowest part of the lens
B. Will influence the size of the lens blank selected to grind the lens
C. Is usually measured from the temporal edge of both lenses and then divided by two
D. All of the above
E. None of the above

12-44. What two values determine the amount the lens blank is decentered to fit the frame?
- **A.** The effective diameter of the lens and the pupillary distance
- **B.** The distance between lenses and the optical center
- **C.** The vertex distance and the effective lens diameter
- **D.** The pupillary distance and the distance between lenses
- **E.** None of the above

12-45. Matching the pupillary distance of the frame to that of the patient:
- **A.** Minimizes decentration errors
- **B.** Maximizes decentration errors
- **C.** Maximizes the cost
- **D.** Maintains the correct visual acuity no matter what the eye position is
- **E.** None of the above

12-46. Which of the following statements is true?
- **A.** Bridge configuration is a major consideration when selecting frames
- **B.** Silicone nosepads are very soft and inert
- **C.** Adjustable nosepads for high dioptric prescriptions allow vertex distance adjustments
- **D.** People with flat bridges are usually fit with nosepads
- **E.** All of the above

12-47. Tortoiseshell has unique natural properties, which include:
- **A.** A granular nature
- **B.** A very high annealing point
- **C.** An ability to form strong bonds with itself under heat and pressure
- **D.** A paucity of naturally occurring colors
- **E.** All of the above

12-48. Match the mechanical PD of the glasses to the patient's PD knowing that the patient's PD is 58 mm and the distance between lenses is 22 mm. The horizontal lens diameter is 44 mm.
- **A.** The total decentration is 8 mm out
- **B.** A decentration of 3 mm in is needed in both eyes
- **C.** A total decentration of 6 mm in is needed
- **D.** A decentration of 2 mm out is needed
- **E.** None of the above

12-49. What decentration is needed to match the mechanical PD to the patient's PD when the patient's PD is 62 mm and the distance between lenses is 18 mm? The horizontal lens diameter is 36 mm:
- **A.** The total decentration is 9 mm
- **B.** A decentration of 4 mm out is required for each eye
- **C.** A total decentration of 6 mm out is required
- **D.** A decentration of 3 mm in is required for each lens
- **E.** None of the above

12-50. Synthetic plastics frames can be made of:
- **A.** Plexiglas
- **B.** CR-39
- **C.** Nylon
- **D.** Celluloid
- **E.** All of the above

12-51. Synthetic plastic frames can originate as:
- **A.** Large granules that are heated and then coated on a wire template
- **B.** A molten liquid that is cast as a dye
- **C.** A block that is chiseled and carved
- **D.** A soft pliable lump that is molded by hand to create the general configuration and then cured in an oven
- **E.** None of the above

12-52. Celluloid and cellulose acetate share which of the following properties:
- **A.** The plasticizer used
- **B.** The flammability
- **C.** The method of preparing the substances (i.e., acetylation versus nitration)

D. The workability
E. None of the above

12-53. Nylon has reentered the market with an improved product that:
A. Is thinner
B. Is stronger
C. Is easier to insert into the frames
D. Has an inherent memory lock for adjustments
E. All of the above

12-54. Metal frames are:
A. The most inexpensive of all frames
B. The most durable of all frames
C. Difficult to work with
D. Obsolete
E. Very light

12-55. Gold is
A. Corrosion resistant
B. Easily tarnished
C. Always electroplated
D. All of the above
E. None of the above

12-56. Aluminum:
A. Does not lose strength with bending
B. Is anodized to make the surface more resistant
C. Cannot be painted or varnished
D. Is well insulated in the winter
E. All of the above

12-57. Titanium:
A. Is rigid
B. Has poor memory retention
C. Is heat resistant
D. Does not resist corrosion very well
E. None of the above

12-58. Stainless steel:
A. Is made up mostly of iron but does not rust
B. Is nonmagnetic
C. Is corrosion resistant
D. Cannot be soldered
E. All of the above

12-59. For every 2° of pantoscopic tilt, the optical centers must be adjusted by:
A. 0.5 mm
B. 1 mm
C. 1.5 mm
D. 2 mm
E. 2.5 mm

12-60. When measuring the pupillary distance, which of the following measurements may prove useful?
A. The distance between the corneal light reflexes fixing a near light
B. Nasal limbus to temporal limbus in other eye
C. Pupillary border to pupillary border
D. All of the above
E. None of the above

12-61. When measuring the vertex distance:
A. We can use a lensmeter
B. We can use a lenscorometer
C. We must adjust for the near measurement
D. Always add 4 mm
E. None of the above

12-62. In the modern lab existing frames are analyzed by a computer to find out:
A. Contour and shape
B. Total circumference
C. The correct lens blank to accommodate the prescription
D. All of the above
E. None of the above

12-63. The working block:
A. Is created by using alloy with a low melting point that fixes a metal working piece to the finished, protected surface
B. Is necessary to fix the lens in position for grinding the uncut back surface
C. Is necessary to hold the lens in place while it is polished
D. All of the above
E. None of the above

CHAPTER 13: CONTACT LENSES

13-1. Which of the following is not an advantage of using contact lenses over spectacle correction?
A. The optical centers of contact lenses follow the visual axes
B. Induced prismatic effects are eliminated

C. All spherical aberration is corrected
D. Fogging does not occur with temperature changes
E. All of the above

13-2. The reduction in vertex distance when using contact lenses:
A. Reduces magnification
B. Reduces minification
C. Reduces the aniseikonic effects on retinal imagery
D. All of the above
E. None of the above

13-3. Which of the following statements is true?
A. A contact lens is an antigenic substance and can interact with the immune mechanism to cause problems
B. The contact lens acts as a barrier preventing bacteria and other microorganisms from being deposited onto the cornea
C. If the refractive difference is small, aniseikonia may worsen with contacts compared to glasses
D. Contact lenses do not provide stable vision in compound myopia
E. None of the above statements is true

13-4. The refraction and K readings for a patient in contact lenses are:

OD: $-3.00 + 3.00 \times 45$
$K = 43 \times 44.5D$
OS: $-3.00 + 2.50 \times 135$
$K = 43 \times 45.5D$

Which of the following is correct?
A. Regular hard contact lenses could correct all of the astigmatism
B. Soft toric contact lenses could not correct the corneal astigmatism
C. Bitoric hard contacts could correct all of the astigmatism
D. No contact lens is appropriate in the presence of lenticular astigmatism
E. With any contact lens, overcorrection with glasses will be necessary for driving

13-5. Hard lenses:
A. Are less than 1% water
B. Are oxygen impermeable
C. Are more comfortable than soft lenses
D. Yield poor visual results
E. None of the above

13-6. Which of the following statements accurately describes cellulose acetate butyrate (CAB) lenses?
A. They require less adaption time than hard lenses
B. Their contact with the lid is less than for hard lenses
C. They have more advantageous optical qualities than hard lenses
D. All of the above
E. None of the above

13-7. Which of the following accurately describes the relationship between the K reading and the radius of curvature?
A. As the radius of curvature decreases, the power increases
B. The two values are exponentially related
C. As the radius of curvature increases, the power increases
D. The more convex the lens, the lower the refractive power
E. None of the above

13-8. Calculate the radius of curvature of a contact lens fit on K, $K = 42.00$:
A. 5.56 mm
B. 8.04 mm
C. 14.18 mm
D. 3.18 mm
E. None of the above

13-9. The conventional way to express contact lens power is in:
A. Spherocylinder form
B. Minus cylinder form
C. Plus cylinder form
D. Any of the above
E. None of the above

13-10. The posterior optical zone is constructed to conform to the:
A. Anterior corneal surface
B. Posterior corneal surface

C. Central corneal contour
D. Peripheral corneal contour
E. None of the above

13-11. The junction of the different radii of curvature is called a:
A. Blend
B. Point cross
C. Joint
D. Any of the above
E. None of the above

13-12. Which of the following is used to fit hard or rigid gas permeable contacts?
A. Fitting on *K*, where the steepest *K* is used
B. Choosing the correct curvature to eliminate any induced tear meniscus between cornea and lens
C. Overrefracting to compensate for a lens that is too steep and inducing minus sphere
D. All of the above
E. None of the above

13-13. What is the eye error if the *K* readings of a patient are 50 @ 90 by 46 @ 180?
A. -4.00×180
B. $+4.00 \times 90$
C. $+4.00 \times 180$
D. -4.00×90
E. None of the above

13-14. Clinically it would not be uncommon to fit a rigid gas permeable lens:
A. Less than 0.50 D flatter than the steepest *K*
B. 1.00 D steeper than the flattest *K*
C. 2.00 D flatter than the steepest *K*
D. 2.00 D steeper than the steepest *K*
E. None of the above

13-15. If a rigid contact lens is fit properly, which of the following should occur?
A. The corneal apex should just be cleared
B. A physiologic gas and fluid exchange should occur
C. Tears should fill the space and create an additional refracting meniscus
D. The power should be altered
E. All of the above

13-16. The rule of thumb is that for every 0.05 mm change in radius an adjustment to the power must be made equal to:
A. 0.5 D
B. 1.0 D
C. 0.25 D
D. 5.0 D
E. None of the above

13-17. If one is fitting 1.00 D steeper than the flattest *K*, the posterior radius of curvature must be:
A. 0.2 mm shorter and the lens corrected by +1.00 D
B. 0.2 mm longer and the lens corrected by −1.00 D
C. 0.2 mm shorter and the lens corrected by −1.00 D
D. 0.2 mm longer and the lens corrected by +1.00 D
E. None of the above

13-18. Advantages of a hard lens include its ability to be:
A. Custom fit
B. Reground
C. Steepened or flattened
D. Polished
E. All of the above

13-19. Which of the following statements is true?
A. If both meridians are the same radius, the lens is spherical
B. If cylinder is ground on the back surface, the lens is a back toric lens
C. If cylinder is added to the front surface, the lens is bitoric
D. BD prism ballast will orient the lens by gravity
E. All of the above

13-20. Lenses are truncated to:
A. Improve oxygenation by reducing the amount of plastic
B. Follow the axis of the lower lid angle
C. Temporarily stabilize the lens in the desired axis until mild corneal edema holds it in position
D. Create equal image displacement in both eyes to eliminate prismatic effects
E. None of the above

13-21. If one is fitting +1.00 D steeper than

the flattest K, which of the following statements is true?

A. The posterior curve must be made 2 mm flatter
B. +1.00 D should be added to the lens power
C. The posterior curve should be made 2 mm steeper
D. −1.00 D should be added to the lens power
E. None of the above

13-22. A lenticular bevel is formed when:

A. The edges of a high minus lens are thinned
B. The center of a high plus lens is ground flatter
C. A minus carrier of a plus lens is removed
D. Ridging occurs on the edge of a high plus lens
E. None of the above

13-23. For a lens to become steeper:

A. The chord diameter is increased
B. The radius of curvature is increased
C. The apical vault of the lens decreases
D. The epithelial surface shrinks
E. None of the above

13-24. Which of the following are among the effects if the lens diameter of a contact lens is reduced?

A. The apical vault is increased
B. The lens is made steeper
C. The corrected flattest K becomes 36.00 D
D. All of the above
E. None of the above

13-25. Soft toric lenses have:

A. The comfort of soft lenses
B. The power to correct corneal astigmatism
C. The power to correct lenticular astigmatism
D. Less lens rotation than regular soft lenses
E. All of the above

13-26. The corneal index of refraction used to standardize the keratometer is:

A. 1.3333
B. 1.3375
C. 1.3475
D. 1.3760
E. None of the above

13-27. An aphakic patient desires a contact lens. Her spectacle correction is +9.00 +2.00 × 90 at a vertex distance of 10 mm. K readings are 40.0 × 44.0 horizontally and vertically. What power of contact lens is required and at what base curve if a hard lens is chosen which is 1.00 D steeper than K?

A. 8.65 mm/+11.36 D
B. 8.23 mm/+11.36 D
C. 8.23 mm/+13.36 D
D. 8.65 mm/+12.11 D
E. 8.23 mm/+10.11 D

13-28. An aphakic patient desires a contact lens. Her spectacle correction in minus cylinder form is +12.00 −5.00 × 90 at vertex distance 8 mm. K readings are 58 × 63 horizontally and vertically. What power of contact lens is required and at what base curve, if a soft contact lens is chosen which is 2.00 D flatter than the flattest K?

A. 6.03 mm/+15.28 D
B. 4.17 mm/+15.28 D
C. 5.63 mm/+11.28 D
D. 6.03 mm/+11.28 D
E. 5.63 mm/+15.28 D

13-29. For contact lenses whose base curves are in the range 40 to 45 D, which of the following statements is true?

A. Over this range r changes by 2 mm
B. For each millimeter the radius decreases, 5.32 D of power are added
C. A lens of 42.00 D has a radius equal to 7.5 mm
D. All of the above
E. None of the above

13-30. The relative gas permeability of a contact lens depends on the:

A. Diffusion coefficient
B. Solubility constant of the lens material
C. Corneal index of refraction
D. All of the above
E. None of the above

13-31. Which of the following statements is true?
A. A thicker plus lens would have a lesser *DK* value than a thin lens
B. The partial pressure of oxygen across the lens will influence the oxygen flux at the corneal level
C. The thickness factor gives an index of oxygen transmissibility
D. The corneal integrity depends on the aqueous delivery of glucose
E. All of the above

13-32. Which factor adversely affects corneal oxygenation?
A. Increasing the *DK* value
B. Increasing aqueous pO_2
C. Increasing ambient pO_2
D. Increasing center thickness
E. None of the above

13-33. HEMA is a low flux material. If a lens is 3 mm thick, its *DK* value is 22.0 and its partial pressure of oxygen is 2%, what is its flux?
A. 1466.7
B. 14.7
C. 146.7
D. 3.3
E. 33.3

CHAPTER 14: LOW VISION, PENALIZATION, MALINGERING

14-1. The Amsler grid:
A. Is useful for testing accommodative amplitude
B. Tests the central horizontal and vertical 10° of visual field for evidence of central disruption
C. Tests peripheral visual information in jumps of 10°
D. Checks for eccentricity of the fovea
E. None of the above

14-2. Peripheral visual field defects may result from:
A. Retinal problems
B. Optic nerve problems
C. Neurologic problems
D. Glaucomatous problems
E. All of the above

14-3. If peripheral field defects approach fixation:
A. Images may be projected into nonseeing retina
B. Binocularity becomes difficult
C. Magnification may adversely affect vision
D. All of the above
E. None of the above

14-4. The selection of the type and power of visual aid depends on the:
A. Ocular motility
B. Accommodative amplitude
C. Visual acuity of each eye
D. Age of the patient
E. All of the above

14-5. A 40-year-old has 20/80 *OD* 20/200 *OS* and is having difficulty reading textbook-size print. Which of the following methods of correction is appropriate?
A. Binocular 3× loupe
B. 5× magnifier
C. +4.00 D monocular add *OD*
D. +6.00 D binocular adds *OU*
E. +10.00 D half glasses with BI prism

14-6. If the PD of the patient is 64 mm, what is the convergence required for an object of regard at 10 cm?
A. 6.4 P.D.
B. 32 P.D.
C. 640 P.D.
D. 3.2 P.D.
E. 64 P.D.

14-7. Estimate the amount of add a patient needs to read average newsprint if the patient's visual acuity is 20/100?
A. +5.00 D add
B. +1.00 D add
C. 3× magnifier
D. 5× magnifier
E. None of the above

14-8. A patient requires an add greater than +6.00 D:
A. This is quite expensive
B. A trial with a Fresnel Press-On segment will show whether this add is worthwhile

C. It is a special order to get this lens
D. All of the above
E. None of the above

14-9. Estimate the plus lens necessary to read newspaper print at 40 cm when a patient's vision is 20/200:
A. +5.00 D
B. +10.00 D
C. +15.00 D
D. +20.00 D
E. More than +20.00 D

14-10. With a 3× hand-held telescope, what level of Snellen acuity would a patient with 6/18 acuity in the right eye and 6/30 acuity in the left be expected to resolve?
A. 6/10
B. 6/6
C. 6/8
D. 6/54
E. 6/90

14-11. Which of the following statements is not true?
A. Many older people prefer to read at close distances
B. When using a hand magnifier or a stand magnifier an increased field results
C. A hand magnifier can double as a makeshift monocular reading glass
D. All of the above
E. None of the above

14-12. Which of the following examples would produce a Galilean telescope effect with an aphakic patient?
A. A +4.00 D lens held at 17 cm
B. A +5.00 D lens held at 22 cm
C. A −40.00 D lens held at 13 cm
D. A +25.00 D lens held at 19 mm
E. None of the above

14-13. Which of the following is a property of the Amorphic Lens System?
A. It is a hand-held telescope
B. It minifies the 180° meridian
C. It magnifies the vertical perspective
D. The horizontal field is decreased
E. None of the above or all of the above

14-14. Penalization occurs when:
A. A hemianopic patient suffers from decreased central acuity
B. Distance or near vision is purposefully reduced to treat mild to moderate amblyopia
C. Prismatic correction eliminates the strabismic component of amblyopia
D. A neutral density filter is prescribed for the amblyopic eye
E. None of the above

14-15. Hysteria:
A. Is a psychoneurosis
B. Produces a secondary gain of care and sympathy
C. May entail paralysis and blindness
D. Is amenable to psychotherapy
E. All of the above

14-16. 4 P.D. BO prism introduced in front of a seeing eye is accompanied by:
A. Complete blurring to 20/200
B. A fusional ductional response to maintain binocularity
C. Pincushion distortion
D. Monocular diplopia
E. None of the above

CHAPTER 15: INSTRUMENTS

15-1. The lens measure uses several values to calculate refractive power, which include:
A. Chord diameter
B. Radii of curvature
C. Sagittal height of the chord
D. All of the above
E. None of the above

15-2. The lens measure is also useful for:
A. Determining spherical aberration
B. Irregular chord diameters
C. Determining the extent of lens warpage
D. Calibrating lensmeters
E. None of the above

15-3. A radiuscope is used:
A. When dealing with hard or gas permeable contact lenses

B. To verify the anterior central curve of a contact lens
C. To calculate the radii of curvature of contact lenses
D. To determine lens warpage
E. All of the above

15-4. Hand neutralization occurs when a lens of known calibration is placed:
A. At the far point of the unknown lens
B. At the focal distance of the unknown lens
C. In front of the unknown lens
D. At the near point of the unknown lens
E. None of the above

15-5. The lensmeter with glasses temple down:
A. Measures the total dioptric power
B. Measures the back vertex power
C. Measures the anterior radius of curvature
D. Measures the effective power of the lens
E. None of the above

15-6. The non-Badal lensmeter biases the determination of power by:
A. Endpoint discrimination toward the plus side by the observer
B. Magnifying small changes with plus lenses
C. Nonlinear dioptric scale
D. All of the above
E. None of the above

15-7. Badal discovered that if the standard lens is positioned in such a way that its secondary focal point was at the back vertex of the spectacle lens to be measured, the result:
A. Is a logarithmic dioptric scale
B. Is emergent parallel rays at neutralization
C. Is the convergence of emerging rays at the new focal point that falls on the scale
D. Is the introduction of observer magnification, making endpoint determination easier
E. None of the above

15-8. Which of the following are alterations in technique that must be made when measuring fused bifocals of high strength plus or minus lenses?
A. The spectacle must be turned over and measured temples up
B. The distance front vertex correction should be reread at the front optical center
C. The difference between the front vertex correction measured at distance and in the segment is the power of the add
D. All of the above
E. None of the above

15-9. The problem measuring the power of a contact lens with a lens meter arises because:
A. The apical vault falls within the focal plane of the standard lens
B. The front and back vertex powers are very different
C. The prismatic effect of these lenses is too great to ignore
D. All of the above
E. None of the above

15-10. According to the Scheiner principle, when an object of regard is placed conjugate to the retina:
A. A double image is perceived
B. A magnified image is seen
C. A single clear image is seen
D. An inverted, double image is observed
E. None of the above

15-11. Systems currently developed for automated refraction include:
A. Automation of a standard phoropter
B. Automation of a normal refracting sequence with special cross cylinder testing
C. Refraction without any lenses in front of the patient
D. All of the above
E. None of the above

15-12. Which of the following statements accurately describes the direct ophthalmoscope?
A. The field of view is large

B. The field of view is limited by the aperture
C. The magnification is independent of the eye error
D. The minification is similar to that of a Galilean telescope
E. None of the above

15-13. The indirect ophthalmoscope produces an image of the fundus, which then becomes:
A. The object of the condensing lens, which forms an aerial image that is larger and inverted
B. The image of the condensing lens, which forms an aerial image that is smaller and inverted
C. The aerial image of the condensing lens, which is smaller and inverted
D. The object of the condensing lens and later the aerial image, which is smaller and erect
E. None of the above

15-14. Describe the image produced of the retina by a monocular indirect ophthalmoscope with a condensing lens of power +10.00 D examining a emmetropic eye:
A. The image is minified 6×
B. The image is perceived erect
C. The image is magnified 10×
D. The image is blurred
E. None of the above

15-15. A +16.00 D indirect ophthalmoscope condensing lens is held 6 cm from a patient's cornea to achieve proper illumination through the pupil. Where is the aerial image of the retina formed for +10.00 D aphakia? Assume the refractive error is measured with respect to a spectacle plane 10 mm anterior to the cornea.
A. 6.25 cm to the left of the condensing lens
B. 10 cm from the cornea
C. 15 cm from the far point plane
D. 10.72 cm in front of the condensing lens
E. None of the above

15-16. Which of the following would be true of the magnification using direct ophthalmoscopy?
A. An aphakic eye of +50.00 D has magnification of 18.75×
B. Relative to an emmetrope, the image of the fundus of a +75.00 D myope appears 25% larger
C. A myopic eye of +75.00 D would have magnification of 15×
D. Relative to that in emmetropia, the image of the fundus in +50.00 D aphakia appears 23% smaller
E. None of the above

15-17. Describe the magnification of a binocular indirect ophthalmoscope with a +15.00 D condensing lens viewing an emmetropic person. The PD is reduced to one fourth its normal distance:
A. The angular magnification is 4×
B. The axial magnification is 44×
C. The effective axial magnification is 16×
D. All of the above
E. None of the above

15-18. The most accurate method of determining the line of sight involves having the patient:
A. Fix a nonluminous target on the objective lens mount and sighting the center of the pupil with the surgeon using monocular vision
B. Fix a bright nonaccommodative target and then centering the light reflex binocularly
C. Fix the center of a placido disk and mark the center with binocular viewing
D. Fix a light at infinity and align the first two Purkinje images
E. None of the above

15-19. Which of the following statements is true regarding corneal topographic analyzers?
A. Images are digitized and analyzed to give each radius of curvature a value
B. A topographic map can be in color or gray scale

C. These instruments are important for refractive alteration
D. Coupling the information to contact lens manufacturing equipment provides custom fit contacts
E. All of the above

15-20. Sound can be:
A. Refracted
B. Reflected
C. Scattered
D. Absorbed
E. All of the above

15-21. In contact ultrasonography:
A. The near field extends to the posterior lens capsule, and details posterior to this are magnified
B. The far field extends to the anterior lens capsule, and details anterior to this are lost
C. The far field is extended, and any details anterior to the cornea are blurred
D. The near field extends to the posterior lens capsule, and any details anterior to this are lost
E. None of the above

15-22. Which of the following is not a true statement?
A. As the ultrasound encounters different interfaces, it can be displayed visually with a cathode ray oscilloscope
B. The time delay between emission and detection is a function of distance traveled
C. The time delay between emission and detection is a function of the density of the medium it is traveling in
D. The denser the medium, the shorter the delay
E. None of the above or all of the above

15-23. At a corneal applanation of 3.06 mm, what has been shown to occur?
A. The structural resistance to deformation of the cornea is greater than the attractive forces of the surface tension of the tears
B. The opposing forces of applanation are equal
C. The intraocular pressure equals each nanometer of applanation
D. The distance can be determined with a split image prism
E. None of the above

15-24. If the head of the applanation tonometer is not rotated 43° to the axis of the minus cylinder or to the lowest *K*, the error per 4.00 D of cylinder equals:
A. 1 mm Hg
B. 2 mm Hg
C. 4 mm Hg
D. 5 mm Hg
E. More than 5 mm Hg

15-25. The keratometer determines the radii of curvature and refracting power of the two corneal meridians by using:
A. Only the reflective properties of the lens
B. Only the refractive properties of the cornea
C. Both the refractive properties of the lens and the reflective properties of the cornea
D. Both the refractive and reflective power of the lens
E. None of the above

15-26. If one keeps either the image size or the object size constant, by measuring the size of:
A. The variable, the magnification can be calculated
B. The image distance, the magnification can be calculated
C. The object distance, the magnification can be calculated
D. All of the above
E. None of the above

15-27. Which of the following instruments cannot be used to differentiate between cataractous and noncataractous causes of decreased vision?
A. Potential acuity meter
B. Phoropter
C. Laser interferometer
D. Blue field entoptoscope
E. Slit lamp biomicroscope

CHAPTER 16: LASERS

16-1. LASER is an acronym derived from:
A. Light Associated Stimulation by Emission of Radiation
B. Lengthy Amplification by Stimulated Emission of Radiation
C. Light Associated Striation by Emitted Radons
D. Light Amplification by Stimulated Emission of Radiation
E. None of the above

16-2. Ionization:
A. Occurs only in X-irradiation
B. Involves the absorption of energy
C. Was first discovered by Einstein
D. Is independent of photodisruption
E. None of the above

16-3. If all of the electrons in the same medium go from the same excited state to a nonexcited state:
A. Multiple photons are released at the same time
B. The photons have the same wavelength
C. The photons have the same frequency
D. All of the above
E. None of the above

16-4. Which of the following statements is true?
A. Energy can be absorbed and electrons can go from an excited to a nonexcited state
B. With the release of a photon, an electron can go from its nonexcited to its excited state
C. Spontaneously emitted photons are always amplified once released
D. The absorption of a photon can stimulate the absorption of another photon from a similar atom
E. None of the above

16-5. If more than half of the atoms are in the excited state:
A. Absorption exceeds amplification
B. Energy is acquired through thermal sources
C. Laser formation is favored
D. Destructive interference reduces amplification and the resulting wavefront
E. None of the above or all of the above

16-6. A ruby crystal is formed when an aluminum oxide crystal:
A. Has its aluminum replaced by chromium
B. Has its aluminum replaced by silver
C. Reacts with aqueous silver chloride
D. Reacts with copper to form aluminum chloride
E. None of the above

16-7. A resonance chamber:
A. Generally has mirrored ends
B. Is used to reflect emitted radiation and enhance the amplification of stimulated emission
C. Must be multiples of half or full wavelengths
D. May have an aperture at one end that will allow light to escape
E. All of the above

16-8. Any light that might emerge from a resonance chamber is:
A. Polychromatic
B. Highly directional
C. Out of phase
D. Of low intensity
E. All of the above

16-9. The emission of light from a laser can occur in:
A. A continuous wave
B. Pulses of short duration
C. High-intensity releases
D. Bursts
E. All of the above

16-10. Parameters controllable by the surgeon using a laser include:
A. Power
B. Spot size
C. Duration
D. Number of pulses per burst
E. All of the above

16-11. To increase the power, one can:

A. Increase the time
B. Increase the spot size
C. Decrease the distance
D. Increase the work
E. None of the above

16-12. Which of the following statements is true?
A. Energy density is given in units of watts
B. The same amount of energy over a smaller spot increases the energy density
C. The spot size is exponentially related to the energy density
D. All of the above
E. None of the above

16-13. The neodymium-YAG laser has neodymium ions incorporated into:
A. A metal base
B. A crystal
C. An electrode
D. A chromium base
E. None of the above

16-14. A suprathreshold burst increases the laser energy density until:
A. A threshold is overcome where electrons are stripped from their atoms and a plasma is formed
B. An intense electromagnetic disruption occurs
C. Complex shock and acoustic phenomena are experienced
D. An explosion occurs at the focal point
E. All of the above

16-15. Which of the following statements is correct?
A. A laser that does not cause protein coagulation is called a photocatabolizer
B. By doubling the frequency the wavelength is doubled
C. An infrared laser can be converted to a visible laser with the addition of a frequency doubler
D. Infrared lasers tend to be photocoagulators
E. None of the above

16-16. The THC:YAG laser is doped with:
A. Titanium, holmium, and calcium
B. Titanium, holmium, and copper
C. Thulium, hydrogen, and calcium
D. Thulium, holmium, and chromium
E. None of the above combinations

16-17. Which of the following lasers emits ultraviolet light?
A. Er:YAG
B. Excimer XeCl
C. Er:YLF
D. Tunable MgCaF
E. Alexandrite

16-18. Which of the following statements is true?
A. UV light may have acute endothelial toxicity
B. UV light may have retinal toxicity
C. UV light may have chronic degenerative potential
D. IR light may have thermal toxicity
E. All of the above

16-19. Gas discharge lasers:
A. Work by having gas contained in a narrow tube discharged through a tiny filtered aperture, creating a controlled combustion
B. Are stimulated by electric current, which excites the medium and initiates laser propagation
C. Control the amount of discharge by increasing the amount of pressure within the tube
D. Stimulate laser propagation by means of sparks, which are started within the tube under controlled environmental conditions
E. None of the above

16-20. Which of the following statements is true?
A. Argon lasers produce red and yellow light
B. Carbon dioxide lasers emit in the infrared portion of the spectrum
C. Krypton lasers produce blue and green light
D. All of the above
E. None of the above

16-21. The CO_2 laser:
A. Is the most efficient laser with 30% efficiency

B. Dissipates very little heat
C. Emits radiation that all metallic substances absorb
D. Is used mainly for diagnostic purposes
E. None of the above

16-22. Photocoagulation involves:
A. Tissue whose absorption spectrum is within the range of the emitted laser radiation
B. The absorption of light energy, which necessitates heat dissipation
C. A heat release that coagulates the tissue at the anatomic site of absorption
D. All of the above
E. None of the above

16-23. Which of the following statements is incorrect?
A. Ocular pigments are primarily xanthophyll, melanin, and hemoglobin
B. Macular xanthophyll absorbs xenon
C. Argon green is absorbed by xanthophyll
D. Krypton red is not absorbed by xanthophyll
E. None of the above

16-24. Excimer lasers are gas discharge lasers whose media are:
A. Lanthanides
B. Rare earth metals
C. Noble gas–halogen combinations
D. Nonmetals
E. None of the above

16-25. The term excimer is derived from the terms:
A. Excited meridian
B. Excited dimers
C. Excitable mercury
D. Excitable primers
E. None of the above

16-26. Diatomic rare gas halides release UV light:
A. Which when absorbed by target tissues lyse protein intramolecular bonds
B. Which damages surrounding tissue, stimulating sufficient inflammation to promote healing
C. Which weakens atomic bonding and lowers the activation energy needed to ablate the next tissue layer
D. Which causes a great deal of coagulation
E. None of the above

16-27. Early or late phototoxicity due to UV absorption may appear in surrounding structures such as the:
A. Lens
B. Corneal endothelium
C. Retina
D. All of the above
E. None of the above

16-28. Liquid lasers:
A. Are primarily gas lasers
B. Use electrical current for stimulation
C. Involve liquid inorganic dyes
D. Have wavelengths between 360 and 960 nm
E. All of the above

16-29. The greatest feature of semiconductor lasers is their:
A. Convection air cooling
B. Extensive range of available wavelengths
C. Clinical utility at delivering high power levels
D. Lack of toxicity relative to other light sources working at the same wavelength
E. None of the above

16-30. With the aid of hematoporphyrin derivatives, photoradiation can:
A. Reduce the need for air cooling
B. Increase the specificity of the medium
C. Enhance the absorption of light by target tissues
D. Decrease the amount of interference from hemoglobin, which adversely affects the tissue absorption spectrum
E. None of the above

16-31. Each positioning hole on an IOL optic exposed due to a laser capsulotomy:

A. Creates its own secondary image
B. Decreases the interspace
C. Decreases the transmission of light through the pupil
D. Increases the amount of light reflected
E. None of the above

CHAPTER 17: PRINCIPLES OF REFRACTIVE SURGERY

17-1. Radial keratotomy involves:
A. Adding to the radius of curvature of the cornea surgically
B. Radial corneal cuts that steepen the peripheral cornea
C. Decreasing the radii of curvature of the central cornea
D. All of the above
E. None of the above

17-2. The variables that may affect the amount of correction provided by radial keratotomy include:
A. The depth of the cuts
B. The number of cuts
C. The direction of the cuts
D. The size of the optical zone
E. All of the above

17-3. Which of the following is a true statement?
A. The deeper the cuts, the more hyperopic the shift
B. The number of cuts has no effect on the amount of correction
C. The most common number of cuts is 8
D. As the number of cuts is reduced, the size of the optical zone is increased
E. None of the above

17-4. A patient has a spherical cornea prior to cataract surgery but postoperatively requires -3.00×90 for best visual acuity. What is the likely cause of the astigmatism and what is a possible correction?
A. Tight sutures; wedge resection
B. Poor wound healing; suture cutting
C. Flattening of the vertical meridian: astigmatic keratotomy
D. Bulging wound; wound recession
E. Gaping wound; slab-off technique

17-5. Which of the following statements is correct?
A. The steeper the meridian, the larger the chord diameter
B. The shorter the radius of curvature, the larger the chord diameter
C. Relaxing incisions should be made in the meridian with the largest chord diameter
D. The shorter the radius of curvature, the steeper the meridian
E. None of the above or all of the above

17-6. Radial thermal keratoplasty involves:
A. A 34-gauge microprobe
B. Insertion of a microprobe to 85% to 95% stromal thickness
C. Six to 16 rays of 2 to 4 burns with an optical zone of 5 to 8 mm
D. All of the above
E. None of the above

17-7. Hyperopic lamellar keratotomy:
A. Involves the removal of a lamellar disk 360° around an optical zone
B. Can be achieved with a microkeratome
C. Achieves central corneal steepening if 80% depth is achieved
D. All of the above
E. None of the above

17-8. Intracorneal hydrogels have the advantage of:
A. Attracting lipidlike deposits
B. Interface haze, which reduces reflection
C. No risk of endothelial damage
D. Preserving accommodation
E. None of the above

17-9. Epikeratophakia:
A. Does not require AIDS testing of the donor tissue
B. Involves cryolathing a donor cornea

C. Is useful in contact lens failure myopia
D. Is not reversible once in place
E. None of the above

17-10. Keratomilieusis:
A. Is used when aphakia cannot be corrected by any form of spectacle
B. Is similar in technique to the hexagonal keratotomy but performed on aphakic patients
C. Involves the surgical violation of the intact healthy cornea
D. All of the above
E. None of the above

17-11. Photorefractive keratectomy with the excimer laser involves:
A. Sculpting the central cornea by photoablation
B. Flattening the radius of curvature of the peripheral cornea
C. IR radiation at 193 nm
D. Is most useful and predictable in myopia greater than −5.00 D
E. None of the above

17-12. Which of the following statements is applicable to photorefractive keratectomy?
A. The size of the optical zone and the depth of the ablation control the amount of myopic correction
B. Elliptical optical zones can correct anisometropia
C. Hyperopic correction is very predictable
D. All of the above
E. None of the above

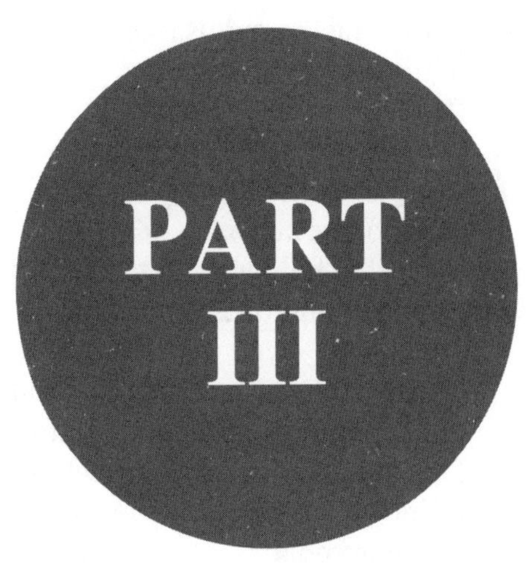

SOLUTIONS

CHAPTER 1: THE BASICS

1-1. (E) The wavelength of UV light is between 280 and 400 nm. Visible light has wavelengths between 380 and 780 nm. Therefore UV light has a shorter wavelength than visible light. (ref. p.2)

1-2. (A) Pseudoexfoliation is not caused by phototoxic damage. (ref. p.2)

1-3. (D) Superoxides, ionized electrons, and free radicals all have electrons that have been removed from their orbitals and are now able to cause phototoxic damage from interactions involving their excess energy. (ref. p.2)

1-4. (C) Anisometropia does not enhance phototoxicity or sensitivity to phototoxicity. (ref. p.2)

1-5. (A) The electric field is perpendicular to the magnetic field. (ref. p.3)

1-6. (D) The amount of divergence is defined by the radius of curvature of the wavefront. This latter entity increases with increasing distance from the source. (ref. p.4)

1-7. (A) As the distance from a source increases to infinity, an advancing plane emerges that is perpendicular to the optical axis and has a vergence of zero. (ref. p.4)

1-8. (E) The diopter is the unit of accommodative amplitude, divergence of a wavefront, vergence at a specific distance from the source, as well as the power of a lens. (ref. p.4)

1-9. (C) The radius of curvature is measured with a radiuscope.

1-10. (D)

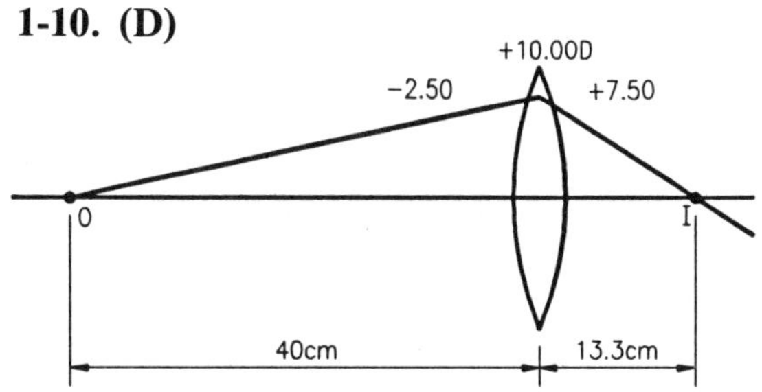

(i) Object vergence: $U = \frac{1}{\mu} = \frac{100}{-40} = -2.50\text{ D}$

(ii) Image vergence: $U + D = V$

$$-2.50\text{ D} + 10.00\text{ D} = V$$
$$+7.50\text{ D} = V$$

(iii) Image distance: $v = \frac{1}{V} = \frac{1}{7.50\text{ D}} = 13.3$ cm to the right of the lens. (ref. p.4-5)

1-11. (B)

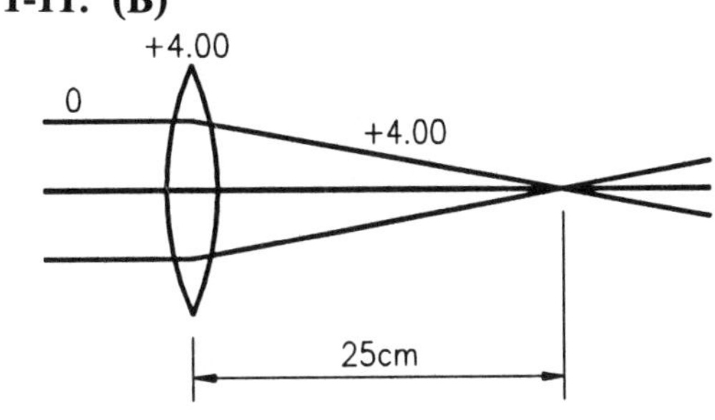

(i) Image vergence: $U + D = V$

$$0 + 4.00\text{ D} = V$$
$$+4.00\text{ D} = V$$

(ii) Image distance: $v = \frac{1}{V} = \frac{1}{+4.00\text{ D}} = 25\text{ cm}$

The image is 25 cm to the right of the lens. (ref. p.4-5)

1-12. (D)

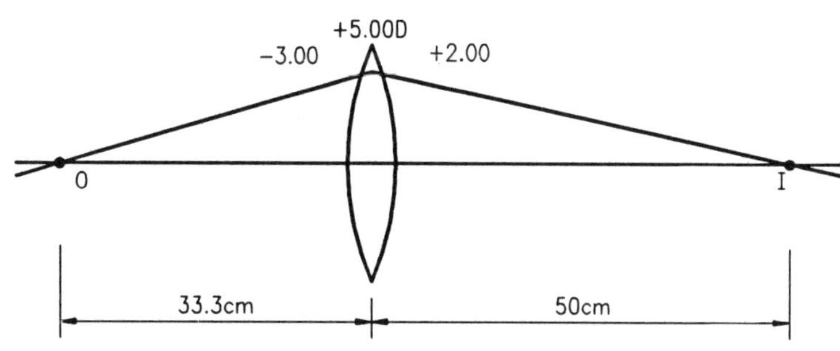

(i) Object vergence: $\frac{-100}{33\text{ cm}} = -3.00\text{ D}$

(ii) Image vergence: $U + D = V$; $-3.00\text{ D} + 5.00\text{ D} = +2.00\text{ D}$

(iii) Image distance: $v = \frac{1}{V} = \frac{1}{+2.00\text{ D}} = 50\text{ cm}$ to the right of the lens

The image is real and erect. (ref. p.4-5)

1-13. (E) An optically active surface can alter vergence by reflection, refraction, diffraction, and convergence. (ref. p.5)

1-14. (D) This simple relationship is true for any interface between two media with a smooth refracting or reflecting surface such as a mirror or lens. (ref. p.5)

1-15. (A) A plus lens always adds vergence, defines a focal point to which image rays are convergent, and produces a real image to the right of the plus lens. (ref. p.5)

1-16. (C) A minus lens always reduces vergence, defines a focal point, and diverges all rays at this point to produce a virtual image to the left of the minus lens. (ref. p.5)

1-17. (B) Spherical lenses have the same power in all meridians (ref. p.5)

1-18. (D) Focal length:

$$U + D = V$$

$$\frac{100}{60} + D = \frac{100}{25}$$

$$D = 4 + \frac{5}{3} = \frac{17}{3}$$

$$\frac{1}{f} = \frac{17}{3},$$

therefore $f = \frac{3}{17}$ m to the right of the lens. (ref. p.5)

1-19. (E) When a ray of light encounters a more dense medium, the frequency remains constant. We know that the speed is reduced compared to that inside a vacuum and thus the wavelength must be reduced to maintain $c = \lambda \times v$. Vergence is inversely related to wavelength and is thus increased. The light ray may emerge with the same frequency, wavelength or be reflected or refracted. (ref. p.6)

1-20. (E) $v = \frac{c}{\lambda} = \frac{3.00 \times 10^8 \frac{\text{m}}{\text{s}}}{589 \times 10^{-9}\text{ m}} = 5.09 \times 10^{14}\text{ Hz}$ (ref. p.6)

1-21. (B) $\lambda_M = \frac{\lambda}{1.24} = \frac{460\text{ nm}}{1.24} = 371\text{ nm}$ (ref. p.6)

1-22. (D) The power of light in a different medium may be called the reduced vergence, the corrected vergence, or the normalized vergence. (ref. p.6,7)

1-23. (C) Refraction is the bending of light between media and is a function of the incident angle. This is based on Snell's law. It is not dependent on speed. (ref. p.7)

1-24. (D) Snell's law is a relationship between the incident and refracted angles of a light ray. It has no bearing on the laws of reflection. (ref. p.7)

1-25. (B) As light travels from a less dense to a more dense medium, it is refracted toward the normal. If it travels from a more dense to a less dense medium, it is refracted away from the normal. (ref. p.7)

1-26. (D) Light perpendicular to the interface between two media and emerging from the more dense medium is transmitted at higher speed but not subject to refraction. (ref. p.7)

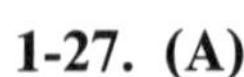

1-27. (A)

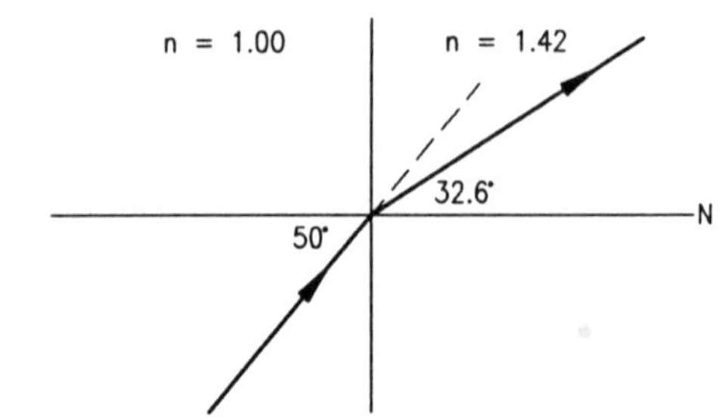

$n \sin i_i = n' \sin i_r$
$1.0 \sin 50° = 1.42 \sin \theta$
$\theta = 32.6°$ from the normal
NOTE: When light travels from a less to a more dense medium, the ray is refracted toward the normal. (ref. p.7)

1-28. (D)

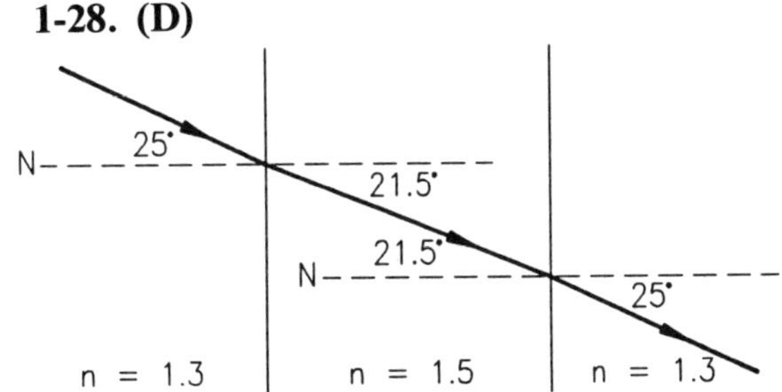

Use $n \sin i_i = n' \sin i_r$
(i) $1.3 \sin 25° = 1.5 \sin \theta$
$\theta = 21.5°$ from the normal
(ii) $1.5 \sin 21.5° = 1.3 \sin \varphi$
$\varphi = 25°$ from the normal
NOTE: Light is displaced but not deviated when it passes through another medium to reemerge in the medium. (ref. p.7)

1-29. (E)

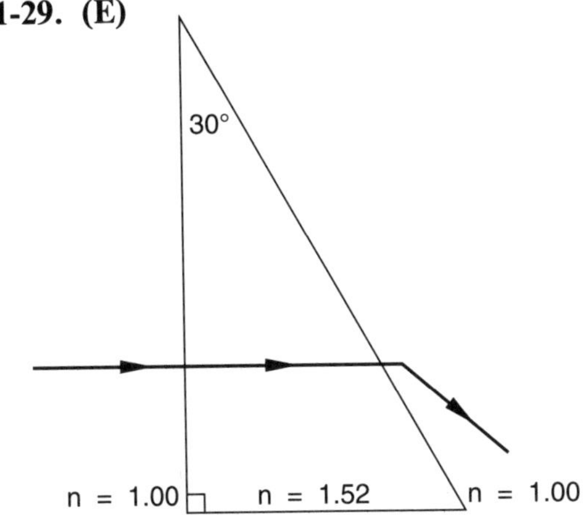

Refraction occurs at the second interface only. There is no deviation at the first interface.

1-30. (D) Reflection of some or all of the incident light occurs whenever light travels between media or the angle is greater than the critical angle. (ref. p.8)

1-31. (E) The critical angle of a surface can be altered by increasing the radius of curvature, altering the vergence or implementing contact lenses. (ref. p.8)

1-32. (C) The critical angle is the basis of fiberoptics, gonioscopy, reflecting prisms, and Goldmann lens fundoscopy. It is not relevant to retinoscopy. (ref. p.8)

1-33. (A) $\sin i_c = \frac{n'}{n} \times \sin 90°$

$$\sin i_c = \frac{1.333}{1.490} \times \sin 90°$$

$i_c = 63.2°$

Any light incident at an angle of greater than 63.2° is reflected. (ref. p.8)

1-34. (A) Reflection traps light in the incident medium. (ref. p.9)

1-35. (D) A plus (concave) mirror would add positive vergence and a minus (convex) mirror would add minus vergence. (ref. p.9)

1-36. (A) The focal length of a mirror is equal to half of the radius of curvature. If the mirror is convergent or plus, the focal point is to the left of the mirror. Similarly, if the focal point is to the right of the mirror, the mirror is divergent or minus. (ref. p.10)

1-37. (E) A single smooth refracting surface affects the velocity of the transmitted light. With reflection there is no change in medium and no change in velocity. (ref. p.10)

1-38. (C)

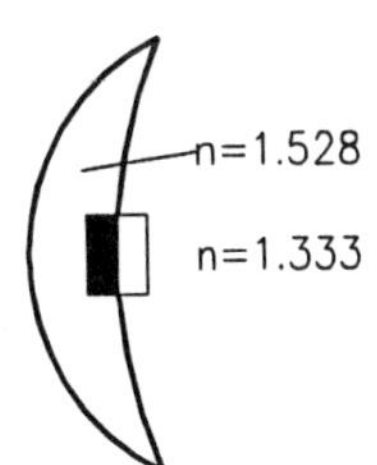

$$D_{IOL} = \frac{n_{IOL} - n_{aq}}{r}$$

$$D_s = \frac{1.528 - 1.333}{-0.015} = -13.00\text{D}$$ (ref. p.10)

1-39. (C)

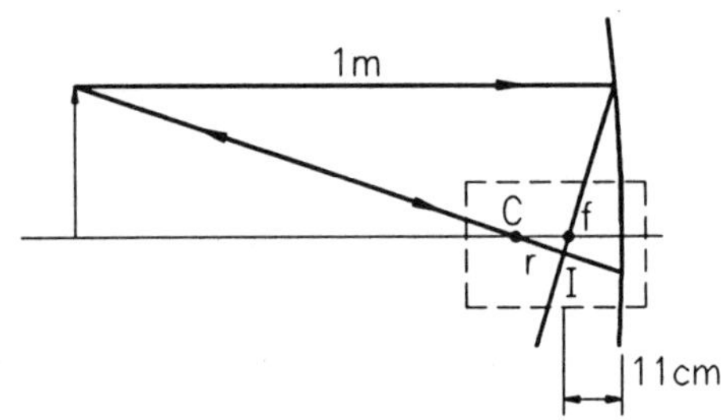

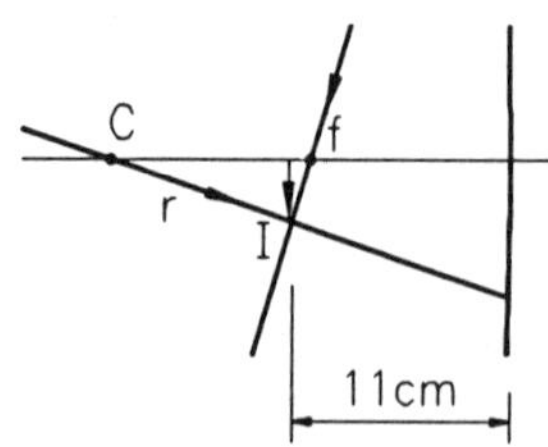

(i) The power of the mirror: $f = \frac{r_m}{2} = \frac{0.2}{2} = 0.10$ m

$$D_m = \frac{1}{f} = \frac{1}{0.10} = +10.00\text{ D}$$

(ii) Image location and nature:

$U + D_m = V$

$-1 + 10.00\text{ D} = V$

$+9.00\text{ D} = V;$

$v = \frac{1}{9} = 11$ cm to the left of the mirror.

(iii) Minification $= \frac{U}{V} = \frac{1}{9}$

The image is real, minified, and inverted. (ref. p.10)

1-40. (D)

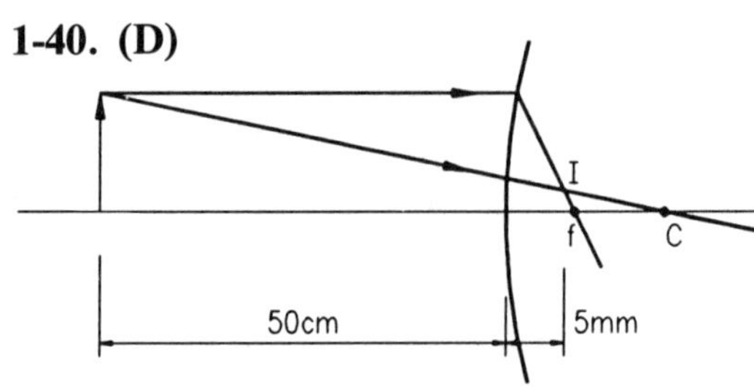

(i) Reflecting power of the cornea: $D_m = \frac{2}{r_m} = \frac{2}{-0.01} = -200.00\text{ D}$

(ii) $U + D = V$

$-2 + (-200) = V$

$V = -202, \frac{1}{v} = -202,$

$v = 4.95$ mm

(iii) $M = \frac{U}{V} = \frac{v}{\mu} = \frac{0.5}{50} = 0.01 \times$

(ref. p.10)

1-41. (A) Ray trace is similar to 1-40.

(i) $U + D = V$

$$-2 - 200 = V;\ v = \frac{1}{V} = \frac{1}{-202} = 0.495\text{ cm} = 4.95\text{ mm}$$

The image coming from the anterior corneal surface is virtual, minified, and erect at 4.95 mm from the cornea. (ref. p.10)

1-42. (E) $U + \frac{2}{r_m} = V$

$$\frac{-100}{40} + \frac{2}{r_m} = \frac{100}{20};$$

$$-2.5 + \frac{2}{r_m} = 5;$$

$$\frac{2}{r_m} = 7.5$$

$r_m = \frac{2}{7.5} = 0.267$ m to the left of the mirror. (ref. p.10)

1-43. (B)

n=1.00

n=1.50

$$D_s = \frac{n' - n}{r} = \frac{0.50}{0.2} = +2.50\text{ D}$$

NOTE: The refracting power is +2.50 D. The sign is determined by the convexity or concavity on the side of the medium with the higher index of refraction. (ref. p.10)

1-44. (A)

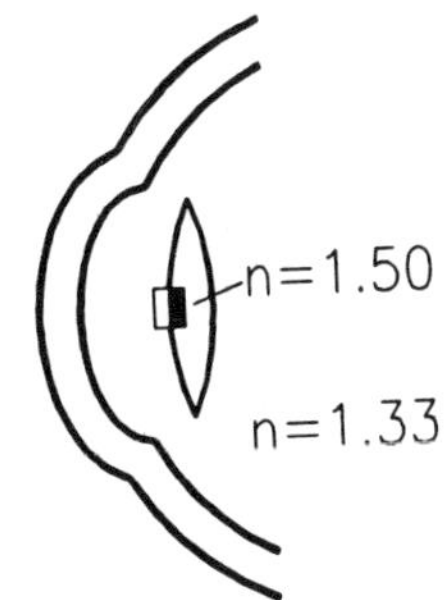

$$nU + \left(\frac{n' - n}{r}\right) = n'\,V \text{ (ref. p.10)}$$

$$1.33 \times \left(\frac{100}{-40}\right) + \left(\frac{1.50 - 1.33}{0.01}\right) = 1.50\,V$$

$$-3.325 + 17 = 1.5\,V$$

$$V = \frac{13.675}{1.5} = +9.12$$

1-45. (C) The vergence formulae can determine the incoming and outgoing vergences as well as the minification, magnification, and power of a lens. They cannot predict the nature of the image. (ref. p.11)

1-46. (A) When defining an optical system, it is conventional to set the incoming rays as object rays, the outgoing rays as image rays, and the light traveling from left to right. (ref. p.11)

1-47. (D)

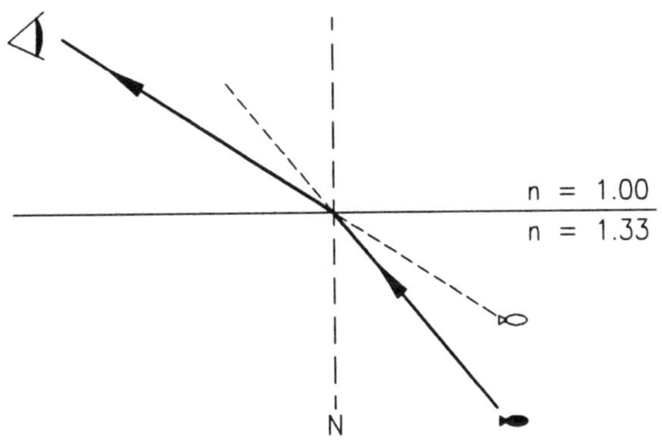

A fisherman looking into the water should spear behind and below the fish. Light from the fish is passing from a more dense to a less dense medium and will be refracted away from the normal. The fisherman therefore sees the virtual image in front of and above the actual fish. (ref. p.12)

1-48. (A)

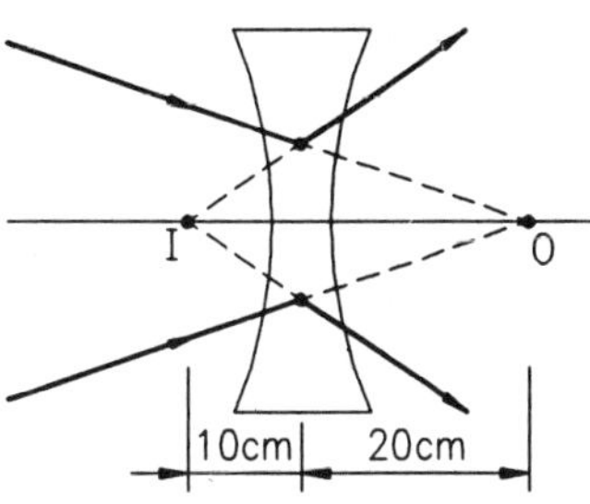

If an object is placed 20 cm behind a concave lens of −15.00 D, the object and image will be virtual and have the following characteristics: (ref. p.12)

(i) Image vergence:

$$U + D = V;$$

$$\frac{+100}{20\text{ cm}} - 15.00\text{ D} = V;$$

$$V = -10.00\text{ D}$$

(ii) Image distance: $v = \frac{1}{V}$; $v = \frac{100}{-10.00\text{ D}} = 10$ cm in front of the lens

1-49. (A)

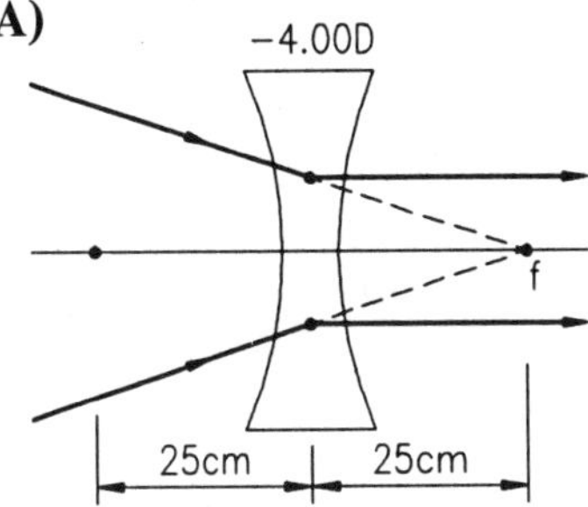

$U + D = V$, where $V = 0$ by definition for a primary focal point

$$+4.00\text{ D} + D = 0;$$

$$D = -4.00\text{ D}$$

$$D = \frac{1}{f}\,f = \frac{1}{D} = \frac{1}{-4} = 25$$

cm behind the lens (ref. p.14)

1-50. (A) In the case of a plane mirror, the image is virtual and lies to the right of the mirror. The magnification is 1 ×. Image and object vergences are equal and the power is zero. (ref. p.16)

1-51. (E) $U = V = +5.00$ D

$$v = \frac{1}{V} = \frac{1}{+5.00} =$$

0.2 m = 20 cm (ref. p.16)

1-52. (C) Magnification:

$$\frac{D}{4} = 2;\ D = +8.00 \text{ D}$$

$$D_s = \frac{n' - n}{r};\ r = \frac{n' - n}{D}$$

$$r = \frac{1.49 - 1}{+8.00} = \frac{0.49}{8.00} =$$

0.0612 m = 6.12 cm (ref. p.16)

1-53. (B) An observer standing directly in front of a plane mirror perceives the magnification differently.

(i) True magnification: $\frac{\mu}{v} = \frac{1.5}{1.5}$ $= 1 \times$

(ii) Perceived magnification:

$$\frac{\mu}{\mu + v} = \frac{1.5}{1.5 + 1.5} = \frac{1.5}{3.0} =$$

$0.5 \times$

(iii) The difference between the two magnifications is a factor of two. (ref. p.16)

1-54. (C) The field of view of a plane mirror is twice the size of the mirror. (ref. p.17)

1-55. (C) Linear magnification (also called lateral magnification) is equal to the image size over the object size. (ref. p.17)

1-56. (C)

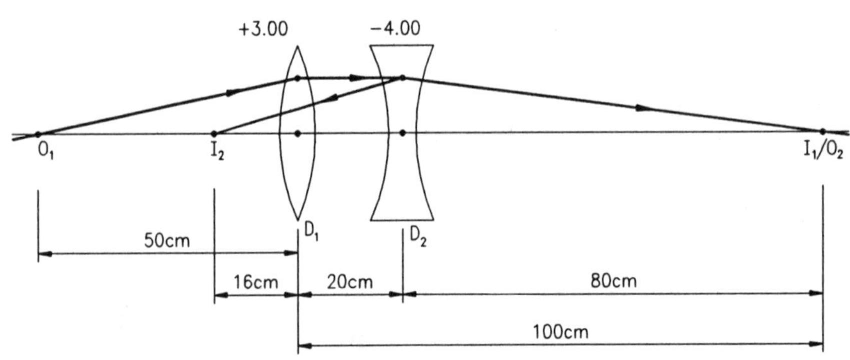

(i) $U_1 + D_1 = V_1$

$$\frac{-100}{50} + 3.00 = \frac{1}{v};$$

$v = +100$ cm behind D_1

(ii) $U_2 + D_2 = V_2$

$$\frac{+100}{80} - 4.00 \text{ D} = V_2;$$

$V_2 = -2.75$ D

$$v_2 = \frac{1}{V_2} = \frac{100}{2.75 \text{ D}} = 36 \text{ cm to}$$

the left of D_2 or 16 cm in front of D_1 (ref. p.17)

1-57. (B)

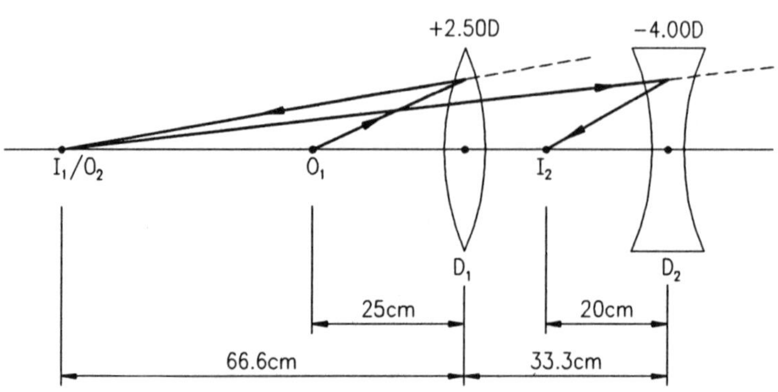

Continued.

1-58. cont'd.

(i) $U_1 + D_1 = V_1$

$$\frac{-1}{0.25} + 2.50 = \frac{1}{v};$$

$$v = -\frac{2}{3} \text{ m in front of } D_1$$

(ii) $U_2 + D_2 = V_2$

$$-1.00 - 4.00 = \frac{1}{v_2} = -0.20$$

m = 20 cm in front of D_2 (ref. p.17)

1-58. (C)

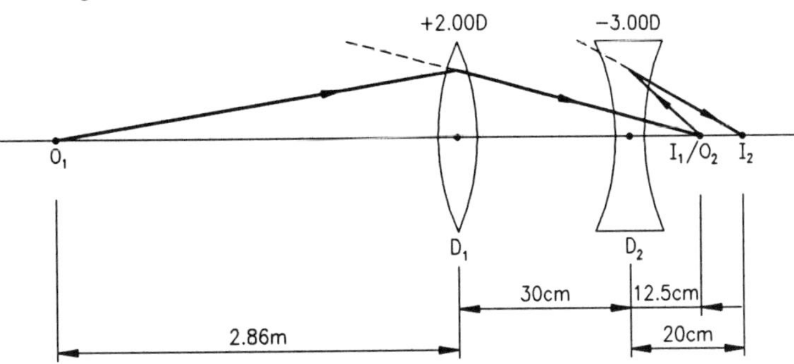

(i) $U_2 + D_2 = V_2; \frac{100}{\mu_2} - 3.00 =$

$$\frac{100}{20}; \frac{100}{\mu_2} = 5 + 3$$

$$\mu_2 = \frac{100}{8} = 12.5 \text{ cm to the}$$

right of D_2

(ii) $U_1 + D_1 = V_1$ where $O_2 = I_1$

$$\frac{1}{\mu_1} + 2.00 = \frac{1}{\mu_1}; \frac{100}{\mu_1} + 2.00$$

$$= \frac{100}{+30 + 12.5}$$

$$\frac{100}{\mu_1} = \frac{100}{42.5} - 2.00 = +2.35$$

$$- 2.00 = 0.35$$

$$\mu_1 = 100 \div 0.35 = 285.7 \text{ cm}$$

= 2.86 m in front of D_1 (ref. p.17)

1-59. (D) The calculations for a multilens system can be simplified by reducing the system to a single theoretical thick lens, or using an optical bench to form two principal planes with two focal points. Depicting the system with ray diagrams is also helpful. (ref. p.18)

1-60. (A) The back vertex power or posterior vertex power is derived with the anterior lens surface facing the examiner and is the measurement taken from the back surface of the lens. (ref. p.18)

1-61. (E) The power of correcting spectacles varies with the index of refraction of the lens material, the vertex distance, the optical center position relative to the visual axes, and the front and back radii of curvature. (ref. p.19)

1-62. (D) The mnemonic CAP stands for "closer add plus" and is used when prescribing correcting spectacles, contact lenses, or implants. (ref. p.19)

1-63. (A) The effective power of an IOL is directly proportional to the differences in refractive indices. (ref. p.19)

1-64. (D)

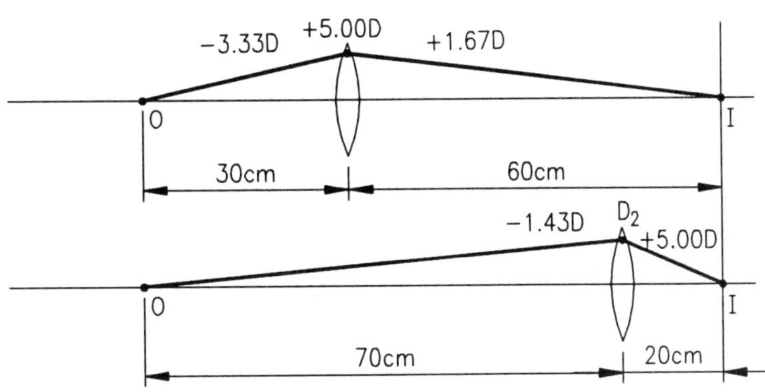

$$\frac{1}{\mu_1} + D_I = \frac{1}{v_I}$$
$$\frac{-1}{0.3} + 5.00 = \frac{1}{v_I};$$
$$v_I = 0.6 \text{ m} = 60 \text{ cm}$$
$$\frac{-100}{70} + D_2 = \frac{100}{20}$$
$$D_2 = 5 + 1.43 = +6.43 \text{ D}$$ (ref. p.19)

1-65. (A) $D_{AIR} = \frac{D_{AIR}}{D_{AQ}} \times D_{AQ}$

$$D_{AIR} = \frac{n_{IOL} - n_{AIR}}{n_{IOL} - n_{AQ}} \times (+12.50 \text{ D})$$
$$D_{AIR} = \frac{1.5 - 1.0}{1.5 - 1.33} \times (+12.50 \text{ D}) = +36.76 \text{ D}$$
(ref. p.20)

1-66. (C)

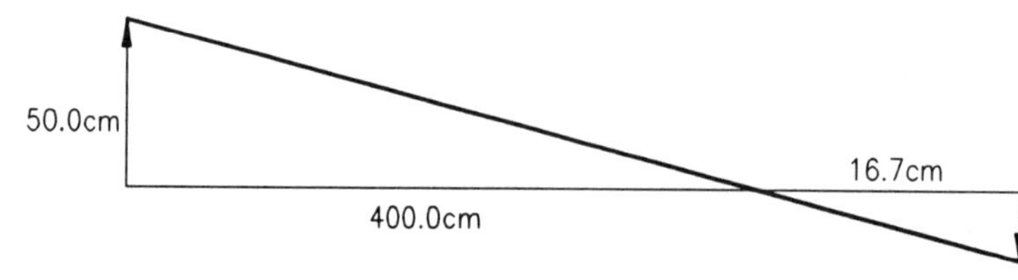

$$D_S = \frac{n' - n}{r}; 60 = \frac{\frac{4}{3} - 1}{r};$$
$$r = 5.55 \text{ cm}$$
$$D = \frac{1}{f}; f = \frac{1}{60}; f = 16.67 \text{ cm}$$
$$\frac{I}{50} = \frac{16.67}{400}; I = 2.08 \text{ cm}$$
(ref. p.20)

CHAPTER 2: LENS ABERRATIONS

2-1. (D) The important lens aberrations for thick lenses do not include diffraction. (ref. p.23)

2-2. (A) A blur interval occurs along the axis when rays approach the periphery of a lens and are subject to an increased prismatic effect and power. (ref. p.21)

2-3. (A) Aspheric surfaces best improve spherical aberrations of high powered spectacle-corrected hyperopia. (ref. p.21)

2-4. (C) Three naturally occurring phenomena which reduce spherical aberration of an eye are the size of the pupil, the radius of curvature of the peripheral cornea, and the index of refraction of the crystalline lens. (ref. p.21)

2-5. (C) Coma relates to off-axis peripheral rays causing distortion to visual imagery. (ref. p.22)

2-6. (E) Astigmatism of oblique incidence results in image distortion, astigmatic imagery, blur circles on the retina, and an astigmatic interval in which the image is blurred. (ref. p.22)

2-7. (C) The only advantageous aberration of the human eye is curvature of field. This causes a curved rather than flat image. (ref. p.22)

2-8. (B) Yellow light is the standard wavelength for calibration. It holds midposition in the chromatic interval of the emmetropic eye and is thus is best focus. (ref. p.23)

2-9. (E) A variety of lens aberrations not included in the ABCs are also associated with thick lenses. These include visual field scotoma, magnification and minification, and aberrant depth perception. (ref. p.23)

CHAPTER 3: PRISMS

3-1. (B) A plane parallel plate will displace a light ray from its initial path but it will not deviate it. (ref. p. 24)

3-2. (D) 1 P.D. is the apparent displacement of a ray 1 cm at 1 m. (ref. p.24)

3-3. (C)

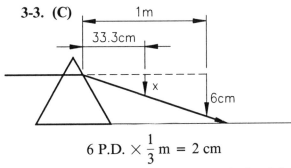

$$6 \text{ P.D.} \times \frac{1}{3} \text{ m} = 2 \text{ cm}$$

of displacement (ref. p.24)

3-4. (B) The base of the prism is clinically used to describe the orientation of the prism power. (ref. p.24)

3-5. (C) A single representative prism corresponding to two prisms presented simultaneously is achieved through vector addition. (ref. p.24)

3-6. (A)

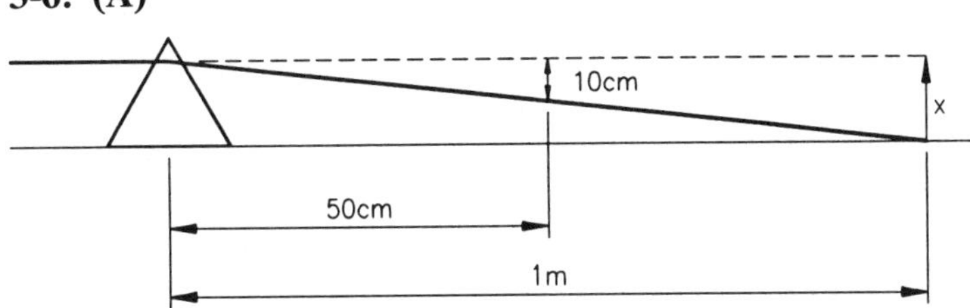

$$\frac{10 \text{ cm}}{50 \text{ cm}} = \frac{x \text{ cm}}{100 \text{ cm}};\ x = 20 \text{ cm}$$

Therefore $P = 20$ P.D. (ref. p.24)

3-7. (D)

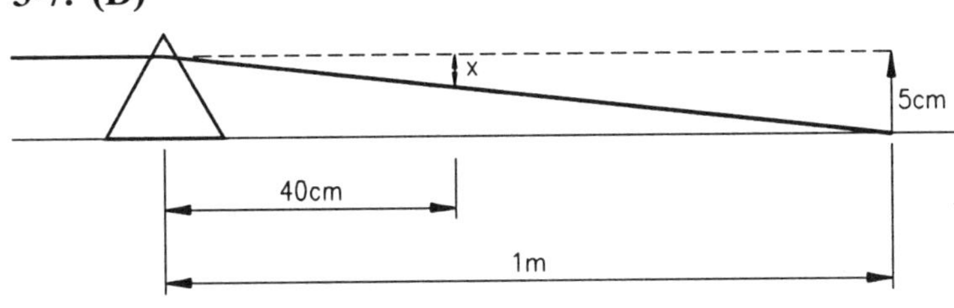

$$\frac{5 \text{ cm}}{100 \text{ cm}} = \frac{x \text{ cm}}{40 \text{ cm}};\ x = 2 \text{ cm}.$$

(ref. p.24)

3-8. (C)

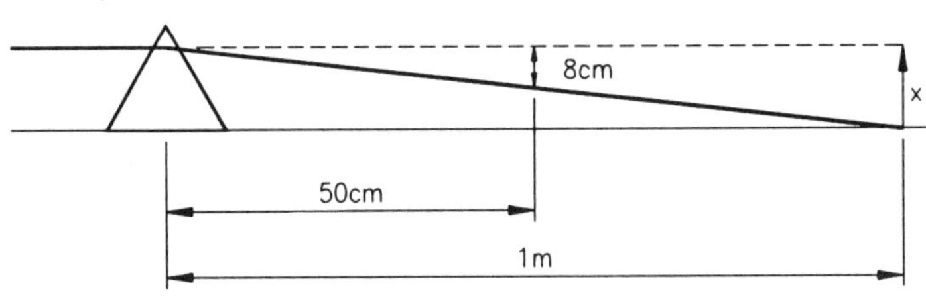

$$\frac{x \text{ cm}}{100 \text{ cm}} = \frac{8 \text{ cm}}{50 \text{ cm}};\ x = 16 \text{ cm}$$

at 1 m

Therefore $P = 16$ P.D. (ref. p.24)

3-9. (D) R

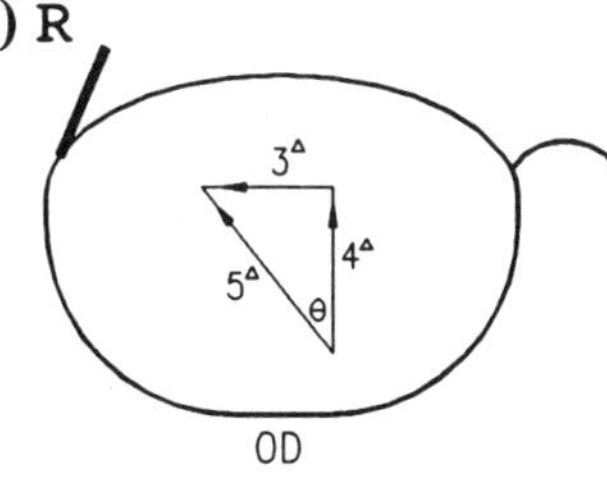

Use Pythagorean theorem to add vectorally:

$R^2 = 4^2 + 3^2 = 25;\ R = 5$ P.D.

Calculate the direction of the vector:

$$\tan\theta = \frac{3}{4};\ \theta = 37°$$

The resultant prism in the right eye is 5 P.D. BO and BU at an angle of 37° with the vertical. (ref. p.24)

3-10. (E) The stenopeic slit is not used to determine the angle at which the combined prism should be placed. (ref. p.25)

3-11. (A) The minimum angle of deviation is achieved at an inclination where equal deviation occurs at both surfaces. (ref. p.25)

3-12. (D) Plastic prisms are calibrated in the position of minimum deviation. (ref. p.25)

3-13. (E) When eye deviations are measured with plastic prisms, the prism should be held in the frontal plane. (ref. p.25)

3-14. (C) A plastic prism should be parallel with the patient's forehead if the measurement is to correspond with the calibration. (ref. p.25)

3-15. (B) Glass prisms are calibrated in the Prentice position. (ref. p.25)

3-16. (D) If the measured deviation is to correspond to the calibrated value for glass prisms, the back or front surface of the prism must be perpendicular to the visual axis. (ref. p.25)

3-17. (D) Prisms can be added to each eye separately. (ref. p.25)

3-18. (A) Radians and degrees are sometimes interchanged with prism diopters. (ref. p.25)

3-19. (B) The angles expressed in prism diopters increase much slower than the corresponding tangents do. (ref. p.26)

3-20. (B) For small angles, the angle of deviation is approximately related to the prism diopter such that 1° ≡ 2 P.D. (ref. p.26)

3-21. (E)

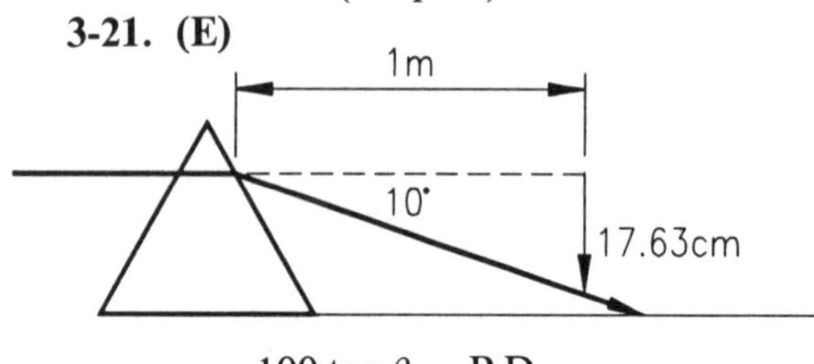

$100 \tan \beta = $ P.D.

$100 \tan 10° = 17.63$ P.D. (ref. p.26)

3-22. (E) The power of a prism to be ground can be verified by means of the apex angle, the lensmeter measurement, the base width, and the prismatic effect of decentration. (ref. p.27)

3-23. (C) When the emergent ray is deviated from the incident ray by 90°, the prism has infinite prism power. (ref. p.27)

3-24. (A) When looking through a prism, the image of a virtual object is virtual and displaced toward its apex. (ref. p.27)

3-25. (B)

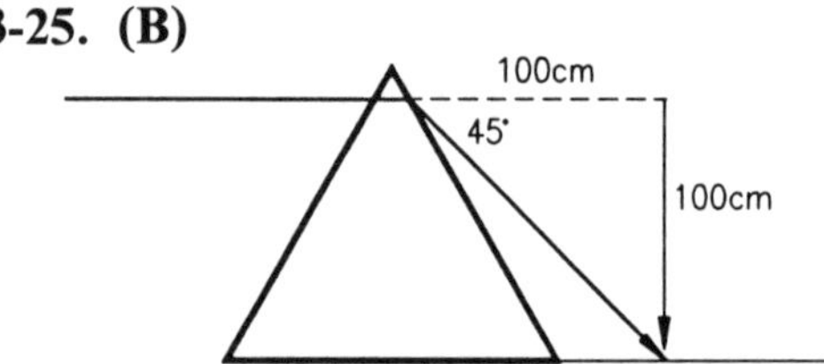

(i) By inspection we can see that the displacement forms an isosceles triangle. The other two angles must be equal, add up to 90°, and therefore are 45° each.

(ii) Approximation formula: 1° ≡ 2 P.D.

Therefore, 45° ≡ 90 P.D. is the approximation

(iii) True value: $\dfrac{100 \text{ cm}}{1 \text{ m}} = 100$

P.D. Error = 10%

The approximation formula yields a less than 10% error for values under 45°. (ref. p.27)

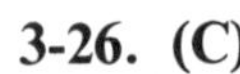

3-26. (C)

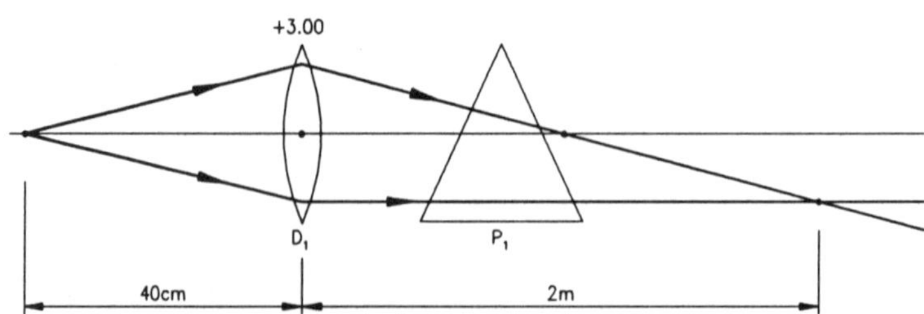

(i) $U + D = V$

$$\frac{-100}{40} + 3.00 \text{ D} = \frac{1}{v};\ v = 2 \text{ m}.$$

The real image is behind the lens.

(ii) Since real images are displaced toward the base of the prism, the image will be displaced downward. (ref. p.27)

3-27. (A) When looking through a prism, both the patient and the examiner see the eye displaced toward the apex. (ref. p.28)

3-28. (C) Heterophoria or heterotropia is a latent or manifest deviation of the eye, respectively. (ref. p.28)

3-29. (E) Esotropia is an eye deviation toward the nose. Exotropia is toward thc temples. Hypertropia is a vertical deviation up, and hypotropia is a vertical deviation down. (ref. p.28)

3-30. (C) If a 30 P.D. BO prism is placed in front of an esotropic eye, objects are focused on or toward the fovea of the deviated eye. (ref. p.28)

3-31. (D) Correcting prism should be placed so the apex points in the direction of deviation. (ref. p.28)

3-32. (A) When prism glasses are placed in front of straight eyes, the induced deviation is pointed out by the direction of the apex of the prism required to correct them. (ref. p.28)

3-33. (B) The prismatic effect of lenses describes lenses as prisms of progressively increasing prismatic power outward from the optical center. (ref. p.28)

3-34. (D) A plus lens can be thought of as an upper BD and lower BU prism. (ref. p.28)

3-35. (D) To calculate the induced prism, we need to know the interpupillary distance of the patient, the distance between optical centers of the glasses, and the power of the lenses. (ref. p.29)

3-36. (B) The induced prismatic effect at the reading position (1 cm down and 0.2 cm in) if one wears a +5.00 D lens over both eyes equals 1 P.D. BO in the right eye. (ref. p.29)

OD p P.D. = (1.0)(+5.00) = 5.00 P.D. *BU OD*
OS p P.D. = (1.0)(+5.00) = 5.00 P.D. *BU OS* = 5.00 P.D. *BD OD*
Net vertical effect: 5.00 P.D. − 5.00 P.D. = 0

(ii) Horizontal effect:
OD p P.D. = (0.2)(+5.00) = 1.00 P.D. *BO OD*
OS p P.D. = (0.2)(+5.00) = 1.00 P.D. *BO OS* = 1.00 P.D. *BO OD*
Net horizontal effect: 1.00 P.D. + 1.00 P.D. = 2.00 P.D. *BO OD*

3-37. (C) *OD p* P.D. = *Dh* = (+5.00) (0.8) = 4.00 P.D. *BU*
OS p P.D. = *Dh* = (+2.00) (0.8) = 1.60 P.D. *BU*
4.00 P.D.*BU OD* = 4.00 P.D. *BD OS*
Net effect = 4.00 P.D. − 1.60 P.D. = 2.40 P.D. *BD OS*
This requires 2.4 P.D. *BU OS* to correct it. This is an induced 2.4 P.D. left hypophoria or 2.4 P.D. right hyperphoria. (ref. p.29-30)

3-38. (C)

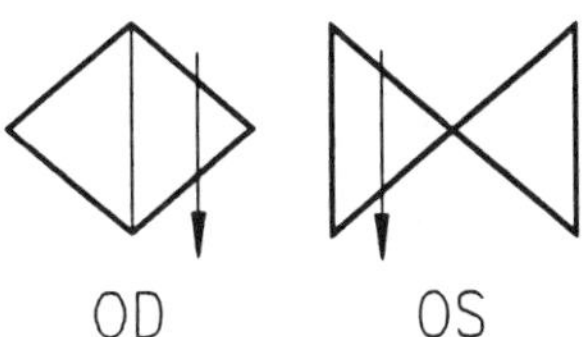

OD: +4.00 + 2.00 × 90 and *OS*: −3.00 D
Horizontal meridian
OD: (+6.00 D) (1.5 cm) = 9.00 P.D. *BO*
OS: (−3.00 D) (1.50 cm) = 4.50 P.D. *BI*
BI OD = *BI OS*
Net effect: 4.50 P.D.*BO OD*
The induced prism may be corrected or neutralized by 4.50 P.D. *BI* apex out. This is an induced exodeviation of 4.5 P.D. (ref. p.29-30)

3-39. (A) (i) Vertical prism:
*OD p*P.D. = *Dh*(cm) = 4 × 0.8 = 3.2 P.D. *BU*
*OS p*P.D. = *Dh*(cm) = 3.2 P.D. *BU*

3.2 P.D. *BU OS* = 3.2 P.D. *BD OD*
Net vertical effect: 3.2 P.D. *BU* + 3.2 P.D. *BD* = 0

(ii) Horizontal prism:
OD *p*P.D. = *Dh*(cm) = 4 × 0.2 = 0.8 P.D. *BO*
OS *p*P.D. = *Dh*(cm) = 0.8 P.D. *BO*
0.8 P.D. *BO OS* = 0.8 P.D. *BO OD*
Net horizontal effect: 0.8 P.D. *BO* + 0.8 P.D. *BO* = 1.6 P.D. *BO* (ref. p.29-30)

3-40. (D) A patient with a right hyperdeviation fixing with the left eye has a left hypodeviation fixing with the right eye except when dealing with a dissociated vertical deviation. (ref. p.30)

3-41. (B) A hyperdeviation in one eye is equivalent to a hypodeviation in the other eye. Similarly, placing a *BU* prism over the right eye is equivalent to placing a BD prism over the left eye. (ref. p.30)

3-42. (A) A patient that requires any prism to correct a deviation requires only the amount of prism to achieve and maintain binocular vision. Under monocular conditions no prism is clearer than some prism. (ref. p.30)

3-43. (E) An anisometropic patient with an induced hypodeviation can be treated with single vision readers, ground-in prism in the appropriate amount, lens decentration, or by lens slab-off to the more minus or less plus lens. (ref. p.30)

3-44. (B) A right hyperdeviation in a straight-eyed patient can be corrected with contact lenses, dropping the optical centers of both lenses (which compensates for some of the vertical imbalance between distance and near vision) and by slabbing off some of the more minus lens from the left lens (this takes away BD prism). (ref. p.30)

3-45. (D)

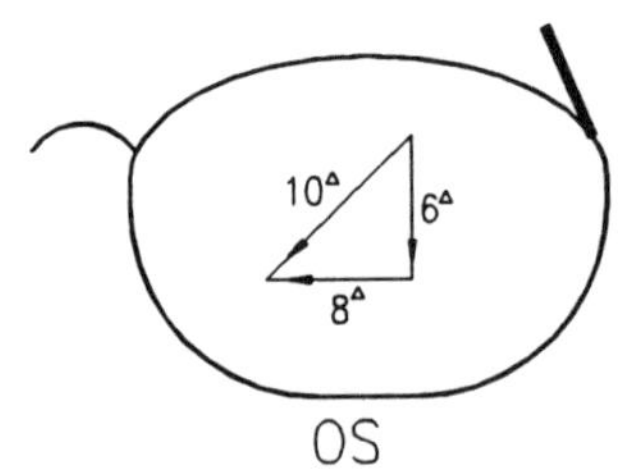

$R^2 = 6^2 + 8^2$
$R = 10$
$\tan\theta = \frac{6}{8}$;
$\theta = 37°$ to the vertical.
Therefore 10 P.D. *BI* and *BD* at 37° to the vertical over the left eye is required. (ref. p.30)

3-46. (D) *OD*: +2.00 + 3.00 × 90 and *OS*: −1.00 D
Vertical meridian:
OD = (+2.00) (1 cm) = 2.00 *BU*
OS = (−1.00) (1 cm) = 1.00 *BD*
Net effect: 3 P.D. *BU OD*
Deviation: 3 P.D. right hyperdeviation or 3 P.D. left hypodeviation (ref. p.30)

3-47. (D) Prescription: *OD*: +4.00; *OS*: +2.00 −1.00 × 180
Vertical meridian:
OD = (+4.00D) (0.5 cm) = 2.0 P.D. *BU*
OS = (+1.00D) (0.5 cm) = 0.50 P.D. *BU* = 0.5 P.D. *BD OD*
Net effect: 1.5 P.D. *BU OD* (ref. p.30)

3-48. (A) **(i)** Vertical meridian:
OD: (+3.00D) (1 cm) = 3 P.D. *BU*
OS: (+3.00D) (1 cm) = 3.00 P.D. *BU* = 3.00 P.D. *BD OD*
Net effect: 0

(ii) Horizontal meridian:
OD: (+3.00D) (0.3 cm) = 0.9 P.D. *BO*
OS: (+3.00D) (0.3 cm) = 0.9 P.D. *BO* = 0.9 P.D. *BO OD*
Net effect: 1.80 P.D. *BO*
The add has no effect because the power, style, and height

are the same in both eyes. (ref. p.30)

3-49. (A)

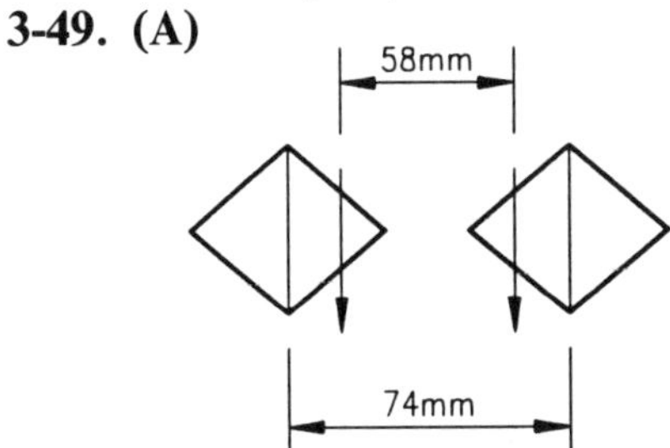

If the pupillary distance is 58 mm and the optical centers are 74 mm apart, the lenses are decentered by 8 mm. (ref. p.30-2)

$$\frac{\textit{Optical center} - \textit{Pupillary distance}}{2} =$$

$$\frac{74 - 58}{2} = 8 \text{ mm}$$

3-50. (B) If one has an esodeviation or an exodeviation, the direction of the correcting prism for the deviation is the same no matter which eye is turned. (ref. p.31)

3-51. (E) When an exodeviation is present, no blur interval exists. *BO* prism does not neutralize an exodeviation. Vertical fusional amplitude has no effect on a horizontal deviation. If horizontal fusional amplitudes are sufficient, no prism is necessary for correction. (ref. p.31)

3-52. (E) Most people have more horizontal than vertical fusional amplitude. The induced deviation is in the direction of the apex of the correcting prism. The magnitude of the net vertical deviation is the difference of the similar vertical prisms. Decentration may be beneficial in some instances where the apex of the induced prism points in the direction of the deviation present. (ref. p.31)

3-53. (D) The maximum power of a cylinder is in the meridian 90° to its axis. (ref. p.31)

3-54. (A) The $+2.00 \times 180$ cylinder has its maximum power at 90°. (ref. p.31)

3-55. (D) *OD* *p*P.D. = (3.00) (0.2) = 0.6 P.D. *BO*
OS *p*P.D. = (4.00) (0.2) = 0.8 P.D. *BO*
Net effect:
0.8 P.D. *BO* + 0.6 P.D. *BO*
= 1.4 P.D. *BO OD* (ref. p.31)

3-56. (B) One can ignore the power of the add for induced deviations if they are equal, set at the same height, and the same style in both eyes. (ref. p.32)

3-57. (B) If the measuring prism is in the same direction as the induced prismatic effect of the spectacle correction, the amount of measuring prism will be less than the true deviation. (ref. p.32)

3-58. (B)

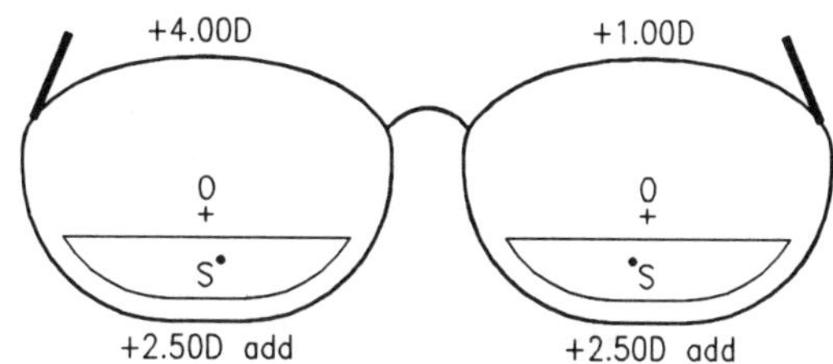

Prescription: *OD*: +4.00 D; *OS*: +1.00 D; add +2.50 *D OU*
Vertical meridian: *OD*: (+4.00 D) (0.8 cm) = 3.2 P.D. *BU*
OS: (+1.00 D) (0.8 cm) = 0.8 P.D. *BU* = 0.8 P.D. *BD OD*
Net effect: 2.4 P.D. *BU OD*
The prism which would correct this deviation is 2.4 P.D. *BD OD*. The add is the same height, power, and style in both eyes, so it is ignored. (ref. p.32)

3-59. (D)

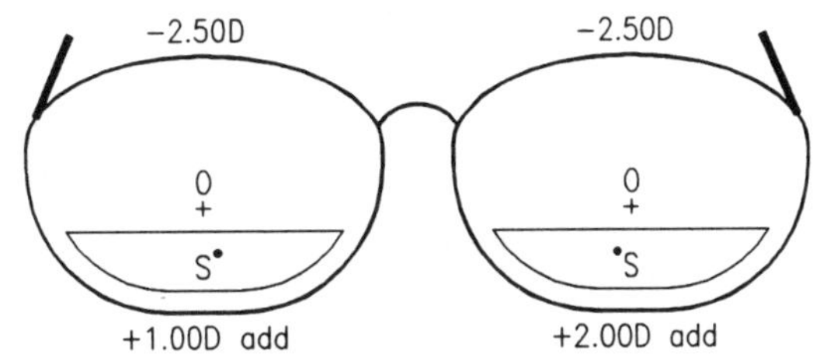

(i) Vertical meridian:
OD: (−2.50 + 1.00)(0.8 cm)
= 1.2 P.D. *BD*

OS: (−2.50 + 2.00)(0.8 cm) = 0.4 P.D. *BD* = 0.4 P.D. *BU OD*
Net vertical effect = 1.2 P.D. −0.4 P.D. = 0.8 P.D. *BD OD*

(ii) Horizontal meridian:
OD: (−2.50 + 1.00)(0.2 cm) = 0.3 P.D. *BI*
OS: (−2.50 + 2.00)(0.2 cm) = 0.1 P.D. *BI* = 0.1 P.D. *BI OD*
Net horizontal effect = 0.3 P.D. + 0.1 P.D = 0.4 P.D. *BI OD* or *OS*

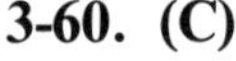

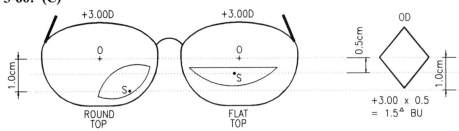

3-60. (C)

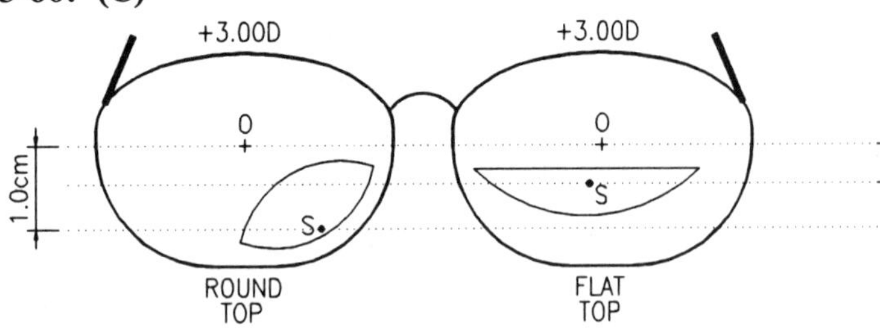

OD
0.5cm
+3.00 x 0.5 = 1.5$^\Delta$ BU
OS
1.0cm
+2.50 x 0.5 = 1.25$^\Delta$ BD
0.5cm

The patient will view through the optical center of the flat top segment 0.5 cm below the distance optical center *OS*. This means there are 2 prism effects to consider *OD*: 0.5 cm down from the distance optical center *OD* and 0.5 cm up from the near optical center.

(i) Vertical meridian
OD: (+3.00)(0.5) = 1.5 P.D. *BU*
(+2.50)(0.5) = 1.25 P.D. *BD*
Net vertical effect *OD*: 0.25 P.D. *BU OD*
OS: (+3.00)(0.5) = 1.5 P.D. *BU* = 1.5 P.D. *BD OD*
Add = 0, since is passes through the optical center of the segment
Net vertical effect: 1.5 P.D. *BD* − 0.25 P.D. *BU* = 1.25 P.D. *BD OD*

(ii) Horizontal meridian:
Ignore the segment and only take into account the decentration.
OD: (+3.00)(0.2) = 0.6 P.D. *BO*
OS: (+3.00)(0.2) = 0.6 P.D. *BO*
Net horizontal effect: 0.6 P.D. + 0.6 P.D. = 1.2 P.D. *BO OD*

3-61. (D)

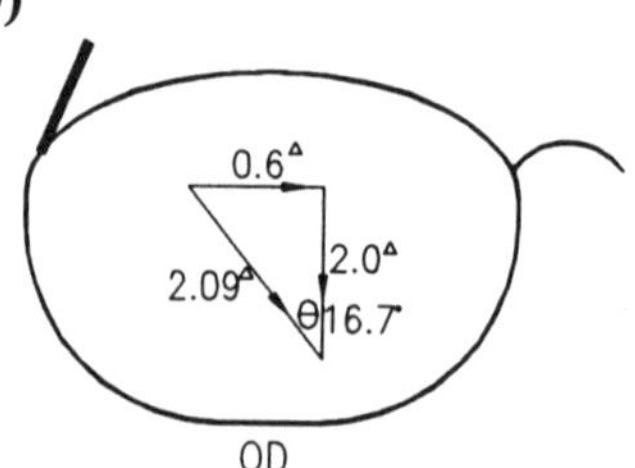

OD: +3.00 + 1.00 × 90;
OS: −2.00 + 1.00 × 180

(i) Vertical effect: *OD*: (+3.00 D)(0.5 cm) = 1.5 P.D. *BU*
OS: (−1.00 D)(0.5 cm) = 0.5 P.D. *BD* = 0.5 P.D. *BU OD*
Net effect: 2.00 P.D. *BU OD*

(ii) Horizontal effect: *OD*: (+4.00 D)(0.3 cm) = 1.20 P.D. *BO*
OS: (−2.00 D)(0.3 cm) = 0.60 P.D. *BI OS* = 0.60 P.D. *BI OD*
Net horizontal effect: 0.60 P.D. *BO*

(iii) Single prism: $R^2 = (2.0)^2 + (0.6)^2$
$R = 2.09$

$$\tan\theta = \frac{0.6}{2};\ \theta = 16.7°$$

The single prism that would correct the above induced prism is 2.09 *BD* and *BI OD* at an angle of 17° to the vertical. (ref. p.32)

3-62. (C)

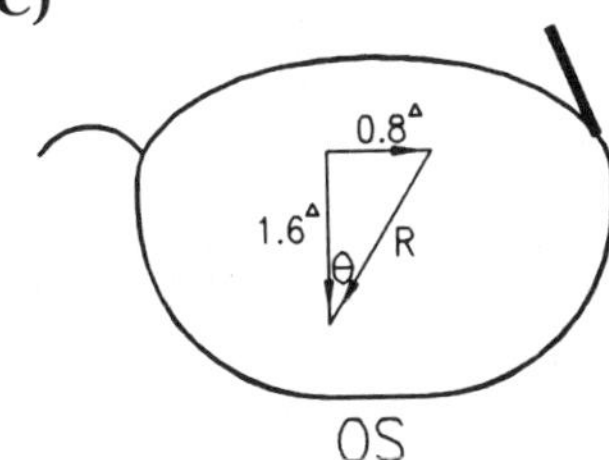

(i) Vertical meridian: *OD*: (+3.00 D)(0.8 cm) = 2.4 P.D. *BU* = 2.4 P.D. *BD OS*
OS: (+1.00 D)(0.8 cm) = 0.8 P.D. *BU*
Net vertical effect = 1.6 P.D. *BD OS*

(ii) Horizontal meridian: *OD*: (+3.00 D)(0.2 cm) = 0.6 P.D. *BO* = 0.6 P.D. *BO OS*
OS: (+1.00 D)(0.2 cm) = 0.2 P.D. *BO*
Net horizontal effect = 0.8 P.D. *BO*

(iii) Single lens: $R^2 = (1.6)^2 + (0.8)^2$
$R = 1.79$
$\tan\theta = \frac{0.8}{1.6}; \theta = 26.6°$
The prism induced at 26.6° is 1.79 P.D. *BD* and *BO* over the left eye. This requires 1.79 P.D. *BU* and *BI* to correct it.

3-63. (E)

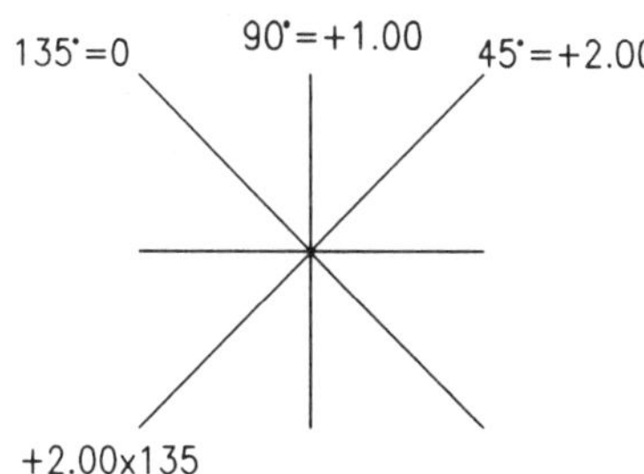

OD = +4.00 + 2.00 × 135 and
OS = +1.00 + 4.00 × 45

(i) Consider *OD* +4.00 + 2.00 × 135:
Consider the cyl +2.00 × 135. Max power is at 45°
At 90° (vertical meridian), it is 45° away
Therefore $\frac{1}{2}$ D; +1.00 × 90
*p*P.D. = (+5.00 D)(0.8 mm) = 4.0 P.D. *BU OD*

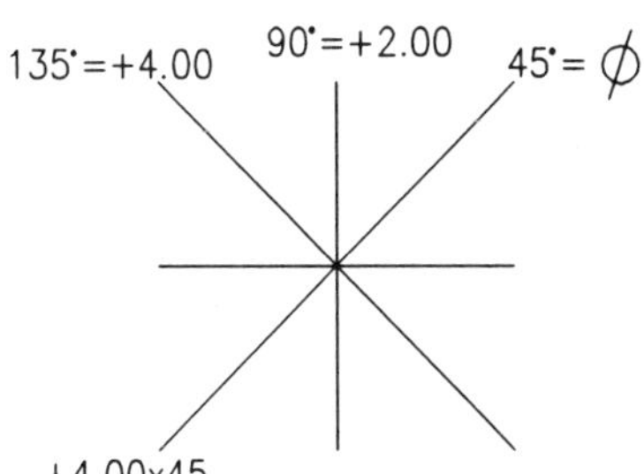

(ii) Consider *OS* +1.00 + 4.00 × 45:
Consider the cyl +4.00 × 45. Max power is at 135
At 90° (vertical meridian), it is 45° away
Therefore $\frac{1}{2}$ D; +2.00 × 90
*p*P.D. = (+3.00 D) × (0.8 mm) = 2.4 P.D. *BU OS*

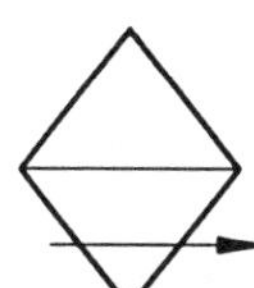

Net vertical effect: 1.6 P.D. *BU OD*
Induced vertical deviation: 1.6 P.D. right hyperdeviation (ref. p.32).

3-64. (B)

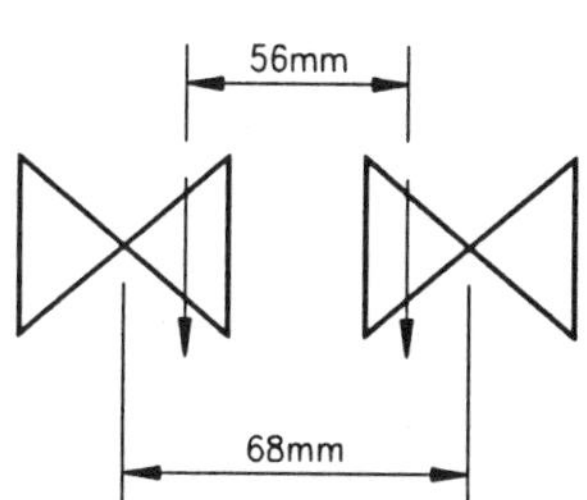

(i) Decentration: $\frac{OD - PD}{2} = \frac{68 - 56}{2} = 6$ mm

(ii) Horizontal meridian:
OD: $(-5.00\text{ D})(0.6\text{ cm}) =$ 3.00 P.D. *BI*
OS: $(-5.00\text{ D})(0.6\text{ cm}) =$ 3.00 P.D. *BI* = 3.00 P.D. *BI OD*
Net effect: 6.00 P.D. *BI* (ref. p.32)

3-65. (A) If the right eye is fixing, the exotropia is equal to 30 P.D. If the left eye is fixing, the exotropia will measure:
Left eye: $2.5 \times 10 = 25\%$ more = 37.5 P.D. (ref. p.32)

3-66. (C) (i) Error: $2.5 \times (-16.00\text{ D}) =$ 40% more (minus measures more)
(ii) True exotropia: $25\text{ P.D.} \times 0.60 = 15\text{ P.D.}$ (ref. p.32).

3-67. (B) (i) The induced error in measurement is:
$(2.50)(+15.00\text{ D}) = 37.5\%$ more esotropia
(ii) The true amount of esotropia is equal to $30 \times 1.375 =$ 41.25 P.D. Minus measures more, so plus measures less than the true value by 37.5% (ref. p.32-3)

3-68. (A) When measuring the primary versus the secondary deviation, the fixing eye becomes the eye without the prism. (ref. p.33)

3-69. (E) Image jump is the sudden shift in the image position when the visual axis descends from the distance optical center to the bifocal segment. (ref. p.33)

3-70. (C) Flat top or executive style bifocals have the least amount of image jump of any bifocal. (ref. p.33)

3-71. (D) Jump and displacement are minimized in a minus lens with a flat top or executive style. (ref. p.33)

3-72. (B) A rotary prism has its maximum power in the base-to-base position. (ref. p.34)

3-73. (C) The Press-On Fresnel Prism is based on the relationship between the apex angle and the power of the prism. (ref. p.35)

3-74. (C) The smaller the prism, the smaller the size of its base and the lighter it is. (ref. p.35)

3-75. (D) One disadvantage of a Fresnel Press-On Prism is chromatic and not spherical aberration. (ref. p.35)

3-76. (D) The Fresnel Press-On Prism can be used to correct static incomitant deviations, nystagmus, visual field defects, as well as other problems. (ref. p.35)

3-77. (D) Prisms of increasing apex angle stacked on top of one another yield an optical system equivalent to a spherical lens. (ref. p.35)

CHAPTER 4: VISUAL IMAGERY

4-1. (C) The human eye can be considered to be a multiple lens system but not a single thin lens. (ref. p.36)

4-2. (A) The anterior air-cornea interface value is 48.80 D. The posterior cornea-aqueous interface value is −5.90 D. The total corneal refractive value is 42.90 D. (ref. p.36)

4-3. (D) The anterior air-cornea interface can act as both a reflecting and a refracting surface. (ref. p.36)

4-4. (E) The cornea is a stronger reflecting than refracting surface. It has a reflecting power of −260.00 D. This is used to advantage in keratometry. (ref. p.36)

4-5. (C) $D_f = \left[\frac{(n' - n)}{(n' + n)}\right]^2 \times 100\%$

$$D_f = \left[\frac{(1.376 - 1.00)}{(1.376 + 1.00)}\right]^2 \times 100\% = 2.5\%$$

The percentage of light that is reflected is 2.5%. (ref. p.36)

4-6. (D)

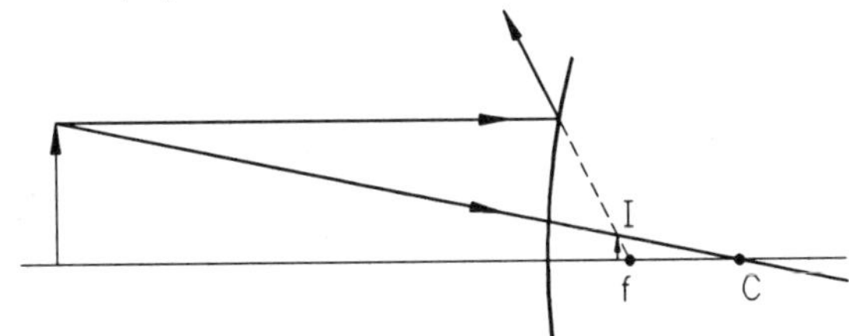

(i) $D_{M_c} = \dfrac{2}{r_m} = \dfrac{2}{-0.0077} =$ -260.00 D

(ii) $f = \dfrac{1}{D} = \dfrac{1}{-260.00\ D} =$ 3.85 mm behind the cornea

As a mirror, the cornea has a power of -260.00 D and a focal point 3.85 mm behind the cornea. (ref. p.36)

4-7. (C) The Purkinje-Sanson images do not include the reflection of the pupil. (ref. p.37)

4-8. (C) The posterior corneal surface and the anterior lens surface are convex mirrors whose images are minified, virtual, and erect. (ref. p.37)

4-9. (A) The posterior lens surface is a concave mirror whose image is real, inverted, and smaller. (ref. p.37)

4-10. (B) The true index of refraction of the lens is 1.42. (ref. p.37)

4-11. (D)

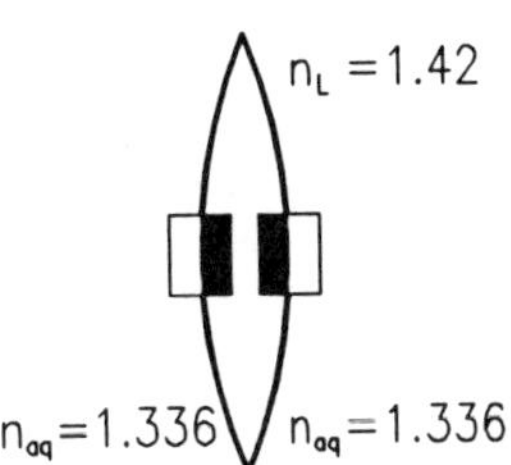

(i) Anterior lens surface:

$$\frac{n_L - n_{aq}}{r_{LA}} = \frac{1.42 - 1.336}{0.0102\ \text{m}} = +8.24\ \text{D}$$

(ii) Posterior lens surface:

$$\frac{n_V - n_L}{r_{LP}} = \frac{1.336 - 1.42}{-0.006\ \text{m}} = +14.00\ \text{D}$$

The total lens surface is equal to $+8.24 + 14.00 = +22.24$ D if it is considered a simple combination thin lens. (ref. p.37)

4-12. (B) The image from the anterior surface reflection of the cornea is virtual, erect, and minified. (mnemonic VERMIN). (ref. p.37)

4-13. (A) $I = \dfrac{30\ \text{mm} \times 17\ \text{mm}}{330\ \text{mm}} = 1.54$ mm (ref. p.38)

4-14. (C) $I = \dfrac{40\ \text{mm} \times 17\ \text{mm}}{330\ \text{mm}} = 2.06$ mm (ref. p.38)

4-15. (A)

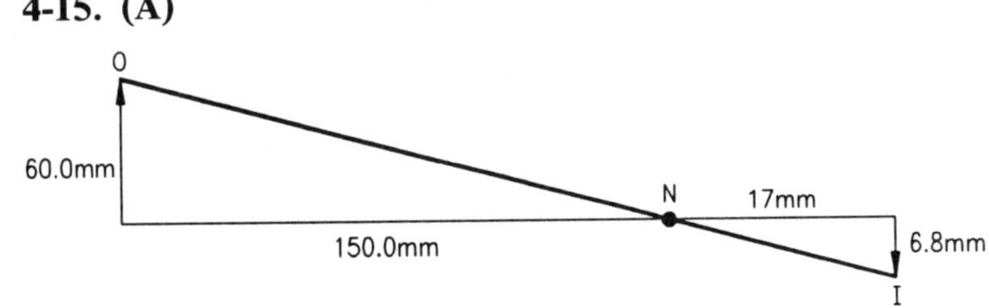

$$\frac{I}{O} = \frac{v}{\mu};$$

$$I = \frac{17\ \text{mm}}{150\ \text{mm}} \times 60\ \text{mm};$$

$I = 6.8$ mm (ref. p.38)

4-16. (C)

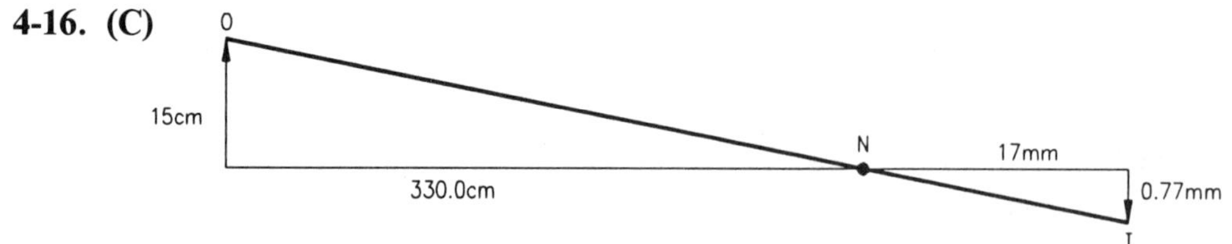

$$\frac{I}{O} = \frac{v}{\mu}; I = \frac{15 \text{ cm}}{330 \text{ cmts}} \times 17 \text{ mm} = 0.77 \text{ mm}$$

When one is using a Goldmann perimeter (330 cm), a scotoma measuring 15 cm corresponds to a retinal lesion 0.77 mm. (ref. p.38)

4-17. (E) Focal point: $\frac{100}{+66} = 1.51$ cm or 15.1 mm, which is 1.9 mm anterior to the retina using this model (ref. p.38)

4-18. (D) Purely axial myopia occurs when the eye is too long with normal refractive power. Image is in front of retina. (ref. p.39)

4-19. (C) If an object moves in one direction, the image moves in the same direction. It must obey the formula $U + D = V$. (ref. p.39)

4-20. (B)

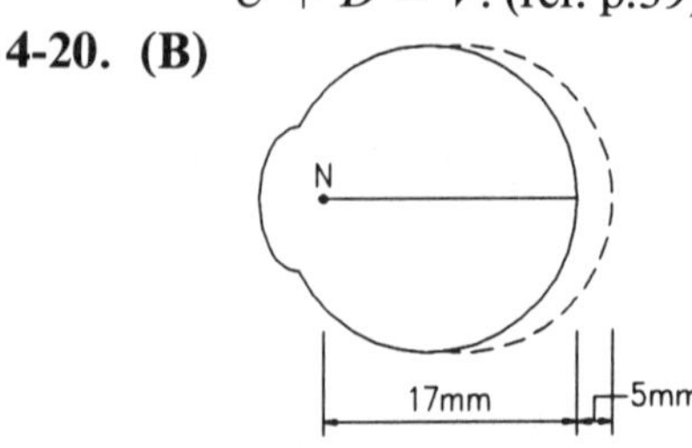

(i) The posterior focal point is 5 mm beyond the retina 1.7 cm + 0.5 cm = 2.2 cm from N.

(ii) In order to bring the image from the posterior focal point to the retina we need:

$$2.2 \text{ cm} = \frac{100}{x}; x = 45.45 \text{ D}$$

$$+60.00 - 14.54 \text{ D} = 45.45 \text{ D}$$

The lens that would correct an eye 5 mm too long has power equal to − 14.54 D. (ref. p.39)

4-21. (D) When power is +55.00 D, focal point is posterior to retina (refractive hyperopia). (ref. p.39)

$\frac{100}{+55} = 18.1$ mm and the focal point is 1.1 mm past the retina.

4-22. (E) If the power of a lens remains the same, a change in object position will always result in a change in image distance in the same direction relative to the light. The rate at which the image moves is dioptrically and not linearly related to object movement. If the power of a lens is changed in the plus direction, the image is pulled against the light. (ref. p.40)

4-23. (A) Image movement is dioptrically related to object movement. (ref. p.40)

4-24. (D) A myopic eye can be corrected by moving the object closer, placing a minus lens in front of the eye, or pushing the image with the light onto the retina. (ref. p.40)

4-25. (B) The far point is the point imaged by the unaccommodated eye on the retina. (ref. p.40)

4-26. (B) If the correcting lens has its secondary focal point coinciding with the far point, the image is in focus. (ref. p.40)

4-27. (D) Accommodation is age dependent, susceptible to fatigue, and closely related to convergence. (ref. p.41)

4-28. (E) Using maximum accommodation we can find a near point, a point beyond which a clear image cannot be maintained on the retina, the amplitude of accommodation, and the interval of clear vision. (ref. p.41)

4-29. (A) In myopia the near point is represented dioptrically by the sum of the myopia and the accommodative amplitude. (ref. p.41)

4-30. (A) Proximal to the near point the chromatic interval would be similar to that of unaccommodated hyperopia and not myopia. (ref. p.41)

4-31. (C) The hyperopic patient uses some accommodative amplitude to bring the image of a near object into focus. This leaves him unable to focus on as near a point as his myopic counterpart. (ref. p.41)

4-32. (D) Hyperopic persons have a near point dioptrically represented by the accommodative amplitude minus the hyperopia. (ref. p.41)

4-33. (C) The emmetropic person has a far point at infinity, a near point related dioptrically to the accommodative amplitude, and normal accommodation. (ref. p.42)

4-34. (C) **(i)** Far point: $\frac{100}{5} = 20$ cm

(ii) Near point: $\frac{100}{8 + 5} = 7.69$ cm

The interval of clear vision for 5.00 D of uncorrected myopia with 8.00 D of accommodative amplitude lies between 7.69-20 cm. (ref. p.42)

4-35. (D) **(i)** Far point: $\frac{100}{5} = 20$ cm in front of the eye

(ii) Near point: $\frac{100}{8 + 5} = \frac{100}{13} =$ 7.69

Without correction the interval of clear vision is 50 cm to ∞ (ref. p.42)

4-36. (A) **(i)** Far point: $\frac{100}{4} = 25$ cm. With $+4.00$ accommodation, infinity is in focus.

(ii) Near point: $\frac{100}{6 - 4} = \frac{100}{2} =$ 50 cm

(iii) Interval of clear vision = 50 cm to infinity

A book at 15 cm is proximal to the interval of clear vision and thus not in focus. (ref. p.42)

4-37. (A) **(i)** Far point: $\frac{100}{4} = 25$ cm for + 4.00 D of hyperopia. It can be brought to infinity with 4.00 D of accommodation.

(ii) Near point: $\frac{100}{10 - 4} = \frac{100}{6} =$ 16.67 cm

(iii) Interval of clear vision = 5.56 cm to 12.5 cm to infinity. (ref. p.42)

CHAPTER 5: ASTIGMATISM

5-1. (C) The fact that two meridians 90° apart have different radii of curvature explains how one meridian of a cylinder can be stronger than the other. (ref. p.43)

5-2. (B) The cornea can be a toric surface. This is corneal astigmatism. (ref. p.43)

5-3. (B) The greatest power of a cylinder is normal to its axis. (ref. p.43)

5-4. (D) The power meridian of a cylinder is dependent on the cylinder radius of curvature. (ref. p.43)

5-5. (C) A power cross is used to depict the power of a spherocylinder and the orientation of the axes. (ref. p.44)

5-6. (C) For the cylindrical lens +5.00 @ 135°, the axis is 45° and the power is at 135°. The power is equal to +5.00 D. (ref. p.44)

5-7. (A) Cylinder notation is in axis form and not according to the power meridian. (ref. p.44)

5-8. (C) Cylinder axis notation is done on a scale ranging between 0° and

180° with reference to the left ear. (ref. p.44)

5-9. (A) If we took multiple small cross-sections of a cylinder, each segment has its own point focus. Joining these foci transcribes a focal line. (ref. p.44)

5-10. (A) The power cross illustrated is equivalent to the following list of notations. (ref. p.44)
Power meridians:
$+3.00 @ 90 = +4.00 @ 180$
Combined cylinder form:
$+4.00 \times 90 = +3.00 \times 180$
Plus cylinder form:
$+3.00 = +1.00 \times 90$
Minus cylinder form:
$+4.00 = -1.00 \times 180$

5-11. (B) The Maddox rod is a device made of high plus cylinders of red or white plastic. (ref. p.45)

5-12. (D) A spherocylinder has a toric surface. (ref. p.45)

5-13. (A) The conoid of Sturm is a complex conical image space bound by the two focal lines of the spherocylinder. (ref. p.45)

5-14. (B) The orientation of the focal lines of a spherocylinder is in the direction of the cylinder axes. (ref. p.45)

5-15. (C) The interval of Sturm is the distance separating the two focal lines. (ref. p.45)

5-16. (C) (i) Vergence: $U + D = V$

$$\frac{-100}{5} + 180 = V$$
$$+160.00 \text{ D} = V$$

(ii) Image location: $\dfrac{100 \text{ cm}}{160 \text{ D}} =$

0.625 cm to the right of the cylinder

The image is real and inverted. (ref. p.45)

5-17. (D) $\dfrac{-100}{40} + 0 = \dfrac{-100}{40}; \mu = v$

The power is zero in the axis meridian. The image in the axis meridian of the cylinder is virtual and in the exact same spot as the object. (ref. p.45)

5-18. (D) The circle of least confusion is a circle located dioptrically midway between the focal lines. The image at this point is least blurred with vertical and horizontal dimensions approximately equal. (ref. p.46)

5-19. (A) The position of the circle of least confusion is described by the spherical equivalent of the spherocylinder. (ref. p.46)

5-20. (E) The spherical equivalent is calculated by adding the sphere to one half of the cylinder. The alternative is half the sum of two combined cylinders. (ref. p.46)

5-21. (C) If the spherical equivalent is the same for any two spherocylinders, the circle of least confusion will be in the same place. (ref. p.45)

5-22. (C) The size of the blur circle depends on the size of the interval of clear vision. The smaller the interval, the smaller the blur circle. (ref. p.46)

5-23. (C) A spherocylinder can be thought of as a combination of two cylinders of different powers. (ref. p.46)

5-24. (C) Contact lenses should always be dealt with in minus cylinder form. (ref. p.47)

5-25. (C) When converting from plus to minus cylinder form, take the sum of the sphere and the cylinder to yield the new sphere. Change the sign of the cylinder and change the axis by 90°. (ref. p.47)

5-26. (D) Conversion of $+2.00 = +1.00 \times 90$ to minus cylinder form (ref. p.47)
Sum of sphere and cylinder: $+2.00 + 1.00 = +3.00$
Change sign of cylinder: -1.00

Change axis by 90°: 90° becomes 180°
The minus cylinder form is $+3.00 - 1.00 \times 180$
Spherical equivalent:

$$+2.00 + \frac{1}{2}(+1.00) = +2.50$$

5-27. (A) Conversion of $+2.00 = -3.00 \times 45$ to plus cylinder form (ref. p.47)
Sum of sphere and cylinder = $+2.00 - 3.00 = -1.00$
Change sign of cylinder = $+3.00$
Change axis by 90° = 45° becomes 135°
The plus cylinder form = $-1.00 + 3.00 \times 135$
Spherical equivalent:

$$+2.00 + \frac{1}{2}(-3.00) = +0.50$$

The power of the plus cylinder is in the 45° meridian.

5-28. (B) The combined cylinder $+2.00 \times 180 = +3.00 \times 90$ can be transposed: (ref. p.47)

$$\begin{array}{l} +2.00 \times 180 = +3.00 \times 90 \\ \underline{-3.00 \times 180 = +3.00 \times 180} \\ -1.00 \times 180 = +3.00 \\ \quad +2.00 + 1.00 \times 90 \end{array}$$

5-29. (A) The spherocylinder $+4.00 \times 90 = +2.00 \times 180$ can also be written as: (ref. p.47)

$$\begin{array}{l} +4.00 \times 90 = +2.00 \times 180 \\ \underline{-2.00 \times 90 = +2.00 \times 90} \\ +2.00 \times 90 = +2.00 \\ \quad +4.00 - 2.00 \times 180 \end{array}$$

5-30. (C) The minus cylinder form is always used when prescribing contact lenses. (ref. p.47)

$$\begin{array}{l} +1.00 \times 90 = +3.00 \times 180 \\ \underline{-3.00 \times 90 = +3.00 \times 90} \\ -2.00 \times 90 = +3.00 \end{array}$$

5-31. (C) Equivalent interconversions: (p.47)
(i) $+1.00 = +1.50 \times 90$ has minus cyl form of $+2.50 = -1.50 \times 180$
(ii) $+4.25 = -1.75 \times 15$ has plus cyl form of $+2.50 = +1.75 \times 105$
(iii) $+1.50 = -2.75 \times 45$ has plus cyl form of $-1.25 = +2.75 \times 135$
(iv) $+3.00 = -4.00 \times 70$ has plus cyl form of $-1.00 = +4.00 \times 160$

5-32. (A) The combined cylinder $+2.00 \times 180 = +3.00 \times 90$ can also be written as $+3.00 - 1.00 \times 180$ arrived at by adding the net zero cylinder $-3.00 \times 180 = +3.00 \times 180$ to the above combined cylinder. (ref. p.48)

5-33. (C) If converting from combined cylinder to spherocylinder form, when a sphere of equal magnitude but opposite sign is placed in the same meridian, the net effect is not zero. (ref. p.48)

5-34. (C) **(i)** Vertical focal line = $\frac{100}{+2}$ = 50 cm to the right of the lens
(ii) Horizontal focal line = $\frac{100}{-1}$ = 100 cm to the left of the lens
The combined cylinder $+2.00 \times 90 = -1.00 \times 180$ has its circle of least confusion $\frac{+2.00 - 1.00}{2}$ = 50 cm to the right of the lens for an object at infinity. (ref. p.48)

5-35. (D) Conversion of
$+3.00 = +3.00 \times 45$
to combined cylinder form:

$0 = +3.00 \times 45$
$+3.00 \times 135 = +3.00 \times 45$
$+3.00 \times 135 = +6.00 \times 45$
combined cylinder form
(ref. p.48)

5-36. (C) If $-3.00 + 6.00 \times 160$ is to have the cylinder reduced by 50% and rotated to 180°, the resultant prescription would be $-1.50 + 3.00 \times 180$. Rotation does not affect the spherical equivalent. When the cylinder is reduced, the spherical equivalent of the original must be preserved by adding $\frac{+3.00}{2} = +1.50$ D to the sphere. (ref. p.48)

5-37. (A) An aphakic patient has K readings of 48.00 @ 70/40 @ 160 six weeks after cataract surgery. This patient's curvature is greater vertically because the 70° meridian has the greatest dioptric power. The astigmatism present is with the rule because the vertical positive axis is the greatest. The 160° meridian has the flattest K = 40.00 D. The 2 o'clock suture is very tight and should be cut. (ref. p.48)

5-38. (B) The resultant combined cylinder $+3.00 \times 180 = +3.00 \times 90$ is a sphere. The interval of Sturm has been collapsed to a stigmatic focal point. (ref. p.49)

5-39. (E)

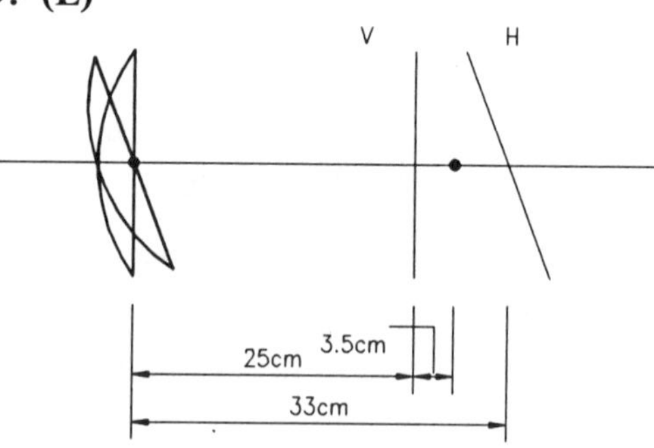

The following are calculations for the combined cylinder $+3.00 \times 180/+4.00 \times 90$ and an object at infinity. (ref. p.49)

(i) $U + D = V$ for $+3.00 \times 180$ is 0 $+ 3 = +3$

$\frac{100}{3} = 33.3$ cm (Horizontal focal line parallel to $+3.00 \times 180$)

(ii) $U + D = V$ for $+4.00 \times 90$ is 0 $+ 4 = +4$

$\frac{100}{4} = 25$ cm (vertical focal line parallel to $+4.00 \times 90$)

(iii) Interval of Sturm = 25 − 33.33 cm

(iv) Circle of least confusion: $\frac{4 + 3}{2} = +3.50$ D, $\frac{100}{+3.50} = 28.5$ cm

---

5-40. (E)

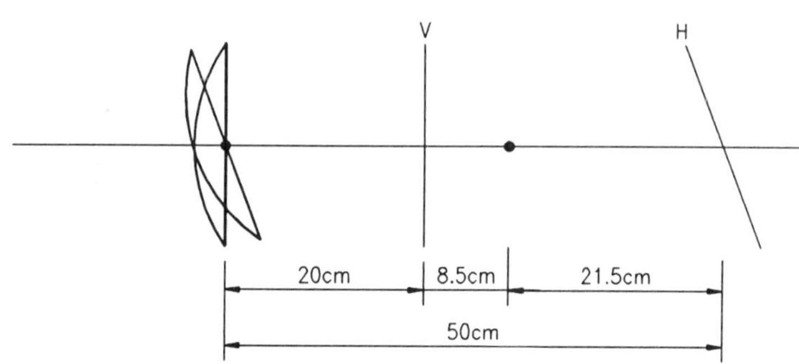

Spherocylinder:
$+2.00 = +3.00 \times 90$

(i) Convert to combined cylinder form

Continued.

5-40. cont'd. $+2.00 \times 180 = +2.00 \times 90$

Add $0 = +3.00 \times 90$

$+2.00 \times 180 = +5.00 \times 90$

(ii) $U + D = V$ for $+2.00 \times 180$

$0 + 2 = 2$

$$\frac{100}{2} = 50 \text{ cm}$$

(horizontal focal line parallel to $+2.00 \times 180$)

(iii) $U + D = V$ for $+5.00 \times 90$

$0 + 5 = 5$

$$\frac{100}{5} = 20 \text{ cm}$$

(vertical focal line parallel to $+5.00 \times 90$)

(iv) Interval of Sturm = 20 − 50 cm

(v) Circle of least confusion: $\frac{5 + 2}{2} = +3.50$ D. $\frac{100}{+3.50}$ = 28.5 cm (ref. p.49)

5-41. (B)

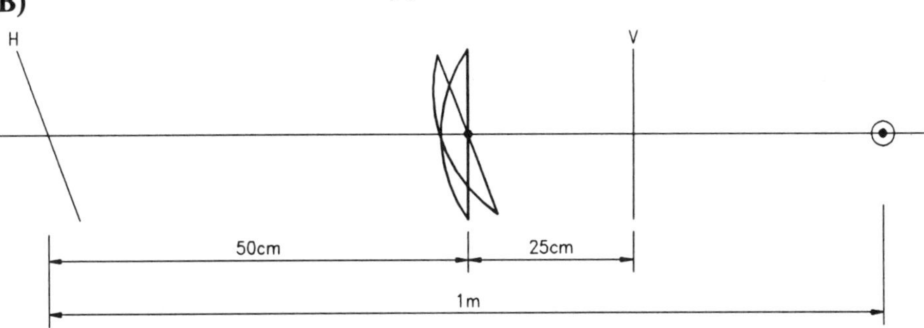

Combined cylinder $+4.00 \times 90 = -2.00 \times 180$:

(i) $U + D = V$ for $+4.00 \times 90$

$0 + 4 = 4$

$$\frac{100}{4} = 25 \text{ cm}$$

(vertical focal line, right of the lens)

(ii) $U + D = V$ for -2.00×180

$0 - 2 = -2$

$$\frac{100}{-2} = -50 \text{ cm}$$

(horizontal focal line, left of the lens)

(iii) Interval of Sturm: in this case the interval of Sturm is not between the lines but instead bridges infinity, extending from the vertical focal line behind the lens to reach the horizontal focal line.

(iv) Circle of least confusion: $\frac{+4 - 2}{2} = +1$ m to the right. (ref. p.49)

5-42. (D) **(i)** Before adding the cylinder:

Horizontal focal line: $\frac{100}{3}$ = 33 cm

Vertical focal line: $\frac{100}{2}$ = 50 cm

(ii) Add the cylinder and the result is a sphere: $+3.00 \times 180 = +3.00 \times 90$

Horizontal focal line: $\frac{100}{3}$ = 33 cm

Vertical focal line: $\frac{100}{3}$ = 33 cm

Circle of least confusion $\frac{3 + 3}{2} = +3.00\text{D} = \frac{100}{3}$ = 33 cm

The interval of Sturm has collapsed and the circle of least confusion is a single stigmatic point 33 cm from the lens. (ref. p.49)

5-43. (A)

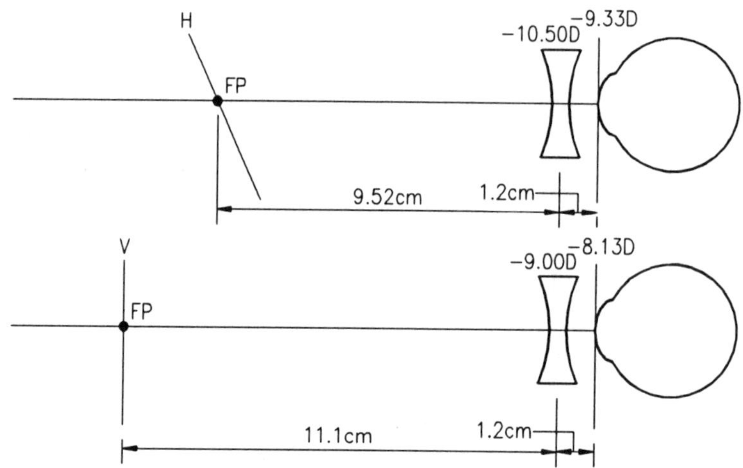

(i) $-10.50 = +1.50 \times 90 =$

$$\begin{array}{rcl} -10.50 \times 180 & = & -10.50 \times 90 \\ & & +1.50 \times 90 \\ \hline -10.50 \times 180 & = & -9.00 \times 90 \end{array}$$

(ii) Horizontal -10.50×180

$$FP = \frac{100}{10.50} = 9.52 \text{ cm at}$$

vertex distance = 1.2 cm

$$-D = \frac{-100}{9.52 + 1.2} =$$

$$\frac{-100}{10.72} = -9.33\text{D at}$$

vertex = 0

(iii) Vertical -9.00×90

$$FP = \frac{100}{-9} = 11.1 \text{ cm at}$$

vertex distance = 1.2 cm

$$-D = \frac{100}{11.1 + 1.2} =$$

$$\frac{100}{12.3} = -8.13\text{D at}$$

vertex = 0

(iv) At the corneal plane

$$\begin{array}{rcl} -9.33 \times 180 & = & -8.13 \times 90 \\ -9.33 \times \ \ 90 & = & +9.33 \times 90 \\ \hline -9.33 & = & +1.20 \times 90 \end{array}$$

An eye's refraction in the spectacle plane 12 mm from the cornea is $-10.50 \times 180 = -9.00 \times 90$ and at the cornea it is $-9.33 = +1.20 \times 90$. (ref. p.49)

5-44. (E) Mixed astigmatism occurs when one focal line is behind and the other is in front of the retina. (ref. p.50)

5-45. (A) One focal line on the retina and the other behind the retina is called simple hyperopic astigmatism. (ref. p.50)

5-46. (B) Simple myopic astigmatism is present if the eye error is +cyl × 180. It requires −cyl × 180 to correct it. (ref. p.50)

5-47. (C) If the eye error is −cyl × 180 and −cyl × 90, then compound hyperopic astigmatism is present. (ref. p.50)

5-48. (E) Mixed astigmatism occurs when the eye error is +cyl × 180 and −cyl × 90. (ref. p.50)

5-49. (B) If the correcting combined cylinder lens is placed in the corneal plane, it will be equal in magnitude and opposite in sign to the eye error. (ref. p.50)

5-50. (A) When sphere is added, both focal lines move an equal amount dioptrically. (ref. p.50)

5-51. (A) Convert $+2.00 = -1.00 \times 90$ to its combined cylinder form. (ref. p.50)

(i)

$$\begin{array}{rcl} +2.00 \times 180 & = & +2.00 \times 90 \\ 0 & = & -1.00 \times 90 \\ \hline +2.00 \times 180 & = & +1.00 \times 90 \end{array}$$

Correcting combined cylinder

(ii) This corrects an eye error of $-2.00 \times 180 = -1.00 \times 90$, which is compound hyperopic astigmatism.

5-52. (D) The combined cylinder that corrects mixed astigmatism is $-3.00 \times 180 = +1.00 \times 90$.

(i) $+4.00 = -3.00 \times 90$ becomes $+4.00 \times 180 = +1.00 \times 90$ in combined cylinder form and corrects compound hyperopic astigmatism.

(ii) $+2.00 \times 90 = +3.00 \times 180$ combined cylinder corrects compound hyperopic astigmatism.

(iii) $+4.00 \times 180 = +1.00 \times 90$ corrects compound hyperopic astigmatism.

(iv) $-3.00 \times 180 = +1.00 \times 90$ corrects an eye error of $+3.00 \times 180 = -1.00 \times 90$ which is mixed astigmatism.

5-53. (B) Convert $-4.00 = +2.00 \times 90$ to combined cylinder form: (ref. p.50-1)

$$\begin{array}{r} -4.00 \times 180 = -4.00 \times 90 \\ 0 = +2.00 \times 90 \\ \hline -4.00 \times 180 = -2.00 \times 90 \end{array}$$

combined cylinder form

This corrects an eye error of $+4.00 \times 180 = +2.00 \times 90$, which is compound myopic astigmatism.

5-54. (A) To selectively move an individual focal line, a cylinder with its axis parallel to the line must be used. (ref. p.51)

5-55. (B) In plus cylinder refracting technique, all forms of astigmatism are converted to simple hyperopic by adjusting the sphere such that the anterior focal line is on the retina. Moving the posterior focal line toward the light and onto the retina collapses the astigmatic interval into a point focus. (ref. p.51)

5-56. (B) Minus cylinder refracting technique requires that sphere is adjusted to obtain simple myopic astigmatism. The anterior focal line is pushed with the light and onto the retina with minus cylinders. (ref. p.51)

5-57. (E) In an astigmatic eye there is no single far point but rather two far planes. The goal of stigmatic imagery is achieved with correction. The two far point planes are coincident with the correcting cylinder focal planes. They in turn correspond to the eye error in the two principal meridians. There are only ever two far point planes. (ref. p.51)

5-58. (C) For the far point planes and the retina to be conjugate, the correcting spherocylindrical lens is placed such that the secondary focal lines of the correcting spherocylinder are coincident with the far point planes of the eye. (ref. p.51)

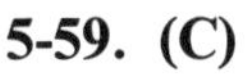

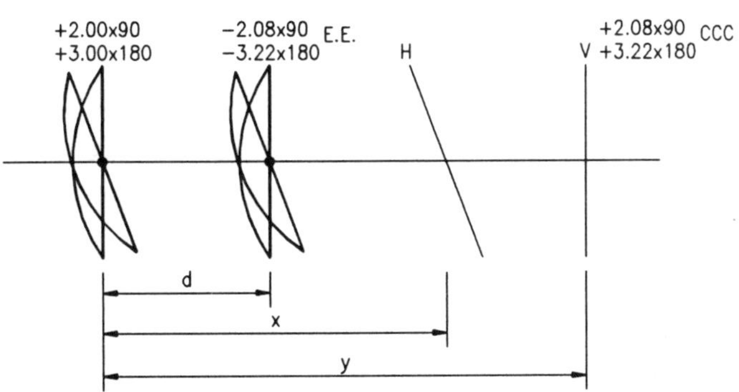

(i) Vertical:

$$\frac{100}{y} = +2.00, y = 50 \text{ cm}$$

(ii) Horizontal:

$$\frac{100}{x} = +3.00, x = 33 \text{ cm}$$

$$\frac{100}{x - d} = +3.22$$

$$\frac{100}{33 - d} = +3.22$$

$$d = 2 \text{ cm} = 20 \text{ mm}$$

An eye error of $-3.22 \times 180 = -2.08 \times 90$ is corrected by the spectacle lens $+3.00 \times 180 = +2.00 \times 90$ at a vertex distance of 20 mm. (ref. p.51)

5-60. (B) Symmetrical astigmatism exists when the axes of the correcting cylinders of both eyes are mirror images of each other. (ref. p.52)

5-61. (B) Regular astigmatism exists when the toricity of the cornea in the visual axis has a uniform refractive surface and measurements of the amount of astigmatism are repeatedly consistent. (ref. p.52)

5-62. (C) Irregular astigmatism occurs when a different astigmatic error is obtained with small excursions from the very central portion of the visual axis. (ref. p.52)

5-63. (B) A contact lens may smooth out the surface of a cornea with irregular astigmatism to yield regular astigmatism. (ref. p.52)

5-64. (D) In keratoconus a degenerative process affects the corneal thickness, resulting in an out-bowing of the central cornea in an irregular fashion. (ref. p.53)

5-65. (D) Irregular astigmatism and all toric surfaces have two principal meridians normal to one another. (ref. p.53)

5-66. (E) If keratometry reveals two principal meridians not normal to each other, two different areas of the visual axis are being tested, two zones of the cornea are being tested, two areas of irregular astigmatism exist, or you made a mistake. (ref. p.53)

5-67. (A) With the rule astigmatism exists when the axis of the correcting plus cylinder is at 90°. (ref. p.53)

5-68. (C) Against the rule astigmatism can be corrected with a minus cylinder axis 90. (ref. p.53)

5-69. (A) Newborns are most likely to develop against the rule astigmatism. There is gradual tendency for it to drift with the rule. After age 50 the drift is again against the rule. (ref. p.53)

5-70. (A) (i) In the corneal plane $-4.00 \times 180 = -6.00 \times 90$ is required.

Horizontal far line plane =

$$\frac{100}{-4} = -25 \text{ cm}$$

Vertical far line plane =

$$\frac{100}{-6} = -16.67 \text{ cm}$$

(ii) Now take into account the vertex distance and calculate the power.

$$D_{HOR} = \frac{-100}{25 - 1} = -4.17 \text{ D} = -4.17 \times 180$$

$$D_{VER} = \frac{-100}{16.67 - 1} = \frac{-100}{15.67} = -6.38 \text{ D} = -6.38 \times 90$$

Combined cylinder form = $-4.17 \times 180 = -6.38 \times 90$

To correct an eye error of $+4.00 \times 180 = +6.00 \times 90$ at vertex distance of 10 mm, spectacle lens with power $-4.17 \times 180 = -6.38 \times 90$ is required. (ref. p.53)

5-71. (C) Eye Error:

$-2.00 \times 90 = +4.00 \times 180$

CCC:

$+2.00 \times 90 = -4.00 \times 180$

Conversion: Add net zero cylinder
$+2.00 \times 90 = -4.00 \times 180$
$+2.00 \times 180 = -2.00 \times 180$
$+2.00 = -6.00 \times 180$
$-4.00 = +6.00 \times 90$, which is with the rule astigmatism. (ref. p.53)

5-72. (E) Eye Error:
$-1.00 \times 90 = -2.00 \times 180$
CCC:
$+1.00 \times 90 = +2.00 \times 180$
Conversion:
$+1.00 \times 90 = +2.00 \times 180$
$+ 1.00 \times 180 = -1.00 \times 180$
Spherocylinder:
$+1.00 = +1.00 \times 180$
This is against the rule compound hyperopic astigmatism. (ref. p.53)

5-73. (E) Once the anterior focal line is on the retina, plus cylinder axis 180 will bring the posterior focal line toward the light and on to the retina. This is against the rule astigmatism. (ref. p.54)

5-74. (C) When a lens is tilted, the amount of induced sphere and cylinder is related to the power of the lens and the amount of lift. (ref. p.54)

5-75. (C) Tilting a minus lens induces a small amount of minus sphere and a larger amount of minus cylinder axis 180. (ref. p.54)

5-76. (D) *K* readings of 40.00 D horizontally and 46.00 D vertically are with the rule astigmatism. The eye error is $+6.00 \times 180$, requiring correcting cylinder in plus cylinder form of $+6.00 \times 90$. (ref. p.54)

5-77. (B) Tilting a plus lens induces a small amount of plus sphere and a larger amount of plus cylinder axis 180. (ref. p.54)

5-78. (E) If a plus lens is tilted, plus cylinder at 180° or minus cylinder at 90° is produced, requiring plus cylinder at 90° to correct it. This is with the rule astigmatism. (ref. p.54)

5-79. (A) The distance separating the III and IV Purkinje-Sanson images is a measure of the amount of implant tilt. (ref. p.54)

5-80. (B) When the pantoscopic tilt is increased by a person with spectacle-corrected myopia raising his temples, the tilt adds minus cylinder axis 180 as well as a small amount of minus sphere. The resultant refractive error is against the rule, compound hyperopic astigmatism needing plus cylinder at 180° to correct it. (Eye error: $-$sph $-$cyl $\times$ 180; CCC: $+$sph, $+$cyl $\times$ 180 = against the rule.) (ref. p.54)

5-81. (A) A patient wearing spectacle correction of $+3.00 = +4.00 \times 90$ has *K* readings of 42.00 by 44.00 D. This patient has 2.00 D of lenticular astigmatism. The total astigmatic error can not be corrected with a regular hard contact lens. A bitoric contact with front cylinder might correct the lenticular component. If not, a soft toric lens is required. (ref. p.54-5)

5-82. (E) A bitoric hard contact lens corrects most forms of astigmatism, including both lenticular and corneal. (ref. p.55)

5-83. (C) A suture at 12 o'clock whose tension is too tight decreases the chord diameter vertically. This reduces the radius of curvature in the same meridian. This increases the power of that meridian. Induced cyl @ 90 = eye error axis 180. (ref. p.55)

5-84. (A) A loose suture will cause plus cylinder astigmatism at 90° to the offending suture. It weakens the power in this meridian by lengthening the chord diameter. This increases the radius of curvature vertically. (ref. p.55)

5-85. (D) Horizontal: 40.00 D =
40.00 D @ 180 = 40.00 × 90
Vertical: 36.00 D =
36.00 D @ 90 = 36.00 × 180
Eye Error: +4.00 × 90
CCC: −4.00 × 90 or
+4.00 × 180
This is against the rule astigmatism. (ref. p.55)

5-86. (B) Horizontal: 42.00 D =
42.00 D @ 180 = 42.00 × 90
Vertical: 45.00 D =
45.00 D @ 90 = 45.00 × 180
Eye Error: +3.00 × 180
CCC: −3.00 × 180 or
+3.00 × 90
This is with the rule astigmatism. (ref. p.55)

5-87. (D) **(i)** The total astigmatic error is +6.00 D
(ii) +5.00 D of the astigmatism is corneal 47.00 D/42.00 D
(iii) The remaining +1.00 D is lens-induced astigmatism.
(iv) The astigmatism is with the rule. (ref. p.55)

5-88. (B) When simple myopic astigmatism is induced in a pseudophakic patient, one focal line is in focus for distance and the other for near. This gives some uncorrected acuity at both distances. (ref. p.56)

5-89. (A) **(i)** Horizontal: 38.00 @ 180 =
38.00 × 90
Vertical: 48.00 @ 90 =
48.00 × 180
Eye Error: +10.00 × 180
CCC: −10.00 × 180
+cyl: +10.00 × 90
This astigmatism is with the rule and can be managed by cutting the suture at 12 o'clock which is too tight. Tight sutures cause plus cylinder astigmatism in the axis of the offending suture. (ref. p.56)

5-90. (E) 44.00 @ 120 = 44.00 × 30
34.00 @ 30 = 34.00 × 120
Eye error = +10.00 × 30
CCC = −10.00 × 30
+cyl = +10.00 × 120
The implications are that a suture may be too tight at 120° or too loose at 30°. The sutures at 30° can be tightened or those at 120° can be cut. (ref. p.56)

5-91. (B) If the axis of astigmatism is different from the axis of the correcting cylinder, two cylinders at oblique axes exist and a new resultant cylinder at a new axis is formed. (ref. p.57)

5-92. (D) When obliquely crossed cylinders of equal power and different sign such as the eye error and correcting cylinder axes are crossed, the new axis is 45° from the eye error axis. (ref. p.57)

5-93. (A) When the spherical equivalent equals zero, this is a cross cylinder. (ref. p.57)

5-94. (E) Subjective refinement of the cylinder power is performed after refinement of the axis. (ref. p.57-8)

5-95. (E) If the circle of least confusion is on the retina, objective or subjective refraction can be refined; the patient could be emmetropic or have mixed astigmatism. (ref. p.58)

5-96. (B) The markings on the cross cylinder denote the axes of the cylinder. (ref. p.58)

5-97. (E) If a correcting minus cylinder is oriented parallel to the posterior focal line and vision diminishes, the interval of Sturm increases and the circle of least confusion is enlarged as the focal line is pushed with the light. (ref. p.58)

5-98. (D) At the endpoint of cross cylinder refinement of the axis and power, the residual astigmatism is from the presence of the cross cylinder. (ref. p.58)

5-99. (C) When the cross cylinder is flipped at the endpoint of subjective refinement of the axis and power, the circle of least confusion remains on the retina. (ref. p.58)

5-100. (A) Power refinement during cross cylinder testing rests on the premise that the circle of least confusion is maintained on the retina. (ref. p.59)

5-101. (C) Adding +0.50 D of cylinder shifts the circle of least confusion by an amount equal to the spherical equivalent +0.25 D; −0.25 D must be added to return the circle of least confusion back onto the retina. (ref. p.59)

5-102. (D) The power of cross cylinder selected for use depends on the visual acuity of the patient. The lower it is, the better the vision of the patient. It determines how precise the refinement will be. (ref. p.59)

5-103. (D) During axis refinement, the cross cylinder is placed such that its two axes straddle the correcting cylinder axis. (ref. p.59)

5-104. (B) The end point of axis refinement occurs when the eye error axis and the correcting cylinder axis are coincident. (ref. p.59)

5-105. (B) If the correcting cylinder is not at the correct axis relative to the eye error, two oblique cylinders exist. If the plus axis position is the same as the induced minus axis, the resultant cylinder is less. The vision is better in this position. (ref. p.60)

5-106. (B) When one is using plus cylinders, the correcting cylinder is rotated toward the plus axis of the cross cylinder in the better of the two positions. (ref. p.60)

5-107. (A) The number of degrees the cross cylinder is rotated at each choice during axis refinement depends on the amount of cylinder present. The greater the amount, the fewer the degrees of rotation. (ref. p.60)

5-108. (C) One property of a cross cylinder is that the spherical equivalent is always zero. (ref. p.60)

(i) $+2.00 = +4.00 \times 90$; spherical equivalent $= 2 + \frac{4}{2} = 4$ (NO)

(ii) $+6.00 = -8.00 \times 180$; spherical equivalent $= 6 - \frac{8}{2} = 2$ (NO)

(iii) $-2.50 = +5.00 \times 180$; spherical equivalent $= -2.50 + \frac{5}{2} = 0$ (YES)

(iv) $-3.00 = -6.00 \times 90$; spherical equivalent $= -3 - \frac{6}{2} = -6$ (NO)

(v) $+2.00 \times 90 = +4.00 \times 180$; spherical equivalent $= \frac{2 + 4}{2} = 3$ (NO)

5-109. (B) If the power is refined before refinement of the axis, the result is the best power for the incorrect axis. (ref. p.61)

5-110. (E) The astigmatic clock is based on the imagery of the extended object as seen at the retina. (ref. p.61)

5-111. (C) In the interval of Sturm, if the vertical focal line is closest to the retina, the vertical aspects of an extended object are in best focus. (ref. p.61)

5-112. (A) When an astigmatic patient looks at 6 equally dark lines in the configuration of a clock, the sharpest line corresponds to the axis of the focal line nearest the retina. (ref. p.61)

5-113. (E) The sharpest line during astigmatic clock testing can be either the anterior or the posterior focal line, whichever is closest to the retina. (ref. p.61)

5-114. (D) Fogging removes any stimulus to accommodation. (ref. p.61)

5-115. (D) If the patient is properly fogged

during astigmatic clock testing, the sharpest line is the posterior focal line, which is perpendicular to the anterior focal line. (ref. p.62)

5-116. (B) For each clock hour between 1 and 6 o'clock, 30° of correcting minus cylinder are added. (ref. p.62)

5-117. (E) The double click method allows the use of plus cylinders for techniques best suited to minus cylinders. (ref. p.62)

5-118. (B) The stimulation of accommodation can be controlled by fogging to about 20/40. This should be maintained at all times. (ref. p.63)

5-119. (B) An IOL tilted about the horizontal meridian induces plus cylinder axis 180°. (ref. Holladay: Avoiding refractive problems)

5-120. (E) The change in spherical power of the lens for a given tilt is one third of the induced cylinder.

CHAPTER 6: MAGNIFICATION

6-1. (D) Meridional magnification is when the image appears taller or wider than the object. Magnification in one meridian has been greater than in the other. (ref. p. 64)

6-2. (D) Linear magnification and minification means the image appears larger or smaller. The word lateral is interchangeable with linear. Axial magnification occurs when the image appears more elevated or depressed than the object. It is not the same as meridional magnification. (ref. p. 64)

6-3. (B) Linear magnification can be calculated by dividing the image size by the object size or the image distance by the object distance. (ref. p. 64)

6-4. (B) Linear magnification of the image, when compared to the object, is measured relative to the distance away from the optical axis of the image and object. (ref. p. 64)

6-5. (A) Axial magnification is measured relative to the distance along the optical axis. (ref. p. 64)

6-6. (B) An object subtends an angle at the nodal point such that the tangent of this angle is equal to the object size over the object distance from the nodal point. (ref. p. 64)

6-7. (A) **(i)**

$$\text{Image size} = \frac{\text{Image distance}}{\text{Object distance}} \times \text{Object size}$$

$$I = \frac{10 \text{ cm}}{40 \text{ cm}} \times 20 \text{ cm}; \quad I = 5 \text{ cm}$$

(ii) Linear magnification $= \frac{\text{Image size}}{\text{Object size}} = \frac{5 \text{ cm}}{20 \text{ cm}} = \frac{1}{4} = 0.25\times$

(iii) Axial magnification = (linear magnification)^2 $= \left(\frac{1}{4}\right)^2 = \frac{1}{16}$; axial minification $16\times$

The image is 5 cm and is linearly minified by a factor of 4 and axially minified by a factor of 16. (ref. p. 64)

6-8. (D) Angular magnification compares the angle subtended with the optical system to the angle subtended without the optical system. (ref. p. 65)

6-9. (D) Simple magnification is related to the power of the magnifier and a reference distance standardised to 25 cm or ¼ m. (ref. p. 65)

6-10. (C) **(i)** $M_{A25} = x\,D = (0.25)\,(60.00 \text{ D}) = 15\times$

(ii) $M_{A30} = x\,D = (0.30)\,(60.00 \text{ D}) = 18\times$

Change in magnification is $18\times - 15\times = 3\times$

The magnification changes by $3\times$ when the standard distance for reference is changed from 25 to 30 cm for the emmetropic eye. (ref. p. 65)

6-11. (B) $M_A = \frac{D_A}{4} = \frac{+28.00 \text{ D}}{4} = 7\times$

The angular magnification of a hand-held magnifier with power equal to +28.00 D is 7×. (ref. p. 65)

6-12. (C) If an object's magnification is calculated for viewing at 40 cm, the image would appear larger by $\frac{40}{25} = \frac{8}{5}\times$ if it was brought 15 cm closer. (ref. p. 66)

6-13. (B) **(i)** $\frac{100}{2.2} = +45.45 \text{ D}$

(ii) $\frac{+45.5 \text{ D}}{4} = 11.4\times$

The magnification of an aphakic eye with an anterior focal point of 22 mm is equal to 11.4×. (ref. p. 66)

6-14. (C) $M = D \times x$ where x = reference distance in meters.

(i) If x = 25 cm or ¼ m (usual standard) then $M = D/4$.

(ii) If x = 50 or ½ m (new reference standard) then M = D/2 +20.00 D lens has $M = +20/2 = 10\times$.

The perceived image size will appear smaller by half. The magnification as a simple magnifier is doubled. (ref. p. 66)

6-15. (A) **(i)** $D_{E_{MYOPE}} = \frac{100}{1.50} = +66.67 \text{ D}$

$M_{A_{MYOPE}} = \frac{+66.67 \text{ D}}{4} =$

16.67× is the magnification of the myope

(ii) $D_{EMM.} = +60.00 \text{ D}$

$M_A = \frac{+60.00 \text{ D}}{4} = 15\times$

is the magnification of the emmetropic eye

(iii) Comparison: $\frac{16.67\times}{15\times} \times 100$

= 11.13% and is therefore 11.13% larger.

A myopic eye with an anterior focal point of 15 mm appears magnified 16.67×. The fundus in myopia appears 11.13% larger than that in emmetropia. (ref. p. 66)

6-16. (D) **(i)** $D_{EYE} = \frac{100}{2} = +50 \text{ D}$

(ii) $M_A = \frac{+50.00 \text{ D}}{4} = 12.5\times$

At 50 cm it would appear half the size again. Magnification is $\frac{12.5\times}{2} = 6.25\times$. (ref. p. 66)

6-17. (A) A Galilean telescope has a plus objective and a minus eyepiece lens. (ref. p. 67)

6-18. (D) The lenses of a Galilean telescope are placed such that the secondary focal point of the first plus objective lens coincides with the primary focal point of the second minus eyepiece lens. (ref. p. 67)

6-19. (D) With a Galilean telescope, an object at infinity forms a real image by the first lens, which becomes a virtual image for the second. This results in a larger, inverted image on the retina and parallel rays emergent from the eyepiece. (ref. p. 67)

6-20. (C) The magnification of a Galilean telescope is calculated using the formula $\frac{-D_E}{D_O}$. (ref. p. 67)

6-21. (C) The separation of the lenses and therefore the length of a Galilean telescope is the difference of the focal lengths of the two lenses. (ref. p. 67)

6-22. (A) If the angular magnification is positive, the perceived image is upright. If it is negative, the perceived image is inverted. (ref. p. 67)

6-23. (C) In the astronomical telescope the eyepiece lens is plus instead of minus, so the image is inverted when perceived. The separation of the lenses is the sum of the focal lengths. (ref. p. 67)

6-24. (E) The astronomical telescope has the following properties:

(i) D_E is plus instead of minus

(ii) The image is inverted when perceived

(iii) f_2 of the objective lens coincides with f_1 of the eyepiece

(iv) Emergent rays are parallel

(v) The separation will be the sum of the focal lengths

6-25. (A) $M_A = \dfrac{-D_E}{D_O} = \dfrac{-\left(\dfrac{-100}{0.5}\right)}{+5.00} = \dfrac{+200}{+5.00} = 40\times$

The image produced on the retina is larger (by a factor of 40), inverted and perceived upright. (ref. p. 67)

6-26. (A)

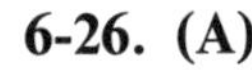

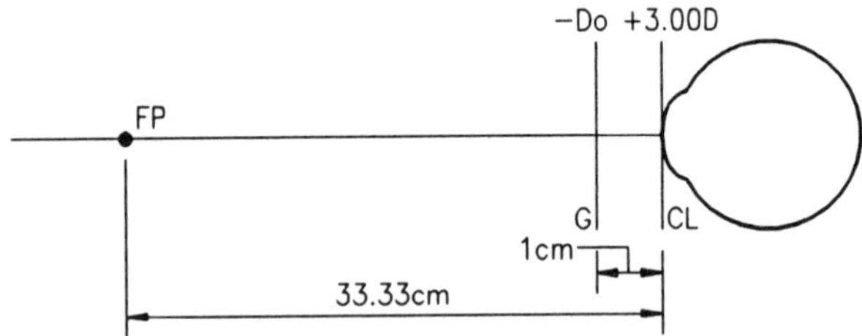

(i) Power $= \dfrac{100}{32.3} = -3.10$ D

(+3.00 D overcorrection with the contact is like converting the patient to a −3.00 D myopia, i.e., it moves the FP

(ii) Minification =

$-\left(\dfrac{3.00\text{ D}}{-3.10\text{ D}}\right) = 0.97\times$ or

minification of 3%

The power of spectacle required is −3.10 D and the minification that occurs is equal to 3%. (ref. p. 67)

6-27. (C) **(i)** $M_A = \dfrac{-D_E}{D_O} = \dfrac{+120.00\text{ D}}{+40.00\text{ D}}$

$= 3\times$ is the magnification of the telescope

(ii) Separation: $\dfrac{100}{40} - \dfrac{100}{120} =$

$2.5 - 0.83 = 1.67$ cm or 16.7 mm

(iii) Perceived image is upright because M_A is positive.

A telescope with a +40.00 D objective and a −120.00 D eyepiece lens has a magnification of 3×, a separation of 16.67 mm and has an image perceived as upright. (ref. p. 67)

6-28. (B) As an object is brought closer for viewing with a telescope, the object vergence is more divergent using the same $U + D = V$. The image vergence is magnified by the telescope and is much greater than the usual $U + D = V$ value. (ref. p. 68)

6-29. (A) Viewing a near object through a telescope demands more accommodation to overcome the increased vergence demands by the telescope such that $A_T = A_N \times M^2$. (ref. p. 68)

6-30. (D) $A_T = \dfrac{100}{25} \times 4^2 = 64.00$ D. The accommodation required for a 4× Galilean telescope and an object 25 cm away is 64.00 D. (ref. p. 68)

6-31. (E) This 4× telescope requires accommodation of $A_T = 2 \times 4^2 = 32.00$ D for an object at 50 cm. A +2.00 D lens in front of the objective lens or a +32.00 D lens behind the eyepiece lens eliminates this demand. (ref. p. 68)

6-32. (C) $M_A^2 = \dfrac{36.00\text{ D}}{(100/25)} = \dfrac{36.00}{4} = 9.00$ D

$M_A = 3\times$

The magnification of a telescope with 36.00 D accommodative demand viewing an object at 25 cm is 3×. (ref. p. 68)

6-33. (D) (i) If the magnification is 5× then, $\frac{D}{4} = 5\times$, $D = +20.00$ D

(ii) $f = \frac{100}{20} = 5$ cm and therefore $(25 - 5) = 20$ cm

Therefore an object viewed by a 5× monocular add must be held 20 cm closer when compared to this 5× loupe. (ref. p. 68)

6-34. (A) (i) $M = \frac{D}{4} = \frac{8}{4} = 2\times$

(ii) $M_T = M_1 \times M_2 = 2 \times 3 = 6\times$

A 6× magnifier yields the same results as +8.00 D readers and a 3× hand-held magnifier. (ref. p. 68)

6-35. (C) The total magnification of a multiple lens system is equal to the product of each component magnifier. (ref. p. 68)

6-36. (C) The correction of ametropia deals with two lenses such that the correcting lens is coincident with the far point of the eye. The focal point of the first lens is coincident with the primary focal point of the second. This is a telescopic system and can be treated thus. (ref. p. 68)

6-37. (B) (i) $A_T = \frac{100}{40} \times 5^2 = +62.50$ D accommodation needed for viewing without the +2.50 D lens but with it, zero

(ii) $M_A = \frac{-D_E}{D_O} = \frac{-D_E}{D_O + 2.50 \text{ D}} = 3.81\times$

(iii) The magnification has changed by $5 - 3.81\times = 1.19\times$

This system requires 62.50 D of accommodation for viewing without the +2.50 D lens. It decreases the magnification by 1.19×, from 5× to 3.81×. (ref. p. 68)

6-38. (E) $A_T = [3.00 \times (4^2)] - 3.00 = +45.00$ D

45.00 D are needed for proper viewing of this object through this telescope. (ref. p. 68)

6-39. (E) (i) $FP = \frac{100}{12} = 8.33$ cm

(ii) $D_E = \frac{-100}{8.33 - 1.5} = -14.7$ D

(iii) $M_A = \frac{-(-14.7)}{12} = 1.22\times$

(iv) $I = 1.5 \times 1.22\times = 1.83$ mm

The optic disk of 1.5 mm would appear to be 1.83 mm when examined with correction. (ref. p. 69)

6-40. (E) As the vertex distance decreases, the simple magnification approaches 1. (ref. p. 69)

6-41. (C) Spectacle-corrected aphakia can be considered a telescopic system with magnification greater than 1×. (ref. p. 69)

6-42. (C) A person with spectacle-corrected +5.00 × 45 astigmatism would see the 135° meridian larger compared to the 45° meridian. (ref. p. 69)

6-43. (B) Aniseikonia is the perception of an image size disparity (i.e., magnification or minification) between the two eyes or when compared to normal seeing. (ref. p. 69)

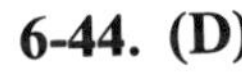

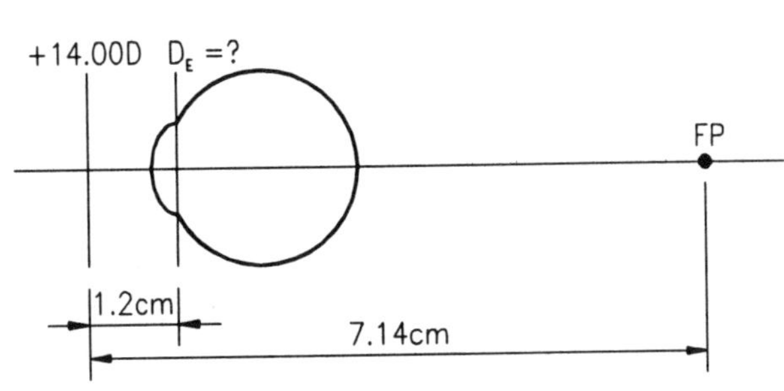

(i) Far point plane: $f_2 = \frac{100}{14} =$ 7.142 cm

(ii) Add the spectacle and the removed lens vertex distances. 7 mm + 5 mm = 1.2 cm

(iii) $D_E = \frac{-100}{7.14 - 1.2} = -16.83$

D is the relative power of the system when compared to emmetropia

(iv) $M_A = \frac{-D_E}{D_O} = \frac{-16.8314}{14} =$ 1.20× or 20% magnification

A person with +14.00 D spectacle-corrected aphakia at a vertex distance of 7 mm has a far point at 7.142 cm behind the eye, an eye error of −16.83 D, and 20% magnification. (ref. p. 69)

6-45. (C)

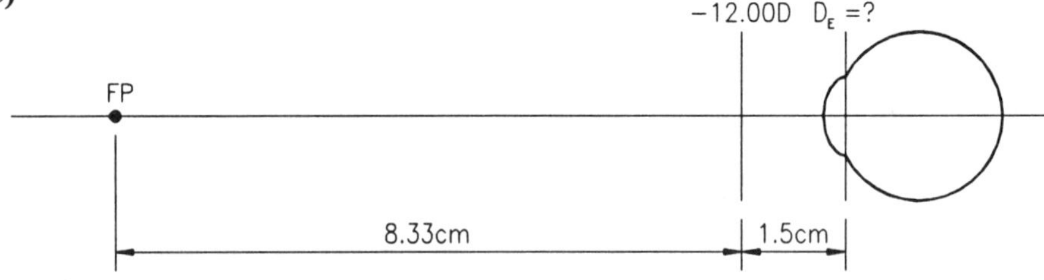

(i) Far point plane: $f_2 = \frac{-100}{12}$ $= -8.33$ cm

(ii) Spectacle vertex distance = 10 mm + 5 mm = 1.5 cm

(iii) $D_E = \frac{-100}{-8.33 - 1.5} = +10.17$

D relative to the power of the system at emmetropia

(iv) $M_A = \frac{-10.17}{-12.00} = 0.85\times$ or minification of 15%

A −12.00 D spectacle correction at a vertex distance of 10 mm minifies 15%. (ref. p. 69)

6-46. (C)

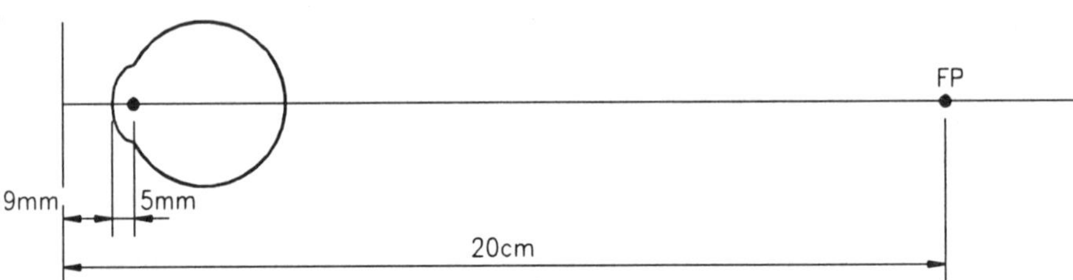

(i) Far point plane: $f_2 = \frac{100}{5} =$ 20 cm

(ii) Spectacle vertex distance: 9 mm + 5 mm = 1.4 cm

(iii) $D_E = \frac{-100}{20 - 1.4} = \frac{-100}{18.6} =$ - 5.38 D is the relative eye error

(iv) $M_A = -\left(\frac{-5.38}{+5.00}\right) = 1.075$ = 7.5% magnification

This person with astigmatism has a far point plane 20 cm from the eye, a vertex distance of 1.4 cm, and magnification of 7.5%. Since the power of the cylinder is at 90° to its axis, the 135° meridian is magnified 7.5%. (ref. p. 69)

6-47. (D) In normal seeing an object of regard falls on corresponding retinal elements and is fused centrally into single binocular vision. (ref. p. 70)

6-48. (A) Diplopia is when the object of regard projects an image that falls on noncorresponding retinal points. Visual confusion is when different objects of regard fall on corresponding retinal points. (ref. p. 70)

6-49. (A) In young children suffering from an eye deviation, visual adaption to diplopia and visual confusion can occur through suppression. (ref. p. 70)

6-50. (C) If the amount of aniseikonia is large, the visually mature patient sees double. If the amount of aniseikonia is small, the plasticity of the occipital cortex will allow adjustment. (ref. p. 70)

6-51. (B) To eliminate or reduce an image size disparity within binocular single vision, an intraocular lens implant in aphakia can be performed. A balance lens over the phakic eye sufficiently blurs the image of facilitate ignoring it but precludes binocular vision. (ref. p. 70)

6-52. (B) A way to reduce some of the image disparity in contact lens–corrected monocular aphakia is to overplus the contact lens and overcorrect with minus spectacle to obtain a reverse Galilean telescopic effect. (ref. p. 70)

6-53. (B) Knapp's rule states that if the correcting lens is placed at the primary focal point, the image will remain the same size no matter what the axial length. (ref. p. 71)

6-54. (E) None of these measurements are exact. (ref. p. 71)

6-55. (B) The myopic person who converts to contact lenses needs to use more accommodation. (ref. p. 71)

6-56. (C) **(i)** Magnification $= \frac{6.38}{6} = 1.06\times$

(ii) $A_T = 4 \times (1.06)^2 = 4.76$ D

(iii) Relative accommodative demand $= \frac{0.76}{4} \times 100\% = 19\%$

A person with +6.00 D spectacle-corrected hyperopia exerts 19% more accommodative demand than their contact lens counterpart if the spectacle vertex distance is 1 cm. (ref. p. 71)

6-57. (D)

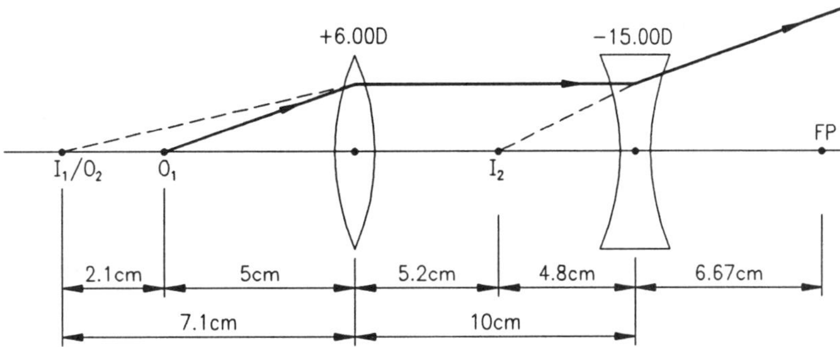

(i) $U_1 + D_1 = V_1$

$$\frac{-100}{5} + 6.00 = \frac{1}{v};$$

$v = -7.1$ cm to the left of the first lens

(ii) $U_2 + D_2 = V_2$

$$\frac{-100}{17} - 15.00 = \frac{-1}{v_2};$$

$v_2 = -4.8$ cm to the left of the second lens

(iii) The image is inside the telescope, virtual and upright.

(iv) $M_{TOT} = M_{TELESCOPE} \times M_{LAT}$

$$= \frac{D_E}{D_O} \times \frac{I_1}{O_1} \times \frac{I_2}{O_2} = \frac{15}{6} \times \frac{7.1}{5} \times \frac{4.8}{171.1} = 0.99\times$$ or minification of 1%

(v) Separation between $D_1 - D_2$

$$= \frac{100}{6} - \frac{100}{15} = 16.67 - 6.67 = 10 \text{ cm}$$ (ref. p. 71)

6-58. (B)

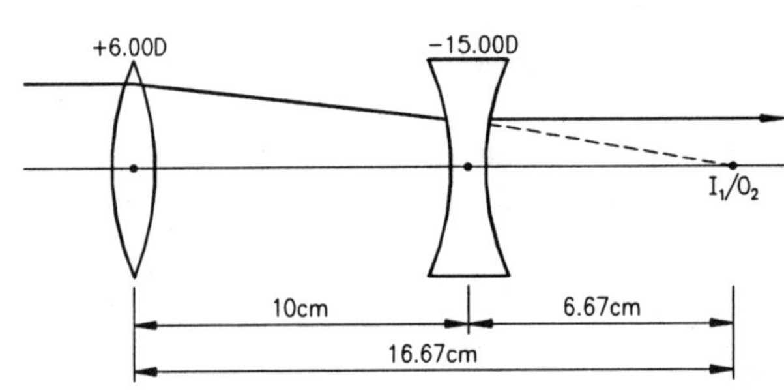

(i) $U + D_O = V$

$0 + 6 = 6$

$$\frac{100}{6\text{ D}} = 16.67\text{ D}$$

(ii) $U + D_E = V$

$$\frac{+100}{6.67\text{ D}} - 15.00 = 0$$

(iii) Image rays emerge parallel

(iv) The image vergence is zero and no accommodation is needed. (ref. p. 71)

6-59. (C)

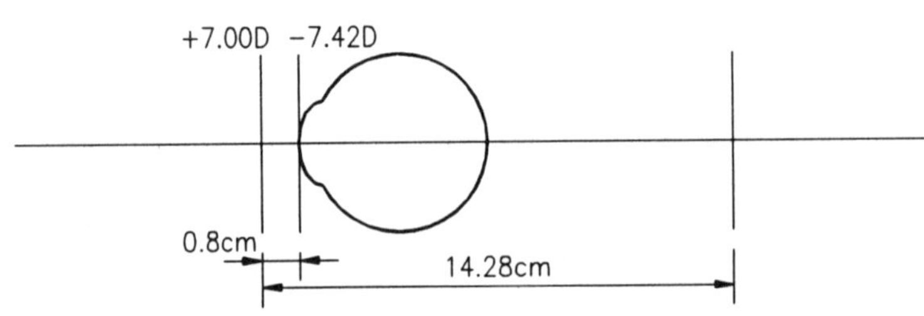

+7.00 D hyperopia

$$\text{FP} = \frac{100}{7} = 14.285\text{ cm}$$

$$-D_E = \frac{100}{14.28 - 0.8} = -7.42\text{ D}$$

$$M_A = \frac{-7.42\text{ D}}{-7.00\text{ D}} = 1.06\times$$

Normal accommodation:

$$A_N = \frac{100}{40} = +2.50\text{ D}$$

$$A_T = 2.50 \times (1.06)^2 = 2.809$$

Accommodation:

$$\frac{2.809 - 2.50}{2.50} \times 100\% = 12.36\%$$

LESS

6-60. (E)

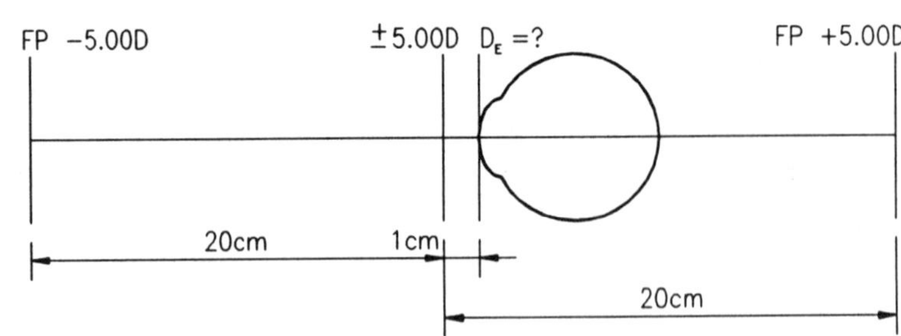

(i) +5.00 D hyperopia

$$\text{FP} = \frac{100}{5} = 20\text{ cm}$$

$$-D_E = \frac{100}{20 - 1} = -5.26\text{ D}$$

$$M_A = \frac{-5.26\text{ D}}{-5.00\text{ D}} = 1.05\times$$

Normal accommodation:

$$A_N = \frac{100}{25} = +4.00\text{ D}$$

$$A_T = 4 \times (1.05)^2 = 4.41\text{ D}$$

Accommodation:

$$\frac{4.41 - 4.00}{4.00} \times 100\% = \frac{0.41}{4.00} \times 100\% = 10.25\%\text{ MORE}$$

(ii) −5.00 D myopia

$$FP = \frac{-100}{5} = -20 \text{ cm}$$

$$D_E = \frac{100}{20 + 1} = +4.76 \text{ D}$$

$$M_A = \frac{(+4.76 \text{ D})}{-5.00 \text{ D}} = 0.952\times$$

Normal accommodation:

$A_N = 4.00$ D

$A_T = 4 \times (0.952)^2 = 3.625$ D

Accommodation:

$$\frac{3.625 - 4.00}{4.00} \times 100\% =$$

$$\frac{0.375}{4} \times 100\% = 9.375\%$$

LESS

A person with hyperopia requires 10.25% more accommodation, and one with myopia saves 9.375% accommodation by using spectacles instead of contacts. (ref. p. 71)

6-61. (C) Persons with myopia who wear spectacles can remove them and eliminate any minification they are experiencing. They see clearly at their far point with NO accommodation. The AC/A ratio must change. The near point is with maximum accommodation by definition (ref. p. 72)

6-62. (A) Magnification, minification, and distortion are all related to the correcting lens. (ref. p. 72)

6-63. (E) A person with uncorrected astigmatism experiences no distortion until he is spectacle corrected. Blur at distance and near occurs without correction. Binocular distortion is much greater than monocular distortion, especially for fore/aft perception. (ref. 72)

6-64. (A) If the correcting cylinder is rotated toward 90° or 180°, it creates a more tolerable form of distortion. (ref. p. 72)

6-65. (C) Distortion can be reduced by using minimal vertex distances and using posterior toric minus cylinder lenses. (ref. p. 72)

CHAPTER 7: RETINOSCOPY

7-1. (E) Retinoscopy can also be called skiascopy. It deals with light reflexes and shadows as they emerge from the eye. It gives an objective estimate to start the subjective refinement of the refraction. (ref. p.73)

7-2. (C) The far point of the emmetropic eye is at infinity. In unaccommodated myopia it is in front of the eye varying with the amount of myopia present. In unaccommodated hyperopia, the far point is behind the eye. (ref. p.73)

7-3. (C) In astigmatism two far line planes exist which are always perpendicular to one another. The position of these lines depends on the type of astigmatism. (ref. p.73)

7-4. (B) When the retina is illuminated with a light source such as a retinoscope, it becomes an object whose image will be formed at its far point. (ref. p.73)

7-5. (E) One can simulate eye errors by placing plus or minus spheres in front of an emmetropic eye. This displaces the far point. Placing objects inside the near point pushes the image behind the retina, simulating hyperopia and stimulating accommodation. (ref. p.73)

7-6. (A) Retinoscopy is based on the direction of movement of light reflexes with different far point positions. (ref. p.73)

7-7. (A) The basis of retinoscopy is the direction of movement of reflected light rays in various directions based on the different far point positions. The retinoscope serves as a light source that illuminates the retina and enables the detection of light movement so as to detect either with or against movement. (ref. p.73)

7-8. (B) A key point exists in retinoscopy when the direction of the light reflex is reversed. This denotes neutralization and the arrival at the far point. (ref. p.74)

7-9. (A) As the streak from the retinoscope descends, the retina is illuminated and becomes imaged at its far point plane. This streak is now the object for the examiner to follow and compare in direction to the intercept on the face. (ref. p.74)

7-10. (A) Less than −1.50 D of myopia yields a with response. (ref. p.74)

7-11. (D) At neutralization the light of the retinoscope fills the examiner's pupil. Beyond this point with motion becomes against motion. (ref. p.74)

7-12. (B) The working lens is +1.50 D, which moves the emmetropic far point to ⅔ m. This redefines emmetropia for retinoscopy purposes as −1.50 D myopia. The working lens causes myopia less than 1.50 D to behave like low hyperopia and yield a with response. (ref. p.74)

7-13. (D) If neutrality is achieved and the examiner moves forward, a with response can be seen. (ref. p.75)

7-14. (A) Against motion is less easily distinguished than with motion. (ref. p.76)

7-15. (C) With a (sleeve-up) streak retinoscope emergent light in the sleeve-down position reverses the traditional motion to against from with. (ref. p.76)

7-16. (D) A refractionist performing streak retinoscopy at 50 cm without a working lens uses a retinoscope adjusted for a plano mirror effect. If the patient has −2.00 D myopia, their far point will be 50 cm in front, which coincides with the working distance. This is neutralization and no motion is seen. (ref. p.76-78)

7-17. (B) If an eye is astigmatic, two far line planes exist perpendicular to one another. Two bands of unequal (or perhaps opposite) motion can be identified. (ref. p.77)

7-18. (C) When one is using plus or minus cylinders in streak retinoscopy, two far line planes exist irrespective of the type of astigmatism. One band will approach neutrality faster than the other. (ref. p.78)

7-19. (A) The second band remains at 90° to the first. The two far line planes are always normal to one another. (ref. p.78)

7-20. (D) During refinement of the cylinder axis, dropping the sleeve helps to point out the axis of the cylinder. (ref. p.78)

7-21. (D) Streak retinoscopy with minus cylinders can use all of the choices. (ref. p.78)

7-22. (B) If only spheres are used to neutralize the two principal meridians, a power cross is formed that must be converted to axis notation. The addition of a stenopeic slit is useful to refine the axis. (ref. p.79)

7-23. (A) Two major sources of inaccuracy in retinoscopy are irregularity of the reflexes studied and loss of accommodative control. (ref. p.79)

7-24. (D) Retinoscopy is usually performed with one eye fogged while the other eye is scoped. (ref. p.79)

7-25. (D) Irregular astigmatism can cause a wider range of neutrality, irregular intervals of myopia, and hyperopia as well as scissor type reflexes. (ref. p.79)

CHAPTER 8: REFRACTION

8-1. (E) Refining the sphere can be achieved by adding +0.25 D sphere in a monocular fashion and asking the patient to rate the change as better or worse, performing the duochrome test, performing binocular balancing with plus sphere or with vectographic techniques and stereo glasses. (ref. p.80)

8-2. (A) During subjective sphere refinement, if the addition of plus sphere is better, the refractionist should keep adding plus until no further improvement is noted. (ref. p.80)

8-3. (A) During subjective sphere refinement, a patient subjectively notes better visual acuity but objectively does not improve when plus is added. The examiner should consider a bias from magnification. (ref. p.80)

8-4. (A) During subjective sphere refinement, a patient states visual acuity is worsened with additional plus sphere. The examiner should add minus sphere and check for a reverse Galilean telescopic effect. (ref. p.80)

8-5. (B) The end point of subjective sphere refinement is achieved when visual acuity is reduced by adding any more plus or minification is achieved by adding more minus. (ref. p.80)

8-6. (B) Chromatic aberration by the crystalline lens results in blue and green light being refracted more than red light. It defines a chromatic interval that bridges the retina for 1.50 to 2.00 D. (ref. p.80)

8-7. (D) Yellow holds the emmetropic position on the retina during clinical duochrome testing. (ref. p.80)

8-8. (A) In aphakia and pseudophakia the duochrome test has no clinical value. The green appears much brighter after removal of the normal crystalline lens with its natural blue-green filter. Implants are corrected for chromatic aberration. (ref. p.81)

8-9. (E) For meaningful results from duochrome testing, the patient must be able to discriminate 0.37 D changes. The patient should be fogged to 20/30 visual acuity with +0.50 D sphere so that the red side appears clearer. The final step should be to ensure that both eyes are equally controlled with respect to accommodation. (ref. p.81)

8-10. (A) Binocular balancing is most valuable when visual acuity is equal in both eyes. (ref. p.81)

8-11. (B) Binocular balancing is best accomplished by prism dissociation and balanced fogging. Polarizing lenses with vectographic slides are also very useful. (ref. p.81)

8-12. (A) In prism dissociation for binocular balancing, the patient is binocularly fogged to 20/40 or so. (ref. p.81)

8-13. (A) +5.25 *OU* +1.00 add would be the bifocal prescription of choice affording 20/20 distance and near acuity with excellent muscle balance. Anything else requires a compromise. (ref. p.82)

8-14. (C) Every alternative is a compromise with this man. With +2.00 *OD* and +1.50 *OS,* 1 P.D. *BD OD,* and 1 P.D. *BU OS* he will blur the distance to 20/30 until he relaxes his accommodation but he sees J_2 (which is important in his occupation). The vertical fusional amplitude is not given but if he has an average amplitude, the vertical prism will bring his into the comfort range. Less plus will not give him sufficient comfort at near nor sufficient acuity (J_3). He has sufficient horizontal fusional amplitudes to ignore the 8 P.D. exophoria at first. With plus correction, this may increase and need some attention. The prism in (E) corrects a left hyperphoria. (ref. p.82)

8-15. (D) The distortion from spectacle correction of this amount of astigmatism will be intolerable. Even cutting down the cylinder may not help because the blur will be sufficient to fail the driver's test. First-time contact lens wear in 48-year-old male taxi drivers is met with a high failure rate. This might be the first modality to attempt but not likely to succeed. Similarly bifocal contacts are unlikely to succeed. The most likely to succeed would be refractive surgery with overcorrection with bifocals or half glasses for near (depending on the postop residual refractive error). A drop of a line of acuity in addition to the bilateral meridional amblyopia may disqualify him from driving. (ref. p.82)

8-16. (A) With an accommodative amplitude of +5.00 D, +2.50 D can be used with the other half held in reserve. For near work at 40 cm, +2.50 D of hyperopic correction plus +2.50 D of accommodation are required. A +2.50 D spectacle would meet the demand. This will blur the distance vision at first but with time, accommodation will relax. This is preferable to bifocals although option (B) may be the second choice if (A) is not tolerated. Contact lenses require less accommodation and can be recommended. (ref. p.82)

8-17. (D) All are possible modalities of treatment but the one with the most chance of success is soft toric contacts. This is not a happy patient. If this is not successful, refractive surgery may be necessary. (ref. p.82)

8-18. (E) If one is to rule out a refractive and accommodative component to the esotropia, full correction must be given. If a residual deviation exists, the child may be a candidate for stronger lenses or surgery. Repeat cycloplegic refraction after about 6 weeks may uncover more latent hyperopia. 2-year-olds have short arms and hold things very close; +3.00 D or stronger adds are appropriate. The bifocal segment should be set high, e.g., bisecting the pupil facilitates its use. (ref. p.82)

8-19. (B) Nuclear cataracts with index myopia occur slowly. Patients adjust to closer reading distances, and stronger adds are better tolerated than otherwise. The equivalent add to the segment in the old glasses would be +4.25 D. If the vision was poorer, one might prescribe this add knowing they already tolerated the proximal focal distance. (ref. p.82, 99)

8-20. (A) The first step is to correct the myopia. This will increase accommodation and accommodative convergence, which may alleviate most of her symptoms. If not, option (D) with some BI prism might be required. She does not yet require bifocals. Bifocals will increase the exodeviation at near relative to distance correction alone. Contacts may precipitate presbyopia and should not be the first choice. (ref. p.82, 105-7)

8-21. (C) Light rays that pass through the pupil but miss the intraocular lens produce a poorly focused secondary image. (ref. Holladay: Evaluating the IOL optic)

8-22. (A) The total magnification produced by a lens is the product of a shape factor $\left(M_S = \dfrac{1}{1 - \dfrac{t}{n} D_l}\right)$ and a power factor $\left(M_P = \dfrac{1}{1 - D_v h}\right)$, where h is the vertex in meters, D_l is the front vertex power, and D_v is the back vertex power. By altering the lens shape, manipulating the lens thickness, index of refraction and front curve (vertex power), the magnification can be altered up to about 5%. Opticians and lens manufacturers use nomograms to de-

termine optimal shape properties. (ref. p.82, 106)
Reference: See Linksz A, Bannon R. Aniseikonia and refractive problems, *Int Ophthal Clin* 5:514-534, 1965.

8-23. (C) It is not desirable to fully correct patients with high hypermetropia. Gradual increases to the convex power of the prescription are recommended. In this case prescribe glasses halfway between full correction and the present prescription, such as *OD* +3.00 D sphere: *OS* + 3.25 D sphere.

CHAPTER 9: VISION TESTING

9-1. (E) Contrast sensitivity with sine gratings is the most sensitive to test for early optic neuropathy. (ref. p.83)

9-2. (E) Testing central visual acuity with uncooperative patients is best with objective testing rather than any of the methods listed. (ref. p.83)

9-3. (B) The Snellen optotype is designed so that at a distance of 20 feet the letter subtends 5′ of arc at the nodal point of the eye. The minimum separable or visual angle is 1′ . (ref. p.83)

9-4. (D) When the visual angle is 2′ of arc, the Snellen fraction would be $\frac{6}{12}$. The object must be held twice as far as the standard Snellen "E" to subtend only 1′ of arc. (ref. p.84)

9-5. (B)
$$\frac{\text{Distance the Snellen letter subtends } 1'}{\text{Distance } 1' \text{ of minimum separable angle is discriminated by the patient}} = \frac{20}{5} = 4$$

The minimum discernible angle is 4′. (ref. p.84)

9-6. (D) (i) Visual angle: $\frac{20 \text{ feet}}{5 \text{ feet/minute}} =$ 4′ of arc

(ii) Visual acuity: $\frac{1}{4} \times \frac{20}{20} = \frac{20}{80}$

The minimum visual angle is 4′ of arc and the acuity is 20/80. (ref. p.84)

9-7. (B) A visual acuity of 20/100 means that one can resolve at 20 feet what the normal patient with 20/20 acuity can resolve at 100 feet. (ref. p.84)

(i) Visual angle: $\frac{1}{VA} = \frac{1}{20/100} = \frac{100}{20} = 5'$ of arc

(ii) The Snellen letter must be held five times as far to subtend 1′ of arc.

9-8. (D) Visual angle $= \frac{100}{20} = 5'$ of arc.

The visual angle is not age dependent. (ref. p.85)

9-9. (E) Glare occurs when patients are sensitive to bright and reflected light. These patients often have media opacities, corneal astigmatism, posterior subcapsular cataracts, or lens aberrations. (ref. p.85)

9-10. (C) Opacities degrade the axial and immediate paraxial rays, but in bright photopic conditions the pupil is smaller and the impairment is worse. (ref. p.85)

9-11. (B) Contrast sensitivity is the ability to detect slight changes in luminance in regions without sharp contours. (ref. p.85)

9-12. (E) Testing contrast sensitivity can be in projected, oscilloscope, or printed chart form, all of which are subjective methods. (ref. p.85)

9-13. (C) The diffractive implant employs multislope concentric diffractive rings on the back of a conventional implant, especially designed to establish two distinct orders of diffraction. (ref. p.86)

9-14. (A) When using refractive or diffractive bifocal implants, one must be concerned with whether the light defocused by the unused portion of the lens degrades the contrast of the one focused on the object of regard. (ref. p.86)

9-15. (D) Stereopsis (or stereoacuity) is the binocular ability of the visual system to appreciate depth. It is reduced with optic neuritis and the monofixation syndrome. (ref. p.86)

9-16. (A) Stereopsis within the confines of single binocular vision can only be perceived if an axial or horizontal disparity in the object of regard can be appreciated within Panum's fusional space. (ref. p.86)

9-17. (B) Fine stereopsis is a function of the slightly different and disparate images of an object presented to each eye. This perspective difference is related to the distance the eyes are apart or the interpupillary distance. (ref. p.86)

9-18. (A) The image disparity generated by angle θ can be fused if the image disparity still falls on corresponding retinal points and as long as x falls within Panum's space. (ref. p.86)

9-19. (D) As the distance away from the eye increases, the stereoacuity decreases. As the depth of the object increases, the angle it subtends increases. The larger the pupillary distance, the greater the stereoacuity. Pupil size does not alter stereoacuity. (ref. p.86)

9-20. (A) Certain materials are structurally arranged so that only those electric fields with their orientation in the same direction as the light are transmitted. (ref. p.87)

9-21. (E) Glass, water, plastic, and mirrors can all have polarizing properties. (ref. p.87)

9-22. (D) The Haidinger brush entoptic test is used to determine macular position and function and is clinically determined by rotating a polarizing filter in a uniform blue field. (ref. p.87)

9-23. (E) Placing a horizontal polarizing filter over one eye and a vertical polarizing filter over the other enables the examiner to perform stereotesting and sphere refinement, determine the fixing eye for penalization, as well as to selectively project polarized objects to either eye. (ref. p.87)

9-24. (D) The perifoveal region is rich in capillaries, contains photoreceptors that are relatively dark adapted beneath the blood column, and has a red blood cell column queued single file interrupted only by white blood cells. (ref. p.87)

9-25. (B) The blue field entoptoscope produces white spots when an intact capillary network is present in the foveal region. (ref. p.87)

9-26. (A) Constructive interference occurs when two light waves of equal magnitude are in phase and interact. (ref. p.88)

9-27. (B) A parallel plate of glass, when coupled with a monochromatic light source, will produce two wavefronts that will interfere with each other. (ref. p.88)

9-28. (E) The pattern of interference rings results in interference fringes; a bright band indicates constructive interference, a dark band destructive interference. Coherence is the measurement of how well the two light beams interact. (ref. p.88)

9-29. (B) The potential acuity meter projects a visual acuity chart through an aerial aperture of 0.1 mm and focuses the chart on the retina with an optometer to neutralize the refractive error. It can also determine the Snellen fraction visual acuity. (ref. p.88)

9-30. (E) Uncorrected visual acuity is standardized for military service, aviation, law enforcement, and fire fighting. Standardization applies where public safety is a major concern. (ref. p.88)

9-31. (D) Visual maturity is reached between the ages of 6 and 10 years. (ref. p.89)

9-32. (C) A 3-year-old emmetropic eye has a normal visual acuity of 20/30. (ref. p.89)

CHAPTER TEN: ACCOMMODATION AND CONVERGENCE

10-1. (A) Accommodation is a response stimulated by blurred retinal imagery, which may be contributed to by the reversal of the color blur circles secondary to chromatic aberration, bitemporal retinal disparity as an object of regard approaches, and the sensation of near. (ref. p.90)

10-2. (A) Bitemporal retinal disparity may affect the orientation and effectivity of the photoreceptors. It is also a potent stimulus for convergence. (ref. p.90)

10-3. (D) Accommodation, convergence, and miosis form the synkinetic triad of the near response. (ref. p.90)

10-4. (A) Each step in the synkinetic triad can occur independently of the other parts. (ref. p.90)

10-5. (B) Accommodation causes movement of the iris, lens, retina, and vitreous but does not cause any corneal movement. (ref. p.90)

10-6. (D) When accommodation occurs, the structural changes include contraction of the ciliary muscles, producing an anterior lens shift, and the tension of the zonules of the lens is relaxed. The lessened stress on the equatorial capsule causes an increase in the anteroposterior diameter of the lens and a decrease in the transequatorial diameter. The radii of curvature of the anterior and posterior refracting surfaces are reduced, the former more than the latter. (ref. p.90)

10-7. (B) Relaxation of the zonules increases the effectivity of the lens. Miosis increases the depth of field and decreases spherical aberration. An increase in convexity of both surfaces results in an increase in power being added to the lens, and an anterior shift in the lens position may provoke angle closure in a susceptible patient. (ref. p.90)

10-8. (B) Accommodation decreases with age because the lens proteins are structurally altered and become more rigid and less deformable. (ref. p.90)

10-9. (C) An increase in the anteroposterior and transequatorial girth of the lens leads to a shift toward myopia. (ref. p.90)

10-10. (B) Presbyopia is the reduction of accommodation due to age. (ref. p.90)

10-11. (C) The accommodative amplitude decreases by 1.50 D every 4 years between the ages of 40 and 48. (ref. p.91)

10-12. (D) With distance correction in place, the far point of the eye is at infinity. In emmetropia the near point can be directly converted to accommodative amplitude. When the eye is overplussed, the refractive error affects both the far and the near points but the difference will always equal the amplitude. (ref. p.91)

10-13. (B) The Prince rule measures, on a ruler, the near point and far point with +3.00 D lenses. (ref. p.91)

10-14. (E) Half of the accommodative amplitude should always remain in reserve. If less than half is in reserve, fatigue will occur. If only a fourth is held in reserve, recession of the near point can occur. Corrective lenses can be prescribed to maintain half of the accommodative amplitude in reserve. (ref. p.91)

10-15. (B) **(i)** Far point $= \frac{100}{3} = 33$ cm

(ii) Near point $= \frac{100}{3 + 5} = 12.5$ cm

The interval of clear vision is between 12.5 and 33 cm. (ref. p.92)

10-16. (A) Cycloplegia has great diagnostic importance in the identification of latent hyperopia and other deficiencies not listed. (ref. p.92)

10-17. (A) The basis of action of cycloplegics is their inhibition of the postganglionic response associated with acetylcholine. (ref. p.92)

10-18. (B) Cycloplegics are absorbed into the nasal mucosa and have similar effects to the administration of atropine—the systemic side effects of the anticholinergic variety. (ref. p.92)

10-19. (D) Distribution and dosage of cycloplegics should be based on body weight, surface area, and the planned method of administration. (ref. p.92)

10-20. (B) Accommodative amplitude (AA) = 4.00 D. Store half = +2.00 D

Additional distance requirement +2.00 D with the use of the accommodative amplitude.

For near at 50 cm require $\frac{100}{50} =$ +2.00 D

Therefore +4.00 D is needed for comfort. This allows clear distance vision and holds half of the AA in reserve.

R_x: single vision glasses +4.00 D

The prescription for comfortable work at 50 cm should be +4.00 D single vision glasses. (ref. p.92)

10-21. (D) **(i)** Accommodative amplitude = +3.00 D

Save one half for comfort = +1.50 D

(ii) +1.50 D remaining but + 7.00 D hyperopia

Additional requirements are +5.50 D for distance

For near at 40 cm need +2.50 D more

For comfort +8.00 D

R_x: single vision glasses of +8.00 D or bifocals of +6.50 with a +1.50 D add.

Single vision glasses of +8.00 D would enable reading at 40 cm, but distance would be blurred. +6.50 + 1.50 add as a bifocal would fit the bill as well. (ref. p.92)

10-22. (A) Common side effects of atropine 1% include nausea, dry mouth, flushing, fever, and others. (ref. p.93)

10-23. (B) The time for maximum cycloplegia in the shorter acting agents is crucial if residual accommodation is to be effectively reduced. (ref. p.93)

10-24. (A) **(i)** Far point: $\frac{100}{4} = 25$ cm

(ii) Near point: myopia + amplitude = 4.00 + 5.00 = 9.00 D; $\frac{100}{9} = 11.1$ cm

(iii) Interval of clear vision is between 11.1 and 25 cm.

The interval of clear vision without correction is between 11.1 and 25 cm. (ref. p.93)

10-25. (E) **(i)** Accommodative convergence = 20 P.D. − 15 P.D. = 5 P.D.

(ii) Accommodation $= \frac{100}{33} =$ 3.00 D

(iii) Therefore the AC/A ratio is 5/3

Using the clinical method, the AC/A ratio is 5/3. (ref. p.93)

10-26. (A) **(i)** Accommodative convergence = 35 P.D. − 10 P.D. = 25 P.D.

(ii) Accommodation = 5.00 − 1.00 = +4.00 D

(iii) Therefore the AC/A ratio is 25/4

The AC/A ratio is 25/4. (ref. p.93)

10-27. (C) When one is using the heterophoria method of AC/A determination, the total accommodative convergence found is equal to the normal accommodative convergence plus the overshoot or undershoot of convergence. (ref. p.95)

10-28. (D) The heterophoria method of AC/A determination yields higher values than the lens gradient method. (ref. p.95)

10-29. (D) When one is determining the AC/A ratio by the heterophoria method, a patient is found to be more exodeviated at near. The exodeviation in this case represents an undershoot and must be subtracted from the normal convergence. (ref. p.95)

10-30. (B) A patient has a 5 cm pupillary distance, a near deviation of 15 P.D. esophoria, and a far deviation of 10 P.D. esophoria. If her accommodation is +6.00 D, the resultant AC/A ratio as found by the heterophoria method is 5.83/1. (ref. p.95)

(i) $\frac{AC}{A} = PD + \frac{P.D_N - P.D_D}{D}$

$= 5 + \frac{15 - 10}{6} = 5.83$

10-31. (B) **(i)** Accommodative amplitude $= \frac{1}{⅔} - \frac{1}{2} = \frac{3}{2} - \frac{1}{2} =$ +1.00 D

(ii) Amplitude in reserve = +0.50 D

(iii) To see clearly at 40 cm = $\frac{100}{40} = +2.50$ D

(iv) The patient is 0.50 D myopic.

(v) Need to supply +2.50 D − 0.50 D = +2.00 D for reading at 40 cm. Use +0.50 D from AA reduces readers to +1.50 D

−0.50 + 2.00 add or +1.50 D readers are needed. (ref. p.95)

10-32. (C)

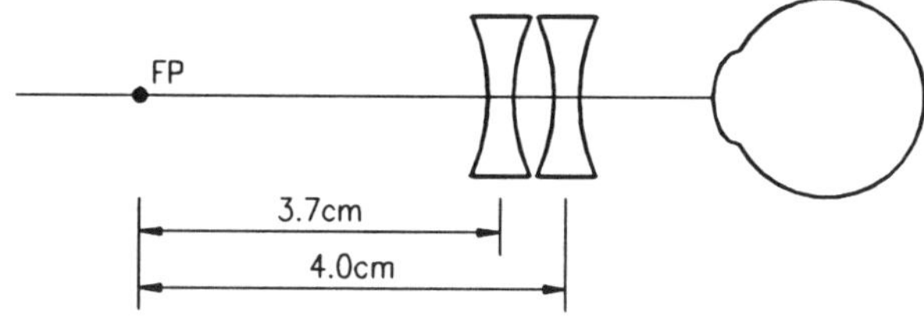

−27.00 D of myopia

Far point $= \frac{100}{-27} = 3.70$ cm = 37 mm

$-25\text{ D} = \frac{1}{f}; f = 4.0\text{ cm} = 40\text{ mm}$

f must be coincident with FP to correct the myopia.

To correct a −27.00 D error with a −25.00 D lens, the secondary focal point of the latter must be placed at the far point of the −27.00 D lens, or in other words moved 3 mm towards the eye. (ref. p.95)

10-33. (D) The clinical method of AC/A determination ignores the pupillary distance, is not numerically accurate enough, and reflects the same abnormalities as the heterophoria method. (ref. p.96)

CHAPTER 11: PRESCRIBING

11-1. (B) Diabetes insipidus does not result in acquired hyperopia. (ref. p.97)

11-2. (C) Orthokeratology corrects myopia by flattening the central portion of the cornea. There probably is some compensatory peripheral steepening. (ref. p.97)

11-3. (E) Astigmatism can be acquired by means of ptosis, pterygia, keratoplasty, lid tumors, and many other diseases. (ref. p.97)

11-4. (D) Manifest hyperopia is that amount of hyperopia which can be accepted by the patient without cycloplegia to maintain or obtain 20/20 visual acuity. (ref. p.98)

11-5. (D) The absolute portion of hyperopia is that part which cannot be compensated for by the available accommodative amplitude. (ref. p.98)

11-6. (A) Latent hyperopia is compensated for by the accommodative amplitude. (ref. p.98)

11-7. (C) The total amount of hyperopia is equal to the sum of the facultative, absolute, and latent components of hyperopia. (ref. p.98)

11-8. (C) In deciding the amount of correction given to a hyperopic person, consideration must be given to the severity of the symptoms, visual needs, occupation, ocular motility status, age and amplitude of accommodation. Gender should not affect correction. (ref. p.98)

11-9. (B) If the hyperopic patient is young, asymptomatic, orthophoric with a good amplitude, no correction is necessary. (ref. p.98)

11-10. (B) The hyperopia is distributed as follows: (ref. p.98)

(i) 0-20/50
(ii) +2.00 – 20/20 absolute (+2.00 D)
(iii) +5.00 – 20/20 facultative (+3.00 D)
(iv) +8.00 – 20/20 latent (+3.00 D)

Manifest = Absolute + Faculatative = +5.00 D
Total = Latent + Manifest = +8.00 D

11-11. (A) If a hyperopic patient is young with an exophoria or exotropia, only the absolute hyperopia is corrected. (ref. p.99)

11-12. (E) Correction to preserve half the amplitude of accommodation is important for presbyopia, accommodative insufficiency, orthophoria, and esophoria. (ref. p.99)

11-13. (B) A person with hyperopia can delay the use of bifocals with contact lenses. (ref. p.99)

11-14. (D) Hyperopic persons are accustomed to very clear distance vision and are intolerant of ANY overcorrection. Undercorrection of hyperopia is better tolerated than any overcorrection. (ref. p.99)

11-15. (B) Myopia is a progressive disease often associated with exodeviations presumably on the basis of reduced accommodative demand and reduced accommodative convergence. (ref. p.99)

11-16. (A) Factors contributing to the progression of myopia include ciliary muscle tonus and accommodation. (ref. p.100)

11-17. (C) Night myopia is an anomalous myopia similar to instrument and empty field myopia. (ref. p.100)

11-18. (A) Laser speckle optometers are used to measure the amount of night myopia by creating reflected laser light from a granular surface whose direction of motion varies with the refractive error. (ref. p.100)

11-19. (D) The movement of speckles when using a laser speckle optometer are one way in myopia (with) and opposite in hyperopia (against). (ref. p.100)

11-20. (B) Both dark retinoscopy and laser speckle optometry converge on the concept of a dark focus, which is a true resting state between distance and near. (ref. p.100)

11-21. (B) Under scotopic conditions it is natural to overaccommodate for distance and underaccommodate for near. (ref. p.100)

11-22. (B) Radial keratotomy was first performed by the Japanese, who approached it from the endothelial side with radial partial thickness incisions designed to flatten the central cornea. Fyodorov's method involves a variable number of 90% thickness radial incisions from the epithelial side of the cornea. (ref. p.100)

11-23. (B) Keratomileusis involves the removal and controlled lathing of a lamellar autolenticule, which is flattened and returned to its original bed. It flattens the cornea but is not without risk. (ref. p.101)

11-24. (E) In astigmatic children full correction is given. (ref. p.101)

11-25. (E) Astigmatic children have little problem with distortion. Cortical readaption is readily accomplished. (ref. p.101)

11-26. (C) In asymptomatic astigmatic adults who have achieved adaption, the practitioner should avoid major changes in the axis of the correcting cylinder. (ref. p.101)

11-27. (B) The correction of the 35-year-old engineer should be rotated toward 90°. (ref. p.101)

11-28. (E) In presbyopic undercorrected myopia the only way to test if full correction for distance will precipitate problems at near is to fully correct with a trial frame and test at near under binocular conditions. (ref. p.102)

11-29. (E) If a previously undercorrected astigmatic person does not tolerate full correction and distortion proves to be the problem, the following approaches might prove to be helpful. The power of the cylinder could be reduced, contacts could be prescribed, correction could be at the minimum vertex distance, and the cylinder axis should be rotated toward 180, 90, or the old axis, whichever is most acceptable. (ref. p.102)

11-30. (A) T, L, and curvilinear keratotomy procedures can be used to reduce or eliminate corneal astigmatism, but they are not as yet very predictable. (ref. p.102)

11-31. (E) When correcting for presbyopia, it is important to consider the accommodative range and amplitude, the image jump and displacement, any induced anisophoria, and contact lenses with their altered accommodative demand. (ref. p.102)

11-32. (C) Bifocals and trifocals are poorly tolerated with neck problems. When prescribing for presbyopia it is common practice to undercorrect rather than overcorrect. Try bifocals if any distance correction is required and handle any induced prismatic effect in anisometropia with slab-off prism or single vision readers. (ref. p.103)

11-33. (D) When measuring high plus or minus bifocal lenses for presbyopia a new reading in the segment should be performed. The distance and near front vertex power should be taken and the glasses reversed from their normal position in the lensmeter. (ref. p.104)

11-34. (D) When nuclear sclerosis produces myopia, the reading distance becomes closer. The patient adjusts to the proximity and magnification of this new reading distance.

If the myopia is corrected for distance, a boost in the add is better tolerated. (ref. p.104)

11-35. (A) Convergence is a disconjugate (nonparallel) monocular or binocular eye movement to maintain the object of regard on corresponding retinal points. (ref. p.105)

11-36. (E) Sheard's criteria for convergence insufficiency state that less than double the phoria is measurable as the horizontal fusional amplitude. (ref. p.105)

11-37. (D) High adds are better tolerated by monocular patients, increase the convergence demands of binocular patients, and can be coupled with prisms. (ref. p.105)

11-38. (A) Amblyopia is very common in young anisometropic persons. It is more common in hypermetropic anisometropia than in myopic anisometropia. Lack of binocularity promotes strabismus. Treatment consists of occlusion, penalization, pleioptics, or orthoptics and stops the progression of the disease. (ref. p.106)

11-39. (D) In adults with anisometropia the amount of correction is that which maintains fusion and single binocular vision. (ref. p.106)

11-40. (C) Nonpresbyopic adults can avert any induced anisophoria by using the optical centers of their distance correction. (ref. p.106)

11-41. (E) Prism therapy should only be given to symptomatic patients and should involve the exact amount of prism needed to control the symptoms. Decentration is effective in high myopia and hyperopia. Prisms may be used to shift the null point in nystagmus patients when a head turn is present. (ref. p.107)

11-42. (A) A BO prism requires BI, apex out to correct it. This induces an exophoria and hence requires more convergence. (ref. p.107)

11-43. (A) There is still hope that fusion is achievable without prisms, but there are limits to patience and sick leave. To get him back to work he will require some BO prism. Give him the least amount to allow fusion. If he wears glasses, use Fresnel Press-On Prisms. If not, ground prism glasses are necessary. (ref. p.107)

11-44. (E) Incomitant strabismus can be treated with surgery, orthoptics, prisms for primary and downgaze as well as Fresnel prisms. (ref. p.108)

11-45. (E) It is true that cyclovertical disorders cannot be corrected with prisms. Combined horizontal and vertical prisms add vectorally. A double Maddox rod test is useful to examine incomitant cyclovertical strabismus. It is also true that patients "eat up" prism as their fusional amplitudes are relaxed. (ref. p.108)

11-46. (E) When binocular aphakia is spectacle corrected, a smaller portion of the visual field of each eye now covers a larger retinal area. Everything appears closer and taller. (ref. p.109)

11-47. (D) The size of the refractive scotoma depends on the power, vertex distance, and the size of the lens. (ref. p.109)

11-48. (E) Through a high plus lens it can be seen that the scotoma corresponding to the blind spot is found closer to fixation, and all isopters of the field appear smaller. (ref. p.110)

11-49. (B) Segment decentration can improve induced prismatic effects of a person with bilateral spectacle-corrected aphakia trying to read inside the distance optical centers. (ref. p.110)

11-50. (C) The advantages of plus aspheric

lenses include weight reduction, cosmetic superiority, and their ability to be set in more modern frames. These lenses do not, however, prevent magnification of the eye or the view. (ref. p.111)

11-51. (A) Each millimeter of anterior displacement of an IOL is equal to a change in implant power equal to 1 D. (ref. p.112)

11-52. (E) Each millimeter error in axial length results in a refractive error of 2.50 D. (ref. p.112)

11-53. (E) The important factors in accurately predicting the correct implant power include the position of the lens implant, the type of lens implant selected, the surgeon, the axial length, and the *K* readings of the patient. (ref. p.112)

11-54. (C) A new term called the "anterior chamber depth factor" estimates the distance from the iris to the principal plane of the IOL to improve the predictability of implant power selection. (ref. p.113)

11-55. (C) $D_{IOL} = P - \frac{R}{1.5} = +15.00 \text{ D} - \left(\frac{-2.00}{1.5}\right) =$

+16.33 D is the required power for the IOL. (ref. p.113)

11-56. (A) $D_{IOL} = P - \frac{R}{1.5} = +22.00 \text{ D} - \left(\frac{-4.50}{1.5}\right) =$

+25.00 D is the strength of IOL required. (ref. p.113)

11-57. (B) $D = +17.00 \text{ D} - (118.7 - 116.2) = +14.50 \text{ D}$ should be the power for emmetropia. (ref. p.113)

11-58. (A) The single most important factor when selecting the power of an implant is the *A* constant. (ref. p.113)

11-59. (B) The shape factor of the implant greatly contributes to both the IOL power and the value of the A constant. (ref. p.113)

11-60. (D) Biconvex implants are currently favored because they minimize spherical aberrations, cause less image degradation when decentered and reduce posterior capsular opacification rates. (ref. p.113)

11-61. (C) When converting from a meniscus to a biconvex lens, the *A* constant usually requires a change of +2.00 D. (ref. p.113)

11-62. (A) $D_{IOL} = P - \frac{R}{1.5} = +16.00 - \left(\frac{-4.00 \text{ D}}{1.5}\right) = +18.67 \text{ D}$

The power of the IOL must be +18.67 D to achieve a refractive error of −4.00 D postoperatively. (ref. p.113)

11-63. (E) $D_{IOL} = IOL - (A_{POST} - A_{ANT})$

$+12.50 = +16.50 - (118 - A_{ANT})$

$A_{ANT} = 118 - 4 = 114$

The *A* constant for the anterior chamber IOL must be 114. (ref. p.113)

11-64. (C) $D_{IOL} = P - \frac{R}{1.5}$

$18.00 = P - \left(\frac{-4.50}{1.50}\right)$

$P = +15.00 \text{ D}$

Under these circumstances the SRK formula predicts +15.00 D for emmetropia. (ref. p.113)

11-65. (D) If the patient preoperatively can tolerate contact lenses (don't forget disposables), I think that it is most reasonable to shoot for emmetropia with a +8.00 D IOL if the patient wishes clear uncorrected distance vision. Many persons with myopia like uncorrected reading ability and might prefer option (A). You should include the patient in the decision making. To fit a contact lens postoperatively is fraught with hazard. If the patient is intolerant, there is intolerable anisometropia and diplopia. Find out preoperatively. For −4.50 D of postoperative myopia, a + 11.00 D IOL is required not + 12.50 D.

$$D_{IOL} = +8.00 - \left(\frac{-4.50}{1.50}\right) = +11.00\ \text{D}$$

It is preferable to implant an IOL even with successful contact lens use. (ref. p.112-13)

11-66. (E) Attempts have been made to produce bifocal contact lenses by diffractive and refractive means by having concentric distance and near bands, Fresnel optics, simultaneous near and distance perception, and asphericity. (ref. p.114)

11-67. (D) Preoperatively a patient comfortably wears −1.00 +4.00 × 90. Postoperatively the refraction is plano. The patient complains of distortion in spite of 6/6 vision because cortical adaption has occurred to correct the distortion but is no longer necessary. (ref. p.114)

11-68. (B) Diffraction means to break apart. (ref. p.114)

11-69. (B) The size of the pupil that has the highest resolving power is 2.5 mm. (There is some dispute about this.) (ref. p.115)

11-70. (D) A patient wearing his best correction improves with a pinhole. This means that any or all of the following are true. The correction is not the best possible; irregular astigmatism is present or the pupil is dilated. (ref. p.115)

11-71. (B) A patient wearing his best correction reduces his acuity with a pinhole. This suggests that retinal problems or diffuse medial opacities may exist. Dilated pupils and mixed astigmatism improve with a pinhole. (ref. p.115)

11-72. (C) When the pinhole is used as a screening process, it can crudely determine if the reduced acuity is on a refractive basis or not. (ref. p.115)

11-73. (A) When one is using a pinhole, diffraction will reduce a 20/20 emmetrope's visual acuity to 20/25. Persons with very high hyperopia or myopia experience minimal improvement. When high plus or minus lenses are used in conjunction with the pinhole, the effect is greater. If the target moves in the same direction (with motion), the patient is myopic. (ref. p.115)

11-74. (D) The method that is currently most accurate for measuring the power of an IOL once implanted is by slit-lamp photography. This method should be used before the implant is exchanged. (ref. Holladay: Determining IOL power within the eye)

11-75. (E) With the slit-lamp beam illuminating the diffusing target, the Purkinje-Sanson I and III images can be visualized as well as the posterior IOL image and the anterior corneal image. (ref. Holladay: Determining IOL power within the eye)

11-76. (C) When measuring the power of an IOL within the eye using the reflected image from the anterior IOL surface, one must take into account the magnifying effect of the cornea. (ref. Holladay: Determining the IOL power within the eye)

11-77. (B) An error of 0.50 D in *K* readings results in an error of 0.25 D in the computed lens power. (ref. Holladay: Determining the IOL power within the lens)

11-78. (A) An error of 0.50 D is induced by an error in the anterior chamber depth of 0.5 mm. (ref. Holladay:

Determining the IOL power within the eye)

11-79. (D) If the magnification ratio of the reflected image is off by 15% the computed lens power is off by 1.50 D. (ref. Holladay: Determining the IOL power within the eye)

11-80. (B) If the decentration of the IOL is greater than 1.00 mm, it is clinically significant in affecting vision. (ref. Holladay: Evaluating the IOL optic)

11-81. (D) The aspheric and meniscus lenses cause the greatest amount of astigmatism with decentration. (ref. Holladay: Evaluating the IOL optic)

11-82. (D) When one is determining the optimal size of a capsulotomy, the main factor is diffraction. (ref. Holladay: The optimal size for a posterior capsulotomy)

11-83. (C) The optimal posterior capsulotomy should equal or exceed the diameter of the pupil in scotopic conditions and remain within the border of the IOL. (ref. Holladay: The optimal size for a posterior capsulotomy)

11-84. (C) The typical scotopic pupil diameter following extracapsular cataract extraction with a posterior chamber lens varies between 3.9 and 5.0 mm. (ref. Holladay: The optimal size for a posterior capsulotomy)

11-85. (B) Holladay has identified criteria to identify those measurements which are unusual and require remeasurement if you wish to avoid unpleasant refractive surprises postoperatively. He recommends repeat measurements if:

1. Axial length <22.0 mm or >25.0 mm
2. Average corneal power <40 D or >47 D
3. Calculated emmetropic IOL power is more than 3 D from the average for that specific IOL style
   A constant with surgeon factor, $K = 43.81$ D, axial length $= 23.5$ mm)
4. Between the eyes, the difference in:
   (a) average corneal power >1 D
   (b) axial length >0.3 mm
   (c) emmetropia IOL power >1 D

(ref. Holladay: A Three-part System for Refining Intraocular Lens Power Calculations)

11-86. (E) The photopic pupil is too small and a capsulotomy this size contributes to glare. Extending a capsulotomy beyond the IOL border can lead to vitreous prolapse. According to Holladay, the optimal capsulotomy size equals or exceeds the scotopic pupil and remains within the border of the IOL.
(ref. Holladay: The optimal size of a posterior capsulotomy)

REFERENCES

(1) Holladay JT et al: A three-part system for refining intraocular lens power calculations, *J Cataract Refract Surg* 13:17-24, 1988.

(2) Holladay JT, Rubin ML: Avoiding refractive problems in cataract surgery, *Surv Ophthalmol* 30(6):357-359, 1988.

(3) Holladay JT: Determining intraocular lens power within the eye, Am Intraocular Implant Soc J 11:353-363, 1985.

(4) Holladay JT: Evaluating the intraocular lens optic, *Surv Ophthalmol* 30(6):385-390, 1986.

(5) Holladay JT, Bishop JE, Lewis JW: The optimal size of a posterior capsulotomy, Am Intraocular Implant Soc 11:18-20, 1985.

CHAPTER 12: MATERIALS

12-1. (A) Glass is an amorphorous, inorganic substance with atoms that are strongly bound by covalent bonds yet randomly arranged. (ref. p.117)

12-2. (B) Glass has no definite melting point. It has softening and annealing points as its important temperature barriers. (ref. p.117)

12-3. (B) Crown glass is one optical grade of glass with an index of refraction equal to 1.523. Crown glass weighs 50% more than plastic, warps less, but does require impact resistance treatment. (ref. p.117)

12-4. (E) High index glass has greater vergence for the same radius of curvature. This allows the lens to be thinner. They are more refractive, have greater color dispersion, are more brittle, and are more difficult to work in the lab. (ref. p.117)

12-5. (D) Photochromic glass changes color on absorption of UV light by chemical dissociation of silver chloride. It darkens at a speed which is inversely proportional to the temperature of the glass. (ref. p.117)

12-6. (C) Antireflection coatings (especially on high index materials) are almost universally accompanied by complaints of difficulty keeping the lenses clean. (ref. p.117)

12-7. (E) With silver chloride photochromic glass one can integrate a tint, put a UV coat on the back (which will not inhibit the dissociation process), perform antireflection treatment, and trap the darkened state permanently under special conditions. (ref. p.118)

12-8. (B) Composite technology binds a central plastic polymer to an outer glass lens without the use of bonding agents. (ref. p.118)

12-9. (A) Plastics are macromolecular, organic polymers that can be shaped when heated. (ref. p.118)

12-10. (C) CR-39 constitutes 80% of the lenses dispensed. The index of refraction is 1.498 with relatively low color dispersion. It is lighter than crown but thicker. It is easy to work with in the lab and is quite cheap.(ref. p.119)

12-11. (E) High index plastics (HIPs) make lenses with flatter curves, thinner, lighter, and with an index of refraction around 1.600 D. (ref. p.119)

12-12. (E) HIPs filter all UV less than 380 nm. The surface is softer than CR-39, so scratch coating is necessary. There is considerably more reflection in HIPs, so AR coating is necessary. Wash coating is also preferable. (ref. p.119)

12-13. (C) Polycarbonate "of old" had many disadvantages including its softness, thinness, and eagerness to flex and warp when mounted in a tight frame. The center thickness required 1.8 mm just for stability. Color dispersion was high. The surface was hard to work, and warpage was significant. (ref. p.119-20)

12-14. (A) The new polycarbonate can be cast in glass molds. It is less flexible, allowing the center thickness to be reduced to 1.3 mm. (ref. p.120)

12-15. (B) Polycarbonates produce edge thickness problems in myopia and center thickness problems in hyperopia. Aspheric lenses reduce the curvature from the center to the periphery of the lens. By reducing the curvature of the polycarbonates, lens thickness is reduced. This in turn increases the field. (ref. p.120)

12-16. (E) New aspheric lenses are available for larger frames, approach a flat front surface, flatten a lens, and reduce oblique astigmatism. (ref. p.120)

12-17. (D) The residual myopic halo rings can be reduced by coloring the edges with Cruxite, selecting darker frames, and polishing the edges with a light pink. (ref. p.120)

12-18. (C) Special high index glass (n = 1.800) is used for x-ray absorption. For x-ray protection, a minimum center thickness must be maintained with or without side shields applied. (ref. p.120)

12-19. (D) The standards for impact resistance vary according to the end use of the lens and for center thickness according to the material. These standards also vary by country of origin. (ref. p.120)

12-20. (A) In the United states the standard test for casual dress wear involves dropping a steel ball of ⅝ inch diameter that weights 16 oz from a height of 50 inches without breaking the lens. (ref. p.120)

12-21. (B) To ensure consumer protection, chemically hardened lenses must have a minimum center thickness of 1.8 mm. (ref. p.120)

12-22. (B) To heat temper glass the glass is heated between its annealing and softening point. This is determined by weighing the polished, ground, and edged lens and heating it for a specified duration according to the finished weight. This is air cooled or quenched, causing the outside lens to toughen and the inside to remain under internal stress. (ref. p.121)

12-23. (A) With heat tempered lenses, breakage results in multiple similar, small, smooth-edged pieces instead of splinters and shards. (ref. p.121)

12-24. (D) A heat treated lens cannot be reworked in the lab. It is left with slightly different indices of refraction in different regions. It is able to polarize light, which can be detected before the lens is inadvertently worked on in the lab. (ref. p.121)

12-25. (D) Chemical tempering involves the exchange of smaller sodium ions on the lens with larger potassium or lithium ions. (ref. p.121)

12-26. (C) Chemical tempering can be used for photochromic lenses. (ref. p.121)

12-27. (D) Tints can be deposited on a lens surface in a vacuum, integrated into the material during its manufacture, or fused or cemented as a layer to white glass. (ref. p.122)

12-28. (D) Any integrated tint will have the depth of color of the tint vary with the distance from the center of the lens, the thickness of the lens, and the degree of anisometropia. (ref. p.122)

12-29. (A) The fusion of an equitint or graduated tint layer to the surface of glass distributes the color as desired irrespective of the prescription. (ref. p.122)

12-30. (E) Metals and metallic compounds can be deposited on the surface of glass by a vacuum deposition process. They can be finished with gold, silver, zinc, or chromium. They alter reflected light rather than the absorption spectrum. Special equipment is required to deposit metals or metallic compounds on plastic lenses. (ref. p.122)

12-31. (A) Plastic lenses in a heated immersion bath can be surface dyed according to the surface characteristics of the material. (ref. p.122)

12-32. (C) UV filtration can be achieved by an integrated chromophore that absorbs UV light. Infrared tints can use ferrous oxides and other absorptive lens materials. UV filtration can be achieved by dipping the lens in a heated, colored bath. Tinted lenses can produce adverse effects on color matching. (ref. p.122)

12-33. (A) **(i)** $\frac{D_{glass}}{D_{plastic}} = \frac{n_{crown} - n_{aq}}{n_{plastic} - n_{aq}} = \frac{1.52 - 1.33}{1.49 - 1.33} = \frac{0.19}{0.16}$

(ii) $D_{glass} = \frac{0.19}{0.16} \times D_{plastic} = \frac{0.19}{0.16}(+18.00\ D) = +21.38\ D$

The power of the plastic IOL is +18.00 D. An IOL made of crown glass with the same thickness and surface curvature is +21.38 D. (ref. p.19, 122)

12-34. (E) The following are calculations for the percentage of incident reflected light for the given materials. The formula used for these calculations is $R = \left(\frac{n' - n}{n' + n}\right)^2$.

(ref. p.123)

(i) Crown glass ($n' = 1.523$):

$$R = \left(\frac{1.523 - 1}{1.523 + 1}\right)^2 \times 100\% = 4.3\%$$

(ii) CR-39 ($n' = 1.490$):

$$R = \left(\frac{1.490 - 1}{1.490 + 1}\right)^2 \times 100\% = 3.9\%$$

(iii) Index 7 ($n' = 1.70$):

$$R = \left(\frac{1.700 - 1}{1.700 + 1}\right)^2 \times 100\% = 6.7\%$$

12-35. (B) Destructive interference would eliminate all reflection if the reflected light from the first surface is 180° out of phase with the reflected light from the second surface. (ref. p.124)

12-36. (B) When one is applying a multilayer AR coating to a lens, the lens must be preheated, not cooled, to improve the coating adherence. This may not apply to magnetron sputtering. (ref. p.124)

12-37. (C) The lens materials that cannot undergo AR coating because of the elevated temperatures include laminates, polarized lenses, thermal segments, and thermal lenticulars. (ref. p.125)

12-38. (C) AR coatings can be predictably stripped chemically from CR-39, crown, and photochromic glass. (ref. p.125)

12-39. (E) Antiscratch coating should be applied before undergoing AR coating, and consists of a cured hard resin, which is baked onto the surface of the lens. (ref. p.125)

12-40. (A) Glazing is the process of mounting lenses into frames. (ref. p.125)

12-41. (C) A hot air blower can be used to safely heat and expand an organic frame. (ref. p.125)

12-42. (A) If a lens is off-axis by a few degrees, an attempt to heat the frame and rotate the lens is recommended (except with bifocals). (ref. p.126)

12-43. (B) The effective diameter of the lens is the widest part of the lens and will influence the size of the lens blank selected to grind the lens. (ref. p.126)

12-44. (D) The pupillary distance (PD) and the distance between lenses (DBL) are the two values that determine the amount the lens blanks are decentered to fit the frame. (ref. p.126)

12-45. (A) Matching the pupillary distance (PD) of the frame to that of the patient minimizes decentration errors. (ref. p.127)

12-46. (E) Bridge configuration is a major consideration when selecting frames. People with flat bridges are usually fit with nosepads. Adjustable nosepads for high dioptric prescriptions allow vertex distance adjustments. Silicone nosepads are very soft and inert. (ref. p.127)

12-47. (C) Tortoiseshell has unique natural properties, which include the ability to form strong bonds with itself under heat and pressure. (ref. p.127)

12-48. (E) The DBL is 22 mm. One half the horizontal diameter is 22 mm *OU*. The mechanical PD is 66 mm. This is 8 mm too long relative to the patient's PD. There must be a 4 mm decentration in each lens for the two to be coincident. (ref. p.127)

12-49. (B)

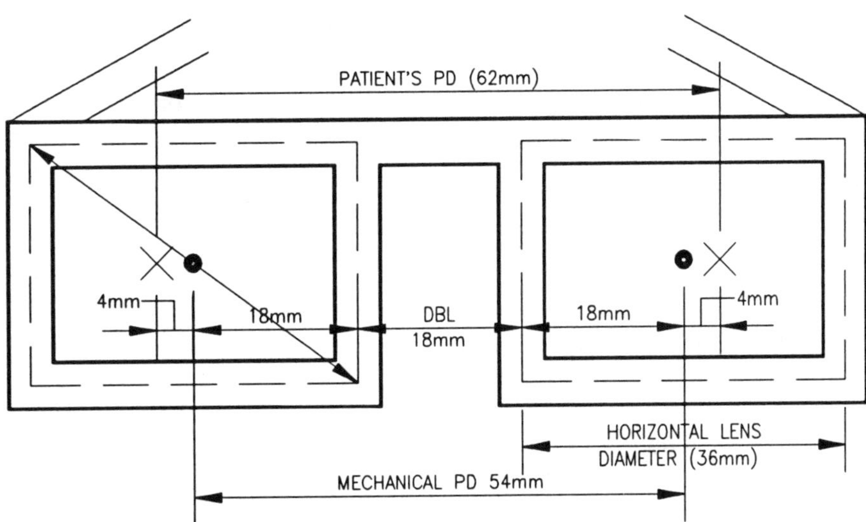

The DBL is 18 mm. One half the horizontal diameter is 18 mm *OU*. The mechanical PD is 54 mm. This is 8 mm shorter than the patient's PD. There must be a 4 mm decentration out of each lens for the two to be coincident. (ref. p.127)

12-50. (E) Synthetic plastic frames can be made of plexiglas, CR-39, nylon, and celluloid. (ref. p.128)

12-51. (B) Synthetic plastic frames can originate as a molten liquid that is cast as a dye. (ref. p.128)

12-52. (D) Celluloid and cellulose acetate share their workability. (ref. p.128)

12-53. (E) Nylon has reentered the market with a thinner, stronger product which has an inherent memory lock for adjustments. It is easier to insert lenses into these new frames. (ref. p.128)

12-54. (B) Metal frames are the most durable product on the market. (ref. p.129)

12-55. (A) Gold is corrosion resistant, acid resistant, tarnishes with difficulty, is easily worked, and can be alloyed to change its color and strength. (ref. p.129)

12-56. (B) Aluminum is light but loses its strength with bending. It is anodized to alter its surface to the oxide form, which is more resistant. It can be painted or colored as desired. It is a high heat conductor and is best insulated with plastic. (ref. p.129)

12-57. (C) Titanium is flexible, corrosion resistant, light, with excellent memory retention, and heat resistance. (ref. p.129)

12-58. (E) Stainless steel is made up of mostly iron but does not rust. It is nonmagnetic and corrosion resistant and cannot be soldered. (ref. p.129)

12-59. (B) For every 2° of pantoscopic tilt, the optical centers must be adjusted by 1 mm to compensate. (ref. p.130)

12-60. (D) When one is measuring the pupillary distance, the distance between the corneal light reflexes fixing a distance or near light, the nasal limbus to temporal limbus of the other eye or similar pupillary border measurements may prove useful. (ref. p.130)

12-61. (B) When one is measuring the vertex distance, a small gauge called the distometer or lenscorometer is used. An adjustment for closed lids is made of about 1 mm but this depends on the instrument being used. (ref. p.130)

12-62. (D) In the modern lab existing frames can be analyzed by a computer. The following measurements can be found: contour and shape, total circumference, and the correct lens blank to accommodate the prescription. (ref. p.130)

12-63. (D) The working block is created by using an alloy with a low melting point that fixes a metal working piece to a finished, protected surface. It is necessary to fix the lens in position for grinding the uncut back surface and for holding the lens in place for polishing. (ref. p.131)

CHAPTER 13: CONTACT LENSES

13-1. (C) The optical advantages of using contact lenses over spectacle correction include the following: the optical centers of contact lenses follow the visual axes; they eliminate any induced prismatic effect, and fogging does not occur. Contact lenses do not correct all spherical aberrations. (ref. p.133)

13-2. (D) When using contact lenses, reducing the vertex distance reduces minification, magnification, and the aniseikonic effects on retinal imagery. (ref. p.133)

13-3. (A) A contact lens and its protein coat are antigenic substances and can interact with immune mechanisms to cause problems. (ref. p.133)

13-4. (C) Lenticular astigmatism can be corrected with a bitoric hard or a soft toric contact lens. The latter corrects both corneal and lenticular astigmatism. (ref. p.101, 133)

13-5. (B) Hard lenses are polymethylmethacrylate. They have less than 3% water content and are virtually oxygen impermeable. They are less comfortable than soft lenses but yield superior visual results. (ref. p.133-4)

13-6. (A) Cellulose acetate butyrate (CAB) lenses and various silicone polymers are gas permeable and require less adaption time than hard lenses. (ref. p.134)

13-7. (A) As the radius of curvature decreases, the refractive power denoted by the K reading increases with the formula $K = \frac{0.3375}{r}$. They are related dioptrically but not linearly. (ref. p.134)

13-8. (B) $K = \frac{n' - n}{r} = \frac{1.3375 - 1}{r} =$ 42.00 D; $r = 8.036$ mm
The radius of curvature of this lens is 8.036 mm. (ref. p.134)

13-9. (B) The conventional way to express contact lens power is in minus cylinder form. (ref. p.135)

13-10. (C) The posterior optical zone is constructed to conform to the central corneal contour. (ref. p.135)

13-11. (A) When different radii of curvature meet to form a junction, this junction is called a blend. (ref. p.135)

13-12. (E) When fitting hard or rigid gas permeable contacts, "fitting on *K*" is where the flattest *K* and the lens are fitted parallel. (ref. p.135)

13-13. (C) 50 @ 90 = 50 × 180
46 @ 180 = 46 × 90
Eye error = +4.00 × 180
This patient's eye error is +4.00 × 180. (ref. p.135)

13-14. (B) It is common clinical practice to fit a rigid gas permeable lens one diopter steeper than the flattest *K*. (ref. p.136)

13-15. (E) If the lens is fit properly, the corneal apex is just cleared. A physiologic gas and fluid exchange occurs. The power is altered by tears filling the space between the contact and the cornea, creating an additional refracting meniscus. (ref. p.136)

13-16. (C) The "rule of thumb" for contact lenses states that for every 0.05 mm change in radius of curvature an adjustment of 0.25 D must be made to the power. If steeper, add minus (SAM). If flatter, add plus (FAP). (ref. p.136)

13-17. (C) **(i)** Difference in length = 0.05 × 4 = 0.2 mm
(ii) Steeper add minus (SAM) = change in power is −1.00 D
If one is fitting 1.00 D steeper than the flattest *K*, the posterior radius of curvature must be 0.2 mm shorter and the lens power corrected by −1.00 D. (ref. p.136)

13-18. (E) The advantages of hard lenses include the ability to be custom fit, reground, steepened, or flattened and polished. (ref. p.136)

13-19. (E) If both meridians of a contact are the same radius, the lens is spherical. If the cylinder is ground on the back surface, the lens is a back toric lens. If it is also ground on the front surface, the lens is bitoric. BD prism ballast will orient the lens by gravity. (ref. p.136)

13-20. (B) Truncation enables the portion of the lens that follows the axis of the lower lid angle to be removed. This stabilizes the lens in the desired axis. (ref. p.136)

13-21. (D) **(i)** Rule of thumb: for every 0.05 mm change in radius, an adjustment of 0.25 D in the appropriate direction must be made.
+1.00 D change = 4 × 0.25
4 × (0.05 mm) = 0.2 mm steeper
(ii) SAM (steeper add minus); therefore add −1.00 D (ref. p.136)

13-22. (A) A lenticular bevel is formed when the edges of a high minus lens are thinned. (ref. p.137)

13-23. (A) To steepen a lens, either the diameter of the lens is increased or the radius of curvature decreased or both. Both of these in turn increase the chord diameter, which will therefore steepen the lens. (ref. p.137)

13-24. (E)

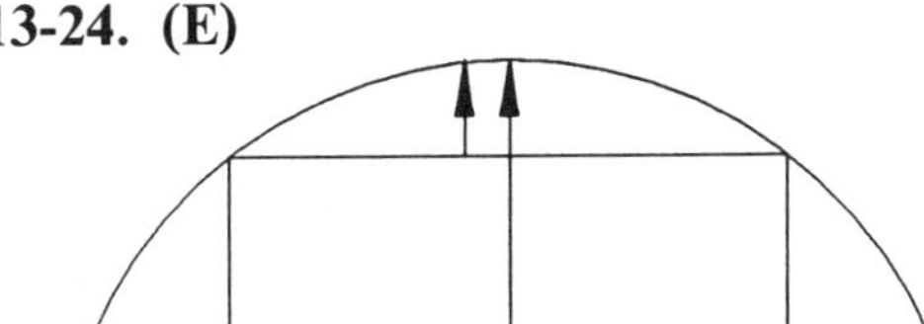

If the lens diameter is decreased, the lens is flattened by decreasing the apical vault. (ref. p.137)

13-25. (E) Soft toric lenses offer the same comfort as regular soft lenses. They can correct corneal and lenticular astigmatism. They are fit tighter resulting in less rotation than regular soft lenses. This often reduces their wear time relative to regular soft lenses. (ref. p.138)

13-26. (B) The index of refraction of the cornea used to standardize the keratometer is 1.3375. (ref. p.139)

13-27. (B)

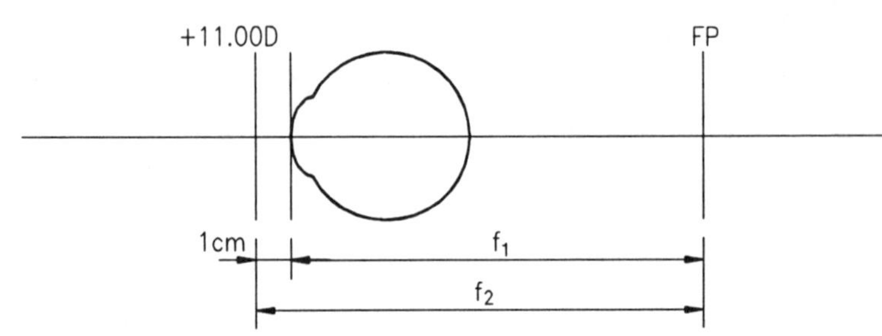

(i) +9.00 + 2.00 × 90 in minus cylinder form
+11.00 − 2.00 × 180 (V_x 10 mm) use only sphere

(ii) At vertex 10 mm: $f_2 = \frac{100}{11}$ = 9.09 cm
At corneal plane vertex = 0:
$f_1 = \frac{100}{9.09 - 1} = \frac{100}{8.09} =$ +12.36 D
For 1.00 D steeper—Add −1.00 D (SAM) − 1.00 D = +11.36 D

(iii) $r = \frac{0.3375}{D}$ (flattest K = 40.00 D, 1.00 D steeper is 41.00 D)
$r = \frac{0.3375}{41.00\ D} = 8.23$ mm
Therefore the hard lens required is 8.23 mm / +11.36 D. (ref. p.139)

13-28. (A) (i) At vertex distance: $f = \frac{100}{12}$ = 8.33 cm
At corneal vertex plane: $f_2 = \frac{100}{8.33 - 0.8} = \frac{100}{7.53} =$ +13.28 D
At 2.00 D flatter, add plus (FAP) +2.00 D = + 2.00 D = +15.28 D

(ii) Flattest K = 58 − 2.00 flatter = 56.00 D
$r = \frac{0.3375}{56.00} = 6.026$ mm
The soft contact lens required is 6.026 mm / +15.28 D. (ref. p.139)

13-29. (B) Using K refractive index 1.3375, the base curve of contact lenses is related to the diopters of power and millimeters of radius of curvature by the formula $D_S = \frac{(n' - n)}{r}$. When solving for r for a given surface, $r = \frac{0.3375}{D_S}$. If the base curves range between 40 D and 45 D, the radii of curvature range is 8.43 mm and 7.50 mm. Over this 5.00 D range, r changes 0.94 mm with power changing at a rate of 5.32D/mm. (ref. p.139)

(i) For D_S = 40.00 D, $r = \frac{0.3375}{40.00\ D} = 8.44$ mm
For D_S = 45.00 D, $r = \frac{0.3375}{45.00\ D} = 7.50$ mm

(ii) Rate of change: $\frac{\text{Change in D}}{\text{\# of mm}} = \frac{5}{0.94} = \frac{5.32\ D}{mm}$

13-30. (A) The relative gas permeability of a contact lens is dependent on the diffusion constant, the solubility of oxygen in the material, and the DK value. (ref. p.140)

13-31. (E) A thicker plus lens has a lesser DK value than a thin minus lens. The partial pressure of oxygen across a lens influences the oxygen flux at the corneal level. The thickness factor gives an index of oxygen transmissibility. The corneal integrity depends on the aqueous delivery of glucose. (ref. p.140)

13-32. (D) Corneal oxygenation depends on oxygen flux, DK value, partial pressure of oxygen, and a thickness factor. Oxygen flux $= \frac{DK}{L} \times \delta P$. Corneal oxygenation increases with an increase in DK value or partial pressure of oxygen but decreases as the thickness increases. The thinner a minus lens, the greater the $\frac{DK}{L}$ value. (ref. p.140)

13-33. (C) Oxygen flux $= \frac{DK}{L} \times \delta P = \frac{22}{0.003} \times 0.02 = 146.67$
HEMA has an oxygen flux of 146.67. (ref. p.140)

CHAPTER 14: LOW VISION, PENALIZATION, MALINGERING

14-1. (B) The Amsler grid tests the central horizontal and vertical 10° of visual field for evidence of central disruption. (ref. p.142)

14-2. (E) Peripheral visual field defects may result from retinal, optic nerve, neurologic, and glaucomatous problems. (ref. p.142)

14-3. (D) When peripheral field defects approach fixation images may be projected into nonseeing retina. This makes binocularity difficult to achieve and may adversely affect vision by altering magnification. (ref. p.142)

14-4. (E) The selection of the type and power of visual aid depends on the ocular motility, accommodative amplitude, visual acuity of each eye, and the age of the patient. (ref. p.143)

14-5. (C) Kestenbaum's rule estimates 80/20 = +4.00 D is required. Monocular correction is appropriate in view of the greater than two line acuity disparity between the eyes. (ref. p.143)

14-6. (E) For an object of regard at 10 cm, 10 meter angles or prism diopters of convergence are required. Therefore with a pupillary distance equal to 64 mm, the convergence of the system is 64 P.D. (ref. p.143)

14-7. (A) **(i)** Kestenbaum's rule says that the initial add should be the reverse of the Snellen fraction: 20/100 becomes 100/20 = +5.00 D

(ii) Magnification produced: $\frac{D}{4} = \frac{5}{4} = 1.25\times$ (ref. p.143)

14-8. (D) Any add greater than +6.00 D is a special order, which makes it more expensive commercially. A trial with a Fresnel Press-On segment will decide if it is worth the price to make this a permanent form of correction. (ref. p.143)

14-9. (B) A patient with 20/200 acuity wants to read newspaper print (J_6, 20/50). This requires an initial add of +10.00 D (Kestenbaum's rule = the reverse of the Snellen fraction) to read. (ref. p.143)

14-10. (B) The patient would hold the telescope over the better (6/18) right eye. The visual angle capable of resolution with a 3× magnifier will be 3× smaller, i.e., from 3° to 1°. This is 6/6 acuity. (ref. p.143)

14-11. (A) Many older people adapt poorly to very close reading distances. A hand or stand magnifier increases the field relative to high-powered monocular adds. A hand magnifier can even double as a makeshift monocular reading glass. (ref. p.144)

14-12. (A) An aphakic patient would experience a Galilean telescopic effect with a +4.00 D lens held at 17 cm from the eye. (ref. p.144)

14-13. (B) The amorphic lens system is a spectacle-mounted telescopic system that minifies the 180° meridian but maintains the vertical perspective. (ref. p.144)

14-14. (B) Penalization occurs when distance or near vision is purposefully reduced to treat mild to moderate amblyopia. (ref. p.145)

14-15. (E) Hysteria is a psychoneurosis in which internal psychologic conflict cannot be adequately dealt with employing ordinary defense mechanisms. Paralysis or blindness are common manifestations, and this condition may be amenable to psychotherapy. (ref. p.146)

14-16. (B) 4 P.D. BO prism introduced in front of a seeing eye is followed by an involuntary fusional ductional response to maintain binocularity. (ref. p.147)

CHAPTER 15: INSTRUMENTS

15-1. (D) The lens measure uses the chord diameter, the radius of curvature, and the sagittal height of the chord to calculate the refractive power of a lens. (ref. p.148)

15-2. (C) The lens measure is useful for determining refractive power and the extent of lens warpage. (ref. p.149)

15-3. (E) A radiuscope is used when dealing with hard or gas permeable contact lenses to determine lens warpage, calculate the radii of curvature, and verify the anterior central curve of contact lenses. (ref. p.149)

15-4. (C) Hand neutralization occurs when a lens of known calibration is placed in front of the unknown lens. (ref. p.149)

15-5. (B) The lensmeter measures the back vertex power of a spectacle lens. (ref. p.149)

15-6. (D) The non-Badal lensmeter biases the determination of power in a nonlinear dioptric scale by magnifying small changes with plus lenses and causing endpoint discrimination toward the plus side by the observer. (ref. p.149)

15-7. (B) Badal discovered that if the standard lens is positioned in such a way that its secondary focal point was at the back vertex of the spectacle lens to be measured, the result is emergent parallel rays at neutralization. (ref. p.150)

15-8. (D) When one is measuring fused bifocals of high strength plus or minus lenses, the spectacle must be turned over and measured temples up. The front vertex should be reread at the front optical center, and the difference between distance and the segment is the power of the add. (ref. p.151)

15-9. (E) The problem in measuring the power of a contact lens with a lensmeter arises because the apical vault falls outside the focal plane of the standard lens of the lensmeter. (ref. p.151)

15-10. (C) The Scheiner principle rests on the fact that the object of regard forms a single clear image when it is placed conjugate to the retina. (ref. p.151)

15-11. (D) The automation of a standard phoropter, the normal refracting sequence with special cross cylinder testing, and the refraction of a patient without the use of trial lenses have all been developed to aid with refraction. (ref. p.151)

15-12. (B) The direct ophthalmoscope field

of view is limited by its small aperture. (ref. p.152)

15-13. (A) The indirect ophthalmoscope produces an image of the fundus, which becomes the object of the condensing lens. This forms an aerial image, which is larger and inverted. (ref. p.153)

15-14. (E) $M_A = \dfrac{-D_E}{D_O} = \dfrac{-60.00}{+10.00} = -6\times$

The image seen through an indirect ophthalmoscope with a condensing lens of power +10.00 D is inverted and magnified 6×. (ref. p.153)

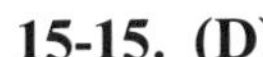

15-15. (D)

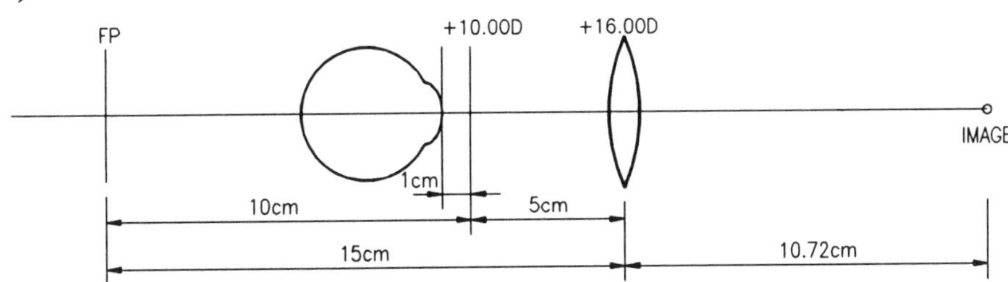

(i) Far point $= \dfrac{100}{10} = 10$ cm from the spectacle plane.

The condensing lens is 6 cm from the cornea, which is 9 cm from the far point.

The far point is the object for the condensing lens.

(ii) $U + D = V$

$$\frac{-100}{15} + 16 = -6.67 + 16 = +9.33$$

$$\frac{1}{v} = \frac{1}{9.33} = 10.72 \text{ cm}$$

The aerial image formed from the retina is 10.72 cm in front of the plus lens. (ref. p.153)

15-16. (B) The following calculations could be performed for a direct ophthalmoscope. (ref. p.153)

(i) Magnification of an emmetropic eye: $\dfrac{+60.00}{4} = 15\times$

(ii) Magnification of a myopic eye of +75.00 D: $\dfrac{+75.00}{4} = 18.75\times$

(iii) Magnification of an aphakic eye of +50.00 D: $\dfrac{+50.00}{4} = 12.50\times$

Relative to emmetropia the fundus in:

(i) Aphakia appears $\dfrac{12.5}{15} \times 100\% \approx 16.67\%$ smaller

(ii) Myopia appears $\dfrac{18.75}{15} \times 100\% \approx 25.00\%$ larger

15-17. (A) **(i)** Angular magnification: $M_A = \dfrac{-D_E}{D_O} = \dfrac{-60}{15} = -4\times$.

The image is 4× larger and perceived inverted

(ii) Axial magnification is $M_A^2 = 16\times$

(iii) Because of the reduction in PD, the effective axial magnification is reduced by the same amount as the PD. Therefore axial magnification $= \dfrac{16\times}{4} = 4\times$. (ref. p.153-4)

15-18. (A) The most accurate method of determining the line of sight involves having the patient fix a nonluminous target on the objective lens mount and sighting the center of the pupil with the surgeon using monocular vision. (ref. p.157)

15-19. (E) Corneal topographic analyzers are important for refractive alterations. They can couple the information received from these to a manufacturing machine to provide custom fit contact lenses. These instruments produce images which are digitized and analyzed to give each radius of curvature a color or grey scale on a topographic map. (ref. p.157)

15-20. (E) Sound can be propagated in waveform and can be reflected, refracted, scattered, or absorbed. (ref. p.157)

15-21. (D) In contact ultrasonography the near field extends to the posterior lens capsule, and any details anterior to this are lost. New ultrasound biomicroscopes regain the anterior field. (ref. p.158)

15-22. (E) As ultrasound encounters different interfaces, it can be displayed visually with a cathode ray oscilloscope. The time delay between emission and detection is a function of the distance travelled and of the density of the medium it is travelling in. The denser the medium, the shorter the delay. (ref. p.158)

15-23. (B) At an applanation of 3.06 mm, the structural resistance to deformation of the cornea is equal to the attractive forces of the surface tension of the tears. These forces thus cancel each other out. (ref. p.159)

15-24. (A) If the applanation head is not rotated 43° to the minus cylinder or lowest *K*, the error per 4.00 D of cylinder equals 1 mm Hg. (ref. p.159)

15-25. (E) The keratometer or ophthalmometer uses both the reflecting and refracting properties of the cornea to determine the radii of curvature and refracting power of its principal meridians. (ref. p.159)

15-26. (A) If one keeps either the image size or the object size constant, the magnification can be calculated by determining the size of the variable. (ref. p.160)

15-27. (B) The phoropter cannot be used to differentiate between cataractous and noncataractous causes of decreased vision. (ref. p.37)

CHAPTER 16: LASERS

16-1. (D) Laser is an acronym derived from light amplification by stimulated emission of radiation. (ref. p.162)

16-2. (B) Ionization is the process by which an atom absorbs quanta of energy and excites an electron into the next energy level or out of the atom. (ref. p.162)

16-3. (D) If all of the electrons in the same medium go from the same excited state to a nonexcited state, multiple photons of the same wavelength and frequency are released at the same time. (ref. p.162)

16-4. (E) When energy is absorbed, electrons go from a nonexcited state to an excited state. When they go from an excited state to a nonexcited state, a photon is released. Energy can be spontaneously emitted with the release of a photon but in a random fashion so that no amplification occurs. The absorption of a photon can stimulate the release of another photon from a similar atom, called stimulated emission. (ref. p.162)

16-5. (C) If more than half of the atoms are in the excited state, laser formation is favored. (ref. p.162)

16-6. (A) A ruby crystal is formed when an

aluminum oxide crystal has its aluminum replaced by chromium. (ref. p.162)

16-7. (E) A resonance chamber generally has mirrored ends, may have an aperture at one end that will allow light to escape, and must have a length that is a multiple of half or full wavelengths. The resonance chamber is used to reflect emitted radiation and enhance the amplification of stimulated emission. (ref. p.163)

16-8. (B) All light that emerges from a resonance chamber is monochromatic, highly directional, in phase, and high intensity. (ref. p.163)

16-9. (E) The emission of light from a laser can occur in bursts, a continuous wave, short pulses, or in high-intensity releases. (ref. p.163)

16-10. (E) The surgeon has control over a number of parameters when using the laser. They include the power, spot size, number of pulses per burst, and duration of the emission. (ref. p.163)

16-11. (D) If the amount of work is increased or the amount of time decreased, the amount of power is increased. (ref. p.163)

16-12. (D) The energy density is given in units of watts and can be increased if the amount of energy is distributed over a smaller area. It is also exponentially related to the energy density. (ref. p.163)

16-13. (B) The neodymium-YAG laser has neodymium ions incorporated or doped into a crystal of yttrium-aluminum-garnet. (ref. p.164)

16-14. (E) A suprathreshold burst increases the laser energy density until a threshold is overcome where electrons are stripped from their atoms and a plasma is formed. It produces an intense electromagnetic disruption, complex shock, and acoustical phenomena, and an "explosion" at the focal point. (ref. p.164)

16-15. (C) An IR laser can be converted to a visible laser with the addition of a frequency doubler. (ref. p.164)

16-16. (D) The THC:YAG laser is doped with thulium, holmium, and chromium. (ref. p.164)

16-17. (B) The excimer XeCl laser uses UV light instead of IR. (ref. p.165)

16-18. (E) UV light may have acute and chronic degenerative potential or any of the following forms of toxicity: acute endothelial, retinal, or thermal. (ref. p.165)

16-19. (B) Gas discharge lasers are stimulated by electric current, which excites the medium and initiates laser propagation. (ref. p.165)

16-20. (B) Carbon dioxide lasers emit in the IR portion of the spectrum. (ref. p.165)

16-21. (A) The carbon dioxide laser is currently the most efficient laser with 30% efficiency. (ref. p.165)

16-22. (D) Photocoagulation involves tissue whose absorption spectrum is within the range of emitted laser radiation, the absorption of which necessitates heat dissipation. This coagulates the tissue at the anatomic site of absorption. (ref. p.165)

16-23. (C) Argon green is not absorbed by xanthophyll and passes through the pigment unaltered. (ref. p.165)

16-24. (C) Noble gas–halogen combinations are the media for excimer gas discharge lasers. (ref. p.166)

16-25. (B) The term excimer is derived from the phrase excited dimer. (ref. p.166)

16-26. (A) Diatomic rare halides release UV light, which when absorbed by target tissues lyses protein intramolecular bonds. (ref. p.166)

16-27. (D) Early or late phototoxicity due to UV absorption may appear in such surrounding structures as the lens, the retina, and the corneal endothelium. (ref. p.166)

16-28. (D) Liquid lasers are primarily tunable dye lasers: they use an argon laser as a pump. Liquid organic dyes and their wavelengths are tunable between 360 and 960 nm. (ref. p.166)

16-29. (A) The greatest feature of semiconductor lasers is their convection air cooling, which allows very small sizes and portability. (ref. p.166)

16-30. (C) The absorption of light by target tissue can be enhanced by photoradiation using hematoporphyrin derivatives. (ref. p.166)

16-31. (A) Each exposed hole will create its own secondary image. (ref. Holladay: Evaluating the IOL optic)

CHAPTER 17: PRINCIPLES OF REFRACTIVE SURGERY

17-1. (B) Radial keratotomy involves radial corneal cuts, which flatten the central cornea and steepen the peripheral cornea. (ref. p.167)

17-2. (E) The variables that may affect the amount of correction provided by radial keratotomy include the depth, number, and direction of the cuts and the size of the optical zone. (ref. p.167)

17-3. (A) The deeper the cuts, the more hyperopic the shift. (ref. p.167)

17-4. (C) This patient had a spherical cornea prior to cataract surgery but postoperatively needs −3.00 D of cylinder axis 90° for better visual acuity. Postoperative astigmatism is most often due to suturing technique or poor wound healing. A gaping wound flattens the central corneal curvature in the vertical meridian. Possible correction is wedge resection, resuturing, or astigmatic keratotomy at 90° to the offending gape. (ref. p.167-8)

17-5. (D) The shorter the radius of curvature, the steeper the meridian. (ref. p.168)

17-6. (D) Radial thermal keratoplasty involves the insertion of a 34-gauge microprobe to 85% to 95% thickness and 6 to 16 rays of 2 to 4 burns with an optical zone of 5 to 8 mm. (ref. p.168)

17-7. (D) Hyperopic lamellar keratotomy involves the removal of a lamellar disk 360° around an optical zone using a microkeratome. To achieve central corneal steepening, 80% depth is necessary. (ref. p.168)

17-8. (D) Intracorneal hydrogels have the advantage of preserving accommodation. (ref. p.168)

17-9. (B) Epikeratophakia involves cryolathing a donor cornea and suturing it to a deepithelialized recipient. (ref. p.169)

17-10. (C) Keratomilieusis involves cryolathing an autolenticule of corneal tissue to correct high myopia. (ref. p.169)

17-11. (A) Photorefractive keratectomy with the excimer laser involves sculpting the central cornea by UV photoablation. (ref. p.169)

17-12. (A) Photorefractive keratectomy is a form of myopic correction that is controlled by the size of the optical zone and the depth of the ablation. (ref. p.169)

APPENDIX C: ANSWERS

CHAPTER 1: THE BASICS

1-1.	E	1-2.	A	1-3.	D	1-4.	C	1-5.	A
1-6.	D	1-7.	A	1-8.	E	1-9.	C	1-10.	D
1-11.	B	1-12.	D	1-13.	E	1-14.	D	1-15.	A
1-16.	C	1-17.	B	1-18.	D	1-19.	E	1-20.	E
1-21.	B	1-22.	D	1-23.	C	1-24.	E	1-25.	B
1-26.	D	1-27.	A	1-28.	D	1-29.	E	1-30.	D
1-31.	E	1-32.	C	1-33.	A	1-34.	A	1-35.	D
1-36.	A	1-37.	E	1-38.	C	1-39.	C	1-40.	D
1-41.	A	1-42.	E	1-43.	B	1-44.	A	1-45.	C
1-46.	A	1-47.	D	1-48.	A	1-49.	A	1-50.	A
1-51.	E	1-52.	C	1-53.	B	1-54.	C	1-55.	C
1-56.	C	1-57.	B	1-58.	C	1-59.	D	1-60.	A
1-61.	E	1-62.	D	1-63.	A	1-64.	D	1-65.	A
1-66.	C								

CHAPTER 2: LENS ABERRATIONS

2-1.	D	2-2.	A	2-3.	A	2-4.	C	2-5.	C
2-6.	E	2-7.	C	2-8.	B	2.9.	E		

CHAPTER 3: PRISMS

3-1.	B	3-2.	D	3-3.	C	3-4.	B	3-5.	C
3-6.	A	3-7.	D	3-8.	C	3-9.	D	3-10.	E
3-11.	A	3-12.	D	3-13.	E	3-14.	C	3-15.	B
3-16.	D	3-17.	D	3-18.	A	3-19.	B	3-20.	B
3-21.	E	3-22.	E	3-23.	C	3-24.	A	3-25.	B
3-26.	C	3-27.	A	3-28.	C	3-29.	E	3-30.	C
3-31.	D	3-32.	A	3-33.	B	3-34.	D	3-35.	D
3-36.	B	3-37.	C	3-38.	C	3-39.	A	3-40.	D
3-41.	B	3-42.	A	3-43.	E	3-44.	B	3-45.	D
3-46.	D	3-47.	D	3-48.	A	3-49.	A	3-50.	B
3-51.	E	3-52.	E	3-53.	D	3-54.	A	3-55.	D
3-56.	B	3-57.	B	3-58.	B	3-59.	D	3-60.	C
3-61.	D	3-62.	C	3-63.	E	3-64.	B	3-65.	A
3-66.	C	3-67.	B	3-68.	A	3-69.	E	3-70.	C
3-71.	D	3-72.	B	3-73.	C	3-74.	C	3-75.	D
3-76.	D	3-77.	D						

CHAPTER 4: VISUAL IMAGERY

4-1.	C	4-2.	A	4-3.	D	4-4.	E	4-5.	C
4-6.	D	4-7.	C	4-8.	C	4-9.	A	4-10.	B
4-11.	D	4-12.	B	4-13.	A	4-14.	C	4-15.	A
4-16.	C	4-17.	E	4-18.	D	4-19.	C	4-20.	B
4-21.	D	4-22.	E	4-23.	A	4-24.	D	4-25.	B
4-26.	B	4-27.	D	4-28.	E	4-29.	A	4-30.	A
4-31.	C	4-32.	D	4-33.	C	4-34.	C	4-35.	D
4-36.	A	4-37.	A						

CHAPTER 5: ASTIGMATISM

5-1.	C	5-2.	B	5-3.	B	5-4.	D	5-5.	C
5-6.	C	5-7.	A	5-8.	C	5-9.	A	5-10.	A
5-11.	B	5-12.	D	5-13.	A	5-14.	B	5-15.	C
5-16.	C	5-17.	D	5-18.	D	5-19.	A	5-20.	E
5-21.	C	5-22.	C	5-23.	C	5-24.	C	5-25.	C
5-26.	D	5-27.	A	5-28.	B	5-29.	A	5-30.	C
5-31.	C	5-32.	A	5-33.	C	5-34.	C	5-35.	D
5-36.	C	5-37.	A	5-38.	B	5-39.	E	5-40.	E
5-41.	B	5-42.	D	5-43.	A	5-44.	E	5-45.	A
5-46.	B	5-47.	C	5-48.	E	5-49.	B	5-50.	A
5-51.	A	5-52.	D	5-53.	B	5-54.	A	5-55.	B
5-56.	B	5-57.	E	5-58.	C	5-59.	C	5-60.	B
5-61.	B	5-62.	C	5-63.	B	5-64.	D	5-65.	D
5-66.	E	5-67.	A	5-68.	C	5-69.	A	5-70.	A
5-71.	C	5-72.	E	5-73.	E	5-74.	C	5-75.	C
5-76.	D	5-77.	B	5-78.	E	5-79.	A	5-80.	B
5-81.	A	5-82.	E	5-83.	C	5-84.	A	5-85.	D
5-86.	B	5-87.	D	5-88.	B	5-89.	A	5-90.	E
5-91.	B	5-92.	D	5-93.	A	5-94.	E	5-95.	E
5-96.	B	5-97.	E	5-98.	D	5-99.	C	5-100.	A
5-101.	C	5-102.	D	5-103.	D	5-104.	B	5-105.	B
5-106.	B	5-107.	A	5-108.	C	5-109.	B	5-110.	E
5-111.	C	5-112.	A	5-113.	E	5-114.	D	5-115.	D
5-116.	B	5-117.	E	5-118.	B	5-119.	B	5-120.	E

CHAPTER 6: MAGNIFICATION

6-1.	D	6-2.	D	6-3.	B	6-4.	B	6-5.	A
6-6.	B	6-7.	A	6-8.	D	6-9.	D	6-10.	C
6-11.	B	6-12.	C	6-13.	B	6-14.	C	6-15.	A
6-16.	D	6-17.	A	6-18.	D	6-19.	D	6-20.	C

6-21. C 6-22. A 6-23. C 6-24. E 6-25. A
6-26. A 6-27. C 6-28. B 6-29. A 6-30. D
6-31. E 6-32. C 6-33. D 6-34. A 6-35. C
6-36. C 6-37. B 6-38. E 6-39. E 6-40. E
6-41. C 6-42. C 6-43. B 6-44. D 6-45. C
6-46. C 6-47. D 6-48. A 6-49. A 6-50. C
6-51. B 6-52. B 6-53. B 6-54. E 6-55. B
6-56. C 6-57. D 6-58. B 6-59. C 6-60. E
6-61. C 6-62. A 6-63. E 6-64. A 6-65. C

CHAPTER 7: RETINOSCOPY

7-1. E 7-2. C 7-3. C 7-4. B 7-5. E
7-6. A 7-7. A 7-8. B 7-9. A 7-10. A
7-11. D 7-12. B 7-13. D 7-14. A 7-15. C
7-16. D 7-17. B 7-18. C 7-19. A 7-20. D
7-21. D 7-22. B 7-23. A 7-24. D 7-25. D

CHAPTER 8: REFRACTION

8-1. E 8-2. A 8-3. A 8-4. A 8-5. B
8-6. B 8-7. D 8-8. A 8-9. E 8-10. A
8-11. B 8-12. A 8-13. A 8-14. C 8-15. D
8-16. A 8-17. D 8-18. E 8-19. B 8-20. A
8-21. C 8-22. A 8-23. C

CHAPTER 9: VISION TESTING

9-1. E 9-2. E 9-3. B 9-4. D 9-5. B
9-6. D 9-7. B 9-8. D 9-9. E. 9-10. C
9-11. B 9-12. E 9-13. C 9-14. A 9-15. D
9-16. A 9-17. B 9-18. A 9-19. D 9-20. A
9-21. E 9-22. D 9-23. E 9-24. D 9-25. B
9-26. A 9-27. B 9-28. E 9-29. B 9-30. E
9-31. D 9-32. C

CHAPTER 10: ACCOMMODATION AND CONVERGENCE

10-1. A 10-2. A 10-3. D 10-4. A 10-5. B
10-6. D 10-7. B 10-8. B 10-9. C 10-10. B
10-11. C 10-12. D 10-13. B 10-14. E 10-15. B
10-16. A 10-17. A 10-18. B 10-19. D 10-20. B

10-21.	D	10-22.	A	10-23.	B	10-24.	A	10-25.	E
10-26.	A	10-27.	C	10-28.	D	10-29.	D	10-30.	B
10-31.	B	10-32.	C	10-33.	D				

CHAPTER 11: PRESCRIBING

11-1.	B	11-2.	C	11-3.	E	11-4.	D	11-5.	D
11-6.	A	11-7.	C	11-8.	C	11-9.	B	11-10.	B
11-11.	A	11-12.	E	11-13.	B	11-14.	D	11-15.	B
11-16.	A	11-17.	C	11-18.	A	11-19.	D	11-20.	B
11-21.	B	11-22.	B	11-23.	B	11-24.	E	11-25.	E
11-26.	C	11-27.	B	11-28.	E	11-29.	E	11-30.	A
11-31.	E	11-32.	C	11-33.	D	11-34.	D	11-35.	A
11-36.	E	11-37.	D	11-38.	A	11-39.	D	11-40.	C
11-41.	E	11-42.	A	11-43.	A	11-44.	E	11-45.	E
11-46.	E	11-47.	D	11-48.	E	11-49.	B	11-50.	C
11-51.	A	11-52.	E	11-53.	E	11-54.	C	11-55.	C
11-56.	A	11-57.	B	11-58.	A	11-59.	B	11-60.	D
11-61.	C	11-62.	A	11-63.	E	11-64.	C	11-65.	D
11-66.	E	11-67.	D	11-68.	B	11-69.	B	11-70.	D
11-71.	B	11-72.	C	11-73.	A	11-74.	D	11-75.	E
11-76.	C	11-77.	B	11-78.	A	11-79.	D	11-80.	B
11-81.	D	11-82.	D	11-83.	C	11-84.	C	11-85.	B
11-86.	E								

CHAPTER 12: MATERIALS

12-1.	A	12-2.	B	12-3.	B	12-4.	E	12-5.	D
12-6.	C	12-7.	E	12-8.	B	12-9.	A	12-10.	C
12-11.	E	12-12.	E	12-13.	C	12-14.	A	12-15.	B
12-16.	E	12-17.	D	12-18.	C	12-19.	D	12-20.	A
12-21.	B	12-22.	B	12-23.	A	12-24.	D	12-25.	D
12-26.	C	12-27.	D	12-28.	D	12-29.	A	12-30.	E
12-31.	A	12-32.	C	12-33.	A	12-34.	E	12-35.	B
12-36.	B	12-37.	C	12-38.	C	12-39.	E	12-40.	A
12-41.	C	12-42.	A	12-43.	B	12-44.	D	12-45.	A
12-46.	E	12-47.	C	12-48.	E	12-49.	B	12-50.	E
12-51.	B	12-52.	D	12-53.	E	12-54.	B	12-55.	A
12-56.	B	12-57.	C	12-58.	E	12-59.	B	12-60.	D
12-61.	B	12-62.	D	12-63.	D				

CHAPTER 13: CONTACT LENSES

13-1	C	13-2.	D	13-3.	A	13-4.	C	13-5.	B
13-6.	A	13-7.	A	13-8.	B	13-9.	B	13-10.	C
13-11.	A	13-12.	E	13-13.	C	13-14.	B	13-15.	E
13-16.	C	13-17.	C	13-18.	E	13-19.	E	13-20.	B
13-21.	D	13-22.	A	13-23.	A	13-24.	E	13-25.	E
13-26.	B	13-27.	B	13-28.	A	13-29.	B	13-30.	A
13-31.	E	13-32.	D	13-33.	C				

CHAPTER 14: LOW VISION, PENALIZATION, MALINGERING

14-1.	B	14-2.	E	14-3.	D	14-4.	E	14-5.	C
14-6.	E	14-7.	A	14-8.	D	14-9.	B	14-10.	B
14-11.	A	14-12.	A	14-13.	B	14-14.	B	14-15.	E
14-16.	B								

CHAPTER 15: INSTRUMENTS

15-1.	D	15-2.	C	15-3.	E	15-4.	C	15-5.	B
15-6.	D	15-7.	B	15-8.	D	15-9.	E	15-10.	C
15-11.	D	15-12.	B	15-13.	A	15-14.	E	15-15.	D
15-16.	B	15-17.	A	15-18.	A	15-19.	E	15-20.	E
15-21.	D	15-22.	E	15-23.	B	15-24.	A	15-25.	E
15-26.	A	15-27.	B						

CHAPTER 16: LASERS

16-1.	D	16-2.	B	16-3.	D	16-4.	E	16-5.	C
16-6.	A	16-7.	E	16-8.	B	16-9.	E	16-10.	E
16-11.	D	16-12.	D	16-13.	B	16-14.	E	16-15.	C
16-16.	D	16-17.	B	16-18.	E	16-19.	B	16-20.	B
16-21.	A	16-22.	D	16-23.	C	16-24.	C	16-25.	B
16-26.	A	16-27.	D	16-28.	D	16-29.	A	16-30.	C
16-31.	A								

CHAPTER 17: PRINCIPLES OF REFRACTIVE SURGERY

17-1.	B	17-2.	E	17-3.	A	17-4.	C	17-5.	D
17-6.	D	17-7.	D	17-8.	D	17-9.	B	17-10.	C
17-11.	A	17-12.	A						

INDEX